D0580321

SECRETS
OF FEEDING
A HEALTHY FAMILY

ALSO BY ELLYN SATTER

Child of Mine:
Feeding with Love and Good Sense

How to Get Your Kid to Eat...
But Not Too Much

ELLYN SATTER'S FEEDING WITH LOVE
AND GOOD SENSE:
Video and Teacher's Guide

ELLYN SATTER'S NUTRITION AND
FEEDING FOR INFANTS AND CHILDREN:
Handout Masters

Ellyn Satter's
Montana FEEDING RELATIONSHIP
Training Package

TREATING THE DIETING CASUALTY:
Training Manual

FEEDING WITH LOVE AND GOOD SENSE:
Training Manual

SECRETS
OF FEEDING
A HEALTHY FAMILY

ELLYN SATTER
MS RD CICSW BCD

KELCY PRESS
MADISON, WISCONSIN

Secrets of Feeding a Healthy Family

Copyright © 1999 Ellyn Satter

Kelcy Press
PO Box 46457
Madison, WI 53744-6457

877-844-0857

ISBN 0-9671189-0-5

All rights reserved. No part of this book may be reproduced or transmitted in any form
or by any means, electronic or mechanical , including photocopying and recording, or by
any information storage and retrieval system, without permission in writing from Ellyn Satter

Library of Congress Cataloging-in-Publication Data

Satter, Ellyn
Secrets of feeding a healthy family/Ellyn Satter.
p. cm.
Includes index
ISBN 0-9671189-0-5
1. Children–Nutrition Popular works. 2. Nutrition Popular works.
3. Diet Popular works. 4. Food habits Popular works. I. Title.
RJ206.S247   1999
613.2–dc21   99-33165

Printed in the U.S.

Distributed in the U.S. by:
Ellyn Satter Associates
4226 Mandan Crescent, Suite 50
Madison, WI 53711

800-808-7976

Developmental editor: Paulette Bochnig Sharkey
Copy Editor: Mary Ray Worley
Layout and Cover Art: Karen Foget
Typesetting: Sherpe Advertising Art
10 9 8 7 6 5 4 3

*Dedicated to the caring people
who work with children,
parents, nutrition and feeding.*

CONTENTS

Preface   ix

Chapter 1   **The Secret in a Nutshell**   2
             Nutrition has a way of falling into place when
             people are the priority rather than the rules that
             govern them.

Chapter 2   **You and *Your* Eating**   16
             There is considerable peace and comfort in
             knowing you are going to be well and
             enjoyably fed.

Chapter 3   **The Feeding Relationship**   32
             Feeding demands a division of responsibility:
             The parent is responsible for the *what, when,* and
             where of feeding; the child is responsible for the
             how much and *whether* of eating.

Chapter 4   **Choosing Food for Your Family**   48
             Avoid negativity. Negativity, fear, and avoidance
             are not good motivators. Optimism, self-trust, and
             adventure are good motivators.

Chapter 5   **How to Get Cooking**   70
             For you to cook, and keep on cooking, food has to
             taste good. Recipes to get you cooking.

Chapter 6   **How to Keep Cooking**   102
             Like eating, cooking can be a creative act that gives
             you a change of pace and restores your energy.
             Recipes to keep you cooking.

Chapter 7   **Enjoy Vegetables and Fruits**   **124**
The point of children and vegetables is not to get
vegetables into your child today, it is to help your
child enjoy vegetables for all his tomorrows.
Recipes to let you enjoy vegetables and fruits.

Chapter 8   **Planning to Get You Cooking**   **146**
Planning can be used or abused. Use planning to
lower your stress level, not to pile on jobs.

Chapter 9   **Shopping to Get You Cooking**   **162**
Foods are your tools. To feed a healthy
family, you have to have good tools.

Chapter 10   **Raising a Healthy Eater in
Your Community**   **178**
The best nutrition education at school helps
children support and extend the intuitive
capabilities with eating they developed at home.

Appendixes   **Appendix A**   **202**
What Surveys Say about Our Eating
Appendix B   **204**
The Dietary Guidelines and Why They
Are Rule Bound
Appendix C   **205**
Grazing, Cue Sensitivity, and Your Weight
Appendix D   **206**
To Diet or Not to Diet—That Is the Question
Appendix E   **208**
Children and Food Regulation
Appendix F   **210**
Children and Food Acceptance
Appendix G   **211**
Dietary Fat and Heart Disease:
It's Not as Bad as You Think
Appendix H   **214**
Children, Dietary Fat, and Heart Disease:
You Don't Have to Panic
Appendix I   **217**
Sodium in Your Diet
Appendix J   **219**
A Primer on Dietary Fat
Appendix K   **221**
Sources Available from Ellyn Satter Associates

Index   **223**

PREFACE

Secrets has been the most willful book I have ever written! It started out to be a simple primer on feeding kids following my golden rule, the division of responsibility in feeding: The parent is responsible for the *what, when,* and *where* of feeding, and the child is responsible for the *how much* and *whether* of eating. The problem is that meals are the cornerstone of that division of responsibility, and today's families have extraordinary difficulty getting meals on the table. It's not for lack of commitment or trying. There are too many barriers, not the least of which is all the rules that have grown up around eating. Thus, *Secrets* turned into a book about providing that cornerstone: about accumulating the knowledge, managing the tasks, and overcoming the barriers that go along with getting a family meal on the table.

Like a beloved child, *Secrets* has taken me places I hadn't expected and maybe hadn't wanted to go. This time, it was into the whole heart disease and diet controversy—a deep, murky, and hazardous place if there ever was one. Along with the confusing and scary parts, there has been pure fun and celebration. *Secrets* took me back to my early-dietitian days and my young-mother roots. This is the book I wish I would have been able to give my children when they left home. I had a fine time writing down recipes, planning menus, giving time-saving tips, and looking up foods in my Food Processor program. I even planned a cycle menu, a task I left behind when I stopped consulting in hospitals and long-term-care facilities. I drew on all my skills as a

dietitian, parent, and family therapist to write this book. It is my conviction that you have to know the rules before you can productively break them. You will see in *Secrets* that I broke a lot of rules.

Once started, a book takes on a life of its own. Secrets seemed to know that it needed to become part of my child feeding trilogy: what to feed your children (*Child of Mine*), how to feed your children (*How to Get Your Kid to Eat*), and now how to get a meal on the table. In *Child of Mine* I made the carefree comment that I wasn't going to give any recipes on the grounds that "you already know how to cook." I can no longer be as carefree. Today's parents don't know how to cook—and plan and shop and keep a kitchen clean. Moreover, while surveys show that we value family meals and want to cook, we are grappling with enormous barriers that we can't seem to get around. It seems nowadays that the first principle of eating is to avoid. Not so. Eating well is one of life's great pleasures. Feeding is the cornerstone of nurturing. Feeding ourselves as well as feeding our children is a legitimate and desperately important priority. In *Secrets* I observe that "you are a family when you start to take care of yourself." Nurturing isn't only for children or for other people. To be mentally, socially, and physically healthy, you must nurture yourself.

In *Secrets*, I take a stand against fat restriction for children and encourage adults to lighten up as well. I have been dismayed at the increasing vehemence about putting children over age two and certainly by age five on modified-fat, low-cholesterol diets. As with fat, recommendations for salt are set so low that they impair cooking and eating. The current population-wide sodium and fat prescriptions make it hard for the busy, ordinary, and frequently low-income young person and family to get a meal on the table. My extensive reading tells me that heart disease is not the national emergency we have been led to believe, nor are dietary restrictions as effective in managing that so-called emergency as we have been told. My goal in *Secrets* was to emphasize variety and satisfaction in menu planning and cooking, using as much fat and salt as you need to make food taste good. On the principle that you can catch more bees with honey than with vinegar, my conviction is that cooking for and feeding ourselves will compete for our time and attention only if it is richly satisfying. Anticipating and eating a wonderful meal is supremely rewarding and soothing. Meeting our needs with flavor, nutrition, and the social and emotional support of regular and satisfying meals provides the necessary backdrop for our busy lives.

The increasing vehemence about body weight provides an ongoing barrier to feeding ourselves well. National health policy makers, advertisers, and many health professionals are adamant that we are too fat and we have to cut back. Doing the research for *Secrets* renewed my conviction that with eating, as with life, you can't control the outcome. You can do the best you can, and you can be healthier if you take good care of yourself. Beyond optimizing and hoping for the best, you can't control. You have to trust. You can try as hard as you can to lower your weight or your cholesterol, and your body just might not cooperate. Instead of adopting ever more drastic methods in the attempt to control, you need to trust: eat well, be active, seek a positive lifestyle, then let your health and weight do what it will in response to your constitutional endowment. Part of the process of learning to trust is distinguishing between what you need and need not manage. What goes on the table can legitimately be managed. What goes into children—or even into adults—can't. No child ever ate according to a formula, and adults who try can't do it for long.

My conclusion? It is more important to eat than to avoid. The failure of current nutrition messages becomes glaringly apparent when we consider that fat avoidance is the nutritional priority of 50 percent of consumers. We emphasize nutritional adequacy only 10 percent of the time. Rather than trying to straighten out our thinking, it seems to me that we have to adjust our attitudes. In my experience, feeding, eating, and the nutritional quality of the diet fall into place when people stop thinking so much about *avoiding* and start putting their energy into *providing*.

I said earlier that *Secrets* took me back to my young dietitian days. On more careful reflection, I realize that *Secrets* goes back further than that—it is woven with the threads of my entire life. I can start with the attitudes and skills I learned from my dear mother, my grandmothers, and a coven of aunts. They cooked and kept on cooking, many times beginning by catching the chickens or climbing ladders to pick the cherries. My high school home economics teacher, Mrs. Beatrice Clark, told me I would go far, and many days must have felt it couldn't possibly have been far enough. Miss Zora Colburn, my South Dakota State University nutrition professor, shared her passion for nutrition. Now in her nineties, Miss Colburn still cooks for me when I visit her. Mrs. Betty Jordan, my University of Wisconsin Hospitals internship director, resisted my diet therapy zeal and indoctrinated me, instead, in not turning my patients into dietary cripples. Dr. Dorothy Pringle, major professor for my masters in nutrition, demonstrated through her discriminating practicality how useful and empowering it can be to cut through complexity to the essential and applicable heart of the matter.

As I turned my emphasis to being a homemaker, I was gifted with three healthy children, Kjerstin, Lucas, and Curtis, who ate and kept on eating. During my mothering years, I had good friends who loved eating, loved cooking and swapping recipes, and loved feeding their families. I am happy to say my children are still capable and enthusiastic eaters, but since most of my friends are dodging some medical calamity, present or threatened, cooking for them isn't as much fun as it used to be. That said, I thank you, dear reader, for providing me an outlet for my frustrated nurturing needs.

My two earlier books, *Child of Mine: Feeding with Love and Good Sense* and *How to Get Your Kid to Eat . . . But Not Too Much*, helped to bring me here. I wrote *Child of Mine* intending it to be a good-bye gift to a part of my life that was very dear—raising young children. My children were in the upper grades, and I was no longer working as a pediatric dietitian. Imagine my surprise when *Child of Mine* gained me a reputation as an authority in child nutrition and kept me in the field. Writing a book is truly the magic carpet ride to wonderful people and opportunities. It was only after I wrote *Child of Mine* that I discovered the area of feeding dynamics, which led me to write *How to Get Your Kid to Eat* and to make feeding dynamics my niche. My curiosity about parent-child interactions around feeding led to graduate school in social work, and graduate school led me to Donald Williams, CICSW, long-time consultant and collaborator who demonstrated how empowering it can be to tell people what is bugging them and let them decide what to do about it.

Many of the people I have encountered on my magic carpet ride helped with *Secrets*. Friends and colleagues discussed, reacted, read, and commented on the manuscript at all stages of preparation. They challenged, applauded, disagreed, thanked, utilized, and even imitated, which I consider to be the most vivid of all stamps of approval. While I appreciate being cited for my work, mostly because it can send readers to more of my information that might be helpful to them, I also realize that it is hard to keep track of where ideas come from. For the record, the division of responsibility in feeding is my brain child—about that, I feel very territorial and want to be cited. I also am careful to cite others for their contributions and will appreciate your drawing my attention to anything in these pages where you feel I have failed to do so.

Having said this, it is hard for me not to give you the names of my many reviewers. They are leaders in the nutrition, health, mental health, and education fields and represent state and federal agencies, health care organizations, and nutrition and health publications. Most hesitated to be thanked by name based on agency policy that such thanking would imply endorsement. So be it. Their names would be a who's who of good people, and I thank them. I have two exceptions to that rule of anonymity. First is my daughter, Kjerstin, now a mother of her own three little girls. Kjestin read and commented on the *Secrets* manuscript at all stages of preparation and gave me a great deal of truly valuable help. Second, I want to recognize and wish all the best to Paulette Sharkey, my developmental editor and generous and creative helper for the last six years.

Many thanks to the parents of the cover children for their generosity in allowing me to use their photos and to the parents who agreed to be pictured as well. They are all beautiful and remind us of the tremendous joy and responsibility that go along with sharing our lives with children. Many thanks as well to Kaj Foget, who allowed me to use as cover art the wonderful valentine strawberry that his wife, Karen, painted for him.

Finally, thanks to my colleagues and helpers. I find much joy in watching excellent people work together to apply their considerable skills to the task at hand. They are all the best: Karen Foget and Howard Sherpe, capable Norwegians who provide entertainment along with design and typesetting; Clio Marsh, charming and tolerant administrative assistant who brings customer service to a higher level of excellence; Matthew O'Brien, steadfast and accurate articles gofer and bibliography database manager, who keeps us current on Irish history; and thoughtful and perceptive Alison Lockeridge, who contributes much and is mostly in charge of order.

And finally, I thank you, dear reader, for giving me the opportunity to write. I often don't know what I think and feel until I do. Like writing a good story, writing *Secrets* has helped me to integrate, understand, and pull together the threads of my life in a most gratifying way.

SECRETS
OF FEEDING
A HEALTHY FAMILY

The Secret in a Nutshell

- The secret of feeding a healthy family is threefold: to love good food, trust yourself, and share that love and trust with your children.
- Parents are responsible for the *what, when*, and *where* of feeding.
- Children are responsible for the *how much* and *whether* of eating.
- Do your job, let your children do theirs, and settle down.

CHAPTER

1

THE SECRET
IN A
NUTSHELL

Secrets of Feeding a Healthy Family aims to help you and your family rediscover the joy and security of sharing good food. Cooking and eating can be about the happiness, comfort, and passion of celebrating wonderful food, enjoying it with others, and leaving the table filled with peace and well-being. Instead, cooking and eating today are too often about applying the rules; about struggling with conflict, shame, and deprivation; and about trying to forgo pleasure in the name of health. Mealtime can be one of the most dreaded parts of parenting, involving struggles with all the parts of managing food to please the big and little people at the table. Many times we are overwhelmed. Instead of going away from the table feeling content, we go away empty, or at least unsatisfied. To get away from the conflict, we try not to think about eating and rush to get it over with and end up with the conviction that anything having to do with food is unrewarding.

Until we recover eating as one of life's great pleasures, it simply is not going to turn out well. Eating is more than throwing wood on a fire or pumping gas into a car. Feeding is more than picking out food and getting it into a child. Eating and feeding reflect our attitudes and relationships with ourselves and others, as well as our histories. Eating is about our regard for ourselves, our connection with our bodies, and our commitment to life itself. Feeding is about the love and connection between you and your child, about trusting or controlling, providing or neglecting, accepting

or rejecting. Eating can be joyful, full of zest and vitality. Or it can be fearful, bounded by control and avoidance.

Secrets of Feeding a Healthy Family is not only about food, eating, feeding, and food preparation but also about emotional health and positive family relationships. The structure of family meals gives you a framework on which to hang the foods and connections that you and your family need. Grazing won't give it; grabbing on the run won't either. Whether your family numbers one or ten (a family is what you are when you start taking care of yourself), meals are essential for nurturing as they are for nutrition. Meals provide us all with reliable access to food, and they provide children with dependable access to their parents and to caring. Without meals, a home is just a place to stay.

The problem, of course, is that there are barriers: lack of skills, time, and money; weight and health prescriptions that make food seem like medicine or, worse, the enemy; lack of food traditions that guide us in fitting food into our ever-changing lifestyles. I offer you my help in finding your way in overcoming the barriers to positive cooking and eating. It won't be easy, but you can do it. You can do it because good eating is normal and natural and because you have the ability inside you—all you have to do is let it out. The secret of feeding a healthy family is to love good food, trust yourself, and share that love and trust with your child. That secret is within you.

I recommend that you savor this book rather

than gobbling it. It contains some fascinating stuff, but there is so much to learn about eating, feeding, cooking, and managing family meals that you may be overwhelmed if you try to do it all at once. Take your time. Begin by browsing through the chapters without trying to apply what you learn right away. Then, as you begin absorbing more, you can turn this book into a how-to manual and begin picking out the changes that you feel will be the most helpful and productive. Remember the 80/20 rule from big business: you get 80 percent of your results from 20 percent of your effort. If you give the information time to sink in, your key areas will emerge and you will develop routines that are comfortable and right for you.

To help yourself, you must remain positive. Throughout the book, my major emphasis is on helping you to adjust your attitude. In my work as an eating therapist, helping with attitude adjustment is my most important task. In my work and on these pages, I approve and encourage: enjoy your food and trust yourself to eat it; enjoy your child and trust your child to eat well. I have found that rather than making the formula or eating plan the priority, people must be the priority. I help people most with their eating when I begin with them and the foods they like and with practical and convenient cooking methods. Surprisingly (or not so surprisingly), nutrition has a way of falling into place when people are the priority rather than the rules that govern them.

Secrets of Feeding a Healthy Family is intended to help you adjust your attitude about eating and feeding. I start with how you can be positive and trusting about your own eating and how to do a good job with feeding your child. Then I talk about taming today's negative food rules to arrive at nutrition principles that support rather than undermine eating. I give you three chapters of fast, simple, and good-tasting recipes that include lots of nifty food selection, cooking, and organizing tips. Then I spend a chapter on how to plan, another on how to shop, and then I wrap up in the last chapter with how to help your child hang on to the healthy eating he learned at home when he gets into the food-crazed outside community. (By the way, I say he because this is a he chapter. With each chapter I alternate between *he* and *she*. The next chapter is a *she* chapter.) Throughout the book my attitude is positive and accepting. There are no goods and bads

here, no rights and wrongs, only what works for you and your family.

I have bent over backward to avoid making you feel guilty and ashamed. There is too much of that going on already. The goal is to help you feel empowered and encouraged. You don't have to go on a campaign to make yourself over, and you don't have to be a zealot about family meals in order to feed a healthy family. However, to make your eating and feeding come out right, you do have to make food important.

Adults at the Table

Start with feeding yourself. Put the emphasis on feeding yourself enjoyably and well. If you find the way with your own eating, you will be able to find the way with feeding your child. Our anxiety and inability to manage our own eating makes us overmanage our children's eating, imposing on them our own controlling and withholding feeding methods—or our anxiety and avoidance. It doesn't work for us, and it doesn't work for our children. Children who are controlled and overmanaged (or, conversely, not given supports or limits) don't learn to be healthy eaters. They learn to take the easy way out—or to fight with their parents rather than taking responsibility for their own eating.

Our children challenge us to do better. By the time your child is 12 or so and has more skills and resources to bring to his eating, he will begin to eat just like you do. If you are a casual grab-and-go eater, your child will become the same. If you don't trust your body and dedicate yourself to trying to make it over (with all the accompanying misery) your child will, too. As I tell you in chapter 2, "You and *Your* Eating," most adults fit into one of three groups in the way they deal with their eating and their nutritional health: the intensely careful and committed, the failing-and-feeling-bad-about-it, and the ones who couldn't care less.

None of those approaches works—either for feeding ourselves or for feeding our children. What does work? Trust. And framework. To have eating turn out well, you need to trust what goes on inside of you. Your hunger, appetite, and satiety can guide you in what and how much to eat. To have your internal signals help you the most, you also need framework. You need the regular and dependable structure of enjoyable and satisfying meals (and equally reliable snacks, if you need them). In my work with adults and their eating, I have developed a new definition of normal eating. Contrast it with the way you and others eat.

WHAT IS NORMAL EATING?

- Normal eating is going to the table hungry and eating until you are satisfied.
- Normal eating is being able to choose food you like and to eat it and truly get enough of it—not just stopping because you think you should.
- Normal eating is being able to give some thought to your food selection so you get nutritious food, but not being so wary and restrictive that you miss out on enjoyable food.
- Normal eating is sometimes giving yourself permission to eat because you are happy, sad, or bored, or just because it feels good.
- Normal eating is three meals a day—or four or five—or it can be choosing to munch along the way.
- Normal eating is leaving some cookies on the plate because you know you can have some again tomorrow, or eating more now because they taste so wonderful.
- Normal eating is overeating at times; feeling stuffed and uncomfortable. And it can be undereating at times and wishing you had more.
- Normal eating is trusting your body to make up for your mistakes in eating.
- Normal eating takes up some of your time and attention but keeps its place as only one important area of your life.

In short, normal eating is flexible. It varies in response to your hunger, your schedule, your proximity to food, and your feelings.

The definition of normal eating is positive, whereas today's eating attitudes and behaviors are negative. Because they are negative, they can't be sustained. Nobody can go through life expecting not to be fed. In chapter 2, "You and *Your* Eating," I grapple with the issues involved in helping you to become more nurturing with yourself.

Children at the Table

If you want to feed a healthy family, everybody has to be offered the same thing to eat—but they don't have to eat it. Because they are young and have natural abilities that haven't yet been distorted, children know more than we do about normal eating. Adults, however, know more about food. Children need to grow up to join the family table. They gradually master the foods that their parents eat. In too many families, it is as if everyone is eating off the high chair tray: the food selection narrows to what the child can readily accept. In the past, family meals were for the adults, and children were expected to join in. Now, family meals are orchestrated primarily on behalf of the children, and adults make do or sneak off to eat other food that is more satisfying. Gearing meals to children is a big mistake. When parents cater to children at the dinner table and limit menus to what children will readily eat, children become increasingly finicky and incapable eaters. Such children are reluctant to eat meals anywhere but at home because they fear they won't be able to manage the food.

Children can't be made the reason for family meals. Families need to be made the reason, including, most importantly, the parents. Expecting children to learn to eat what parents eat is not being mean; it is simply setting up mealtimes so children can learn and grow. It is a child's job to gradually master his environment. It is the parents' job to restrict the environment to what the child can reasonably master, not to make it completely comfortable and familiar to the child. Given proper support, children will cope.

I won't try to cover everything about child nutrition and feeding in *Secrets of Feeding a Healthy Family*. If you want more information, consult my other two books, *Child of Mine and How to Get Your Kid to Eat*. In *Child of Mine* I give step-by-step guidance in food selection for children; in *How to Get Your Kid to Eat* I explain how to raise healthy eaters and solve childhood feeding problems. (See appendix K for information on how to obtain these and other materials from Ellyn Satter Associates.) Here, though, I must be brief in this regard, but in this chapter and in chapter 3, "The Feeding Relationship," I cover enough about feeding children to free you to be successful in managing your family's food.

As I said earlier, the secret of feeding a healthy family involves loving good food, trusting yourself, and sharing that love and trust with your children. Healthy eating has to do with attitudes and feelings as well as choosing nutritious food and getting an appealing meal on the table. Healthy eating for children grows out of a positive feeding relationship with their parents and with other important adults in their lives. To feed your child well, manage what you can and let go of the rest.

I have a golden rule of feeding, and it is this:

> **Parents are responsible for the *what, when,* and *where* of feeding.**
> **Children are responsible for the *how much* and *whether* of eating.**

You are responsible only for what, when, and where you feed your child. After you have fulfilled your responsibility, it is up to your child to decide whether to eat and how much to eat *of what you have put before him*. If you observe this division of responsibility, your child will grow up being what I call a healthy eater. You will enjoy mealtimes with your child and you will avoid 99 percent of the problems parents commonly experience in feeding their children. If you don't follow this golden rule of feeding, you will get into trouble.

Childhood eating problems are getting a lot of attention right now. In the last six months, all three major television networks have called me to ask for interviews on the finicky child. Children become finicky eaters when the family menu is restricted to foods they can readily accept—and when parents hover to get them to eat foods that have been especially prepared for them. Obesity, in children and in adults, is another big concern. Children and adults get fat when struggles about eating or uncertainty about whether they will get enough to eat distorts their ability to eat the right amount to have the body nature intended. In my clinical experience, once people start focusing their efforts on providing appetizing food at predictable times, food regulation falls into place.

But to make the golden rule work, you have to discharge your responsibilities with feeding. You need to get a meal on the table. My sources tell me that many people feel they need help with managing food, so I will help. When you make it your serious business to have a family meal, you will soon realize that your share of work gives you plenty to do. Why would you volunteer for any more by trying to manage your child's eating?*

---

*I have trained other nutrition, health, and mental health professionals in my methods of working with feeding. There may be one of these professionals near you.

What the Healthy Eater Looks Like

It will help organize our discussion about children and their eating to consider what we are working toward. Your child will acquire most of his eating attitudes and behaviors by the time he is 6 years old. By that age, there are certain eating attitudes and behaviors that I would term "healthy." The same evaluation applies to older children as well as to adults and their eating. The healthy eater likes to eat and feels good about eating. He is interested in food and takes charge of his own eating. He is relaxed about picking and choosing from the food on the family table and eating what he wants without making a fuss. Given the support of the family table, over a week or several weeks he can eat a variety of foods—and that variety will add up to a nutritionally adequate diet.

The healthy eater is flexible—once he gets past being a toddler (about age 3), he can eat in places besides home and can let child care providers, the school nutrition program, and friends' parents contribute to his nutritional welfare. He can be around new or strange foods without getting upset and even experiment with new foods and learn to like them. Or he can say "no, thank you" politely if he doesn't want to try something. He can even "make do" with less favorite foods.

The healthy eater knows how much to eat. He knows it by tuning in on what goes on inside of him: how hungry and how full he is. The healthy eater doesn't worry about eating the right amount at any given meal or any given day because he trusts his body to eat the amount of food that is right for him. Because he has that kind of trust, he doesn't get upset if he eats too much or doesn't get enough to eat. If there truly is another meal or another snack coming where he can eat as much or as little as he is hungry for, he can relax because he knows that his body will make up for his mistakes in eating.

Finally, the healthy eater knows how to behave around food and eating. He has pretty good table manners, knows how to be clean with food, and can make a contribution to the comfort and enjoyment of other people at the table.

Raising a healthy eater takes years. Children

learn bite by bite, food by food, meal by meal. The goal of raising a healthy eater is to help your child grow up with positive eating attitudes and behaviors; it is not to get him to eat his peas for tonight's supper. To repeat, because it is important: *Your child's eating attitudes and behavior are more important than what he actually eats on any given day. If his attitudes and behaviors are healthy, he will eat well and get the nutrition he needs.*

It isn't easy, nowadays, to raise a healthy eater. People are upset and anxious about their own eating and confused by lots of advice—much of it destructive—about how to feed their children. Family meals are eroding with too many demands on everyone's time and too little value being placed on seeing that families get this reliable time together. Events get scheduled at dinnertime, and so many rules have piled up about "healthy" eating that meals aren't fun anymore.

To feed your family well, you have to make eating a priority. To be willing to make eating a priority, you have to take the guilt out and put the joy back in. Throughout this book (and especially in chapter 2, "You and *Your* Eating,"), I will tell you how to put the joy back into eating. In chapter 4, "Choosing Food for Your Family," you will learn to select food without being negative and rule bound.

What Children Can Teach Us about Our Eating

Secrets of Feeding a Healthy Family is about trusting not only your *child* but *also yourself* with eating. As I suggested in *How to Get Your Kid to Eat*, when adults let children lead them, they learn what healthy and normal eating is all about. Children intuitively eat what tastes good and what they are hungry for. They intuitively push themselves along to learn to like new foods. We did, too, at one time. We did, that is, until it was educated out of us by well-meaning adults and misguided, puritanical rules about eating. To better understand these intuitive capabilities, let's take a closer look at your child and his eating.

YOUR CHILD KNOWS HOW TO EAT
Even at birth your child knows how to eat, and he knows how much to eat. You trust a newborn by offering food when he is hungry, paying attention to how much he wants to eat, and feeding as fast or as slowly as he wants. When you do that, from the first he will feel good about eating. He will be comfortable and relaxed, and you will get on the same wavelength with each other so he can become more skillful with eating and more clear about telling you what he wants.

If eating has been pleasant for him from the beginning, later in his first year your child will be willing to learn to eat from a spoon and experiment with different tastes and textures. If feeding continues to go well, by age 1 year or even earlier, his desire to grow up will make him want to join the rest of the family at the table and to feed himself soft table food. By around 18 months he will be ready for the structure of planned meals and snacks. Provided no one spoils eating for them by becoming controlling, toddlers, preschoolers, and school-age children push themselves along to get better and better at chewing and swallowing, using utensils, eating in a variety of settings, and learning to like a variety of foods.

When you think of your child learning to eat, think of play, not work. Your child wants to play. He has an enormous drive to touch, to explore, to make things go. The same holds true with eating. You provide the tools, the examples, and the expectations about what he needs to learn. He provides the drive to explore what is available and master new skills. It takes a long time for a child to get all his muscles going so he can learn to ride a bike. But from the first, he is working toward it. Similarly, it takes a long time for your child to grow up to be a healthy eater. He'll work toward that too. But don't hold your breath, and don't worry about tonight's peas.

YOUR CHILD KNOWS HOW TO GROW
Along with trusting your child to want to eat and develop new eating skills, you also can trust him to develop the body that nature intended. Growth has more to do with genetics than feeding. Certainly a child's growth can be disrupted, and he may grow too slowly or too fast. But to be significant, these disruptions have to be major, and they have to go on for a long time. For the most part, children's growth is resilient. They have within them the blueprint for growing in a particular way and the

hunger and appetite to follow that blueprint. It takes a good bit to disrupt that blueprint.

ADULT EATING CAPABILITIES

You had those abilities at one time, and you can have them again—I will teach you how in the next chapter, "You and *Your* Eating." Your inborn drive to master new foods and eat what you need doesn't go away. It simply gets buried—buried under shoulds and oughts, rules and prescriptions. To hang onto eating capability throughout life, people have to be trusted, and they have to trust themselves. Too often, eating gets spoiled by *control*.

How People Lose Eating Capability

The struggle of *trust* versus *control* and the erosion of innate eating capabilities can start at birth. Adults are controlling when they impose a feeding schedule on a baby,* persuade him to finish a bottle, disguise cereal with applesauce to get it to go down, hesitate to let a chubby toddler have seconds, make a preschooler stay at the table until he finishes his vegetables, or lecture a school-age child about nutrition in order to get him to drink his milk. Control is when you worry more about the *food* than the *child*.

During preadolescence, children internalize what parents have taught them and begin to do to themselves what has been done to them. The preadolescent diets if he has been dieted; he is slavishly puritanical about eating if that

---

*A movement called Growing Families International supports parents in forcing infants onto regular schedules. Most professionals believe that this training reinforces parents' fears that if they don't "get the upper hand" early, children will be out of control forever. Infants who have been expected to get by with feeding every three to four hours and who have been expected to sleep through the night too soon are being brought into emergency rooms with poor growth and dehydration. Breastfeeding mothers who schedule feedings are drying up. The occasional child who does well with rigid structure is a child who would have been regular on his own. His parents are lucky, not skillful or successful. When you feed your baby on demand, his demands become more widely spaced and regular as he gets older. By the time he is a year old, he will make a natural transition to the meals and snacks routine of the family table. When children are toddlers, it is time to begin thinking about structure and limits. Doing it when they are babies doesn't work—and it hurts.

is the way he has been raised. (On the other hand, he may be slavishly defiant.) However, the inborn desire to eat satisfying amounts of what tastes good doesn't go away. It simply goes underground. As a consequence, over-controlled adolescents and adults play out both roles: the child who wants to enjoy eating and the adult who makes eating a chore. My adult patients regularly tell me they feel there are two conflicting people inside: the one who wants to eat and the one who tries to put on the brakes. That conflict can become extreme if a person has been raised with rigid and unrealistic standards and has been subjected to disapproval and rejection for failing to live up to those standards. To better understand that conflict, let me tell you about two of my young patients. With children and their parents, the conflict is right on the surface. The parent imposes shoulds and oughts; the child responds based on wants and needs.

TWO CHILDREN WHO WEREN'T TRUSTED

Jeremy's father was controlling, and he wasn't having any success with it. "Come to the table," he insisted, "you have to eat. We can't play catch unless you eat."

"Aargh, I don't want to," whined 5-year-old Jeremy. "Feed me! I want you to feed me!"

"I'm not going to feed you," insisted Father angrily. "You are a big boy! You have to feed yourself!" But eventually Father would give in and feed Jeremy, because he was afraid that if he didn't, Jeremy wouldn't eat. And so it went, weary meal after weary meal, day after day. Jeremy's parents grew to dread meals and hated the fight, but they were afraid to stop. If Jeremy ate this badly when they were putting all this pressure on him, how would he eat if they stopped? The only time Jeremy ate on his own was when he got candy between meals.

To be sure I wasn't missing anything, I did a careful evaluation. I reviewed Jeremy's medical record to be sure there wasn't a health condition affecting his eating. I checked his ability to chew and swallow, watched videotapes of family mealtimes, and talked with both Jeremy and his parents. My diagnosis was that Jeremy and his parents were crossing the lines of division of responsibility. To their credit, the parents were doing a wonderful job of planning and preparing meals, but they were working way too hard. They were making it their responsibility to get food into Jeremy. I told them to stop that part. My prescription was for the parents to do their job—no more, no less—and depend on Jeremy to do his. The parents were skeptical, but they didn't have any better ideas. To their surprise, observing the division of responsibility had the desired result.

Once they concentrated on their own job with feeding and trusted Jeremy to do his, Jeremy's parents were amazed to see him behaving better at the table. They continued to put their efforts into getting a meal on the table. Then they made some rules and enforced them: Jeremy was to sit up to the table; he was not to whine or beg; and he was to politely say "yes, please" or "no, thank you" to food. And they were to take no for an answer. They let him know—in words and behavior—that it was up to him to decide how much or how little he wanted to eat.

As the weeks passed, Jeremy grew up before his parents' eyes. He stopped whining, took an interest in what was on the table, and ever-so-gradually began to experiment with new foods. Jeremy ate enough to do well. But more important, he was pleasant to have around. He made conversation and listened to his parents when they talked. When he was finished eating, he asked to be excused. Between meals, instead of letting him panhandle for candy, his parents gave Jeremy regularly scheduled snacks with nutritious food they picked out. Sometimes they included candy—sometimes they didn't. Candy is all right as long as it doesn't regularly take the place of other nutritious food.

Vicky's mother was controlling, too, but in the opposite direction. Like Jeremy's parents, Vicky's mother cooked good meals, but she, too, worked too hard. She doled food out carefully and tried to restrict the amounts Vicky ate. "Is that all there is?" 6-year-old Vicky would whine as she stood in the kitchen watching her mother dish up her plate. "Isn't there any more?"

"That's all there is," answered her mother through gritted teeth. "I gave you lots more this time. That should be enough." "Every time she starts in on that, I just cringe," confessed Vicky's mother. "It seems like no matter how much I give her, she still wants more. Every time she runs out of something to do, she wants food. I am afraid if I let her eat as much as she wants, she would eat so much she would really get fat. Already she is gaining a lot of weight."

I did the same careful evaluation with Vicky as with Jeremy, and I arrived at the same conclusion. Even though the problems were seemingly opposite, with one child eating what parents thought was too little and the other seemingly eating too much, the solution for Vicky's mother was the same as for Jeremy's parents. She reestablished a division of responsibility with feeding. She put the food in serving dishes on the table and reassured Vicky she could have as much or as little as she wanted to eat. Between meals, instead of bracing herself, waiting for Vicky to beg for snacks, Mother took the initiative. She kept track of the time, and she got the food out at snack time.

At meals, Vicky was careful to remind her mother to use the serving dishes, but it wasn't long before she stopped being so preoccupied with food. Like other 6-year-olds, sometimes she would eat a little, sometimes a lot. The only time she thought a lot about food was when her mother got busy with other things and made less effort to provide meals and snacks. Vicky's mother said that being so reliable about offering regular meals and snacks was a lot of work, but the rewards made it worthwhile. It was such a relief not to have to struggle with Vicky about her eating. She found herself liking Vicky more—and enjoying her own food more. Her struggle with Vicky had been wrecking family mealtimes—and their relationship.

I have concluded from my clinical experience—and research supports my conclusions—that if you try to get children to eat more than they want, they become revolted by food and undereat when they get the chance. If you try to get children to eat less than they want, they become preoccupied with food and overeat when they get the chance. At times the undereating or overeating gets so severe that the child's growth is affected. In a 16-year study that followed almost 200 San Francisco Bay children from infancy through the teen years,[1] when children and parents struggled early on with feeding, children were more likely to be fat when they were teenagers. It seems that struggling with parents about eating made it hard for children to know how hungry and how full they were. They made mistakes in food regulation and grew in a way that wasn't natural for them. Errors in regulation and too much weight gain are serious, but the problems go beyond food regulation and weight. For a child, the struggle isn't about eating—it is about having parents understand and accept them.

CHILDREN WANT TO BE UNDERSTOOD
Why are children so vulnerable to adult interference with their eating? Why didn't we as children hang onto our eating capabilities rather than getting so conflicted and anxious? Because children have an enormous need to be understood and accepted, and they feel their parents are all-powerful. If parents understand them, they feel good about themselves. If adults don't seem to understand them, they feel bad about themselves. For young children, there is no separation between feeding and loving.

If you attend to the *what, when,* and *where* of *feeding* and trust your child to be in charge of the *how much* and *whether* of *eating,* your child concludes that you love and trust him as a *person.* If you overmanage your child's eating, he will doubt your love and trust. If you force your child to eat his peas, his feelings go something like this: "There is something the matter with me for not wanting to eat those peas and that makes me not lovable."

Jeremy put up a good fight, but underneath he felt like something was wrong with him. Vicky felt the same way about herself. Jeremy and Vicky's parents didn't intend to hurt them; they just wanted their children to eat right. The parents were separating feeding and loving. The children were not.

You understand your child when you take his word for how hungry or how full he is and accept it when he tells you whether or not he wants to eat something. You fail to understand when you impose your agenda: when you enforce certain amounts or types of food or you try to get your child to grow in a certain way. Growing out of your early feeding relationships with your parents, you may have developed distorted eating attitudes and behaviors. However, you don't have to be stuck with those distortions. As an adult, you can get enough perspective to give understanding and acceptance to yourself.

Why Parents Control

If control tactics don't work and they make everybody miserable, why do parents persist in using them? Part of the answer is that parents don't trust themselves. Another part of the answer is that feeding lore (most of it false)

is too readily available. Our current social attitudes about eating, health, and weight also contribute to the problem, as does the widespread emphasis on food as medicine and the prevalent, uncomfortable feeling that food is dangerous.

PARENTS DON'T TRUST THEMSELVES
Jeremy's father had grown up at a table where his father pounded his fist and roared, "Eat that!" He ate. He choked down the hated peas and the congealing fried catfish and the dry boiled potatoes. He had long since lost any pleasure in eating and ate pretty much because he knew he had to. Jeremy's father truly did not know that, left to his own natural tendencies, Jeremy would experiment with food and learn to like it. To understand that eating was different for Jeremy than it was for him, his father had to have some help tuning in on feelings and sensations he had long since forgotten: how food tasted to him and whether or not he enjoyed it.

Vicky's mother was not as successful at distancing herself from her feelings. From the time she was small, her mother had been vehement about restricting her food intake and body weight. Vicky's mother started going to Weight Watchers at age 10, and she had been attempting to diet ever since. She wasn't good at it. She would impose food restrictions, then fall off when she got too hungry or food became too appealing, then go back on her diet again. In order to be able to trust her daughter's eating, Vicky's mother had to learn to trust her own. She worked intensively with me for a number of weeks, learning to eat in a positive, tuned-in, self-trusting way.* It was only when she discovered her own intuitive ability to regulate the amount of food she ate that she was able to lighten up with Vicky. In the process, the mother discovered that she loved highly flavored, well-prepared food. She knew how to cook but had avoided making all the foods she loved because she was afraid she

---

*I call my method *How to Eat.* I have trained other nutrition, health, and mental health professionals in my methods in a workshop called *Treating the Dieting Casualty.* There may be one of these professionals near you. Call the nutrition services department at your local hospital or medical clinic and ask whether they have a trained *How to Eat* specialist. Also, see appendix K for information on how to obtain helpful books and other materials from Ellyn Satter Associates.

would go out of control when she ate them. To her surprise, she discovered that when she ate what she really liked, it was so satisfying that she didn't have to overeat to really enjoy it.

These parents were able to end the generational curse of distorted eating attitudes and behaviors because they were different from *their* parents in two vitally important ways. First, they were sensitive to their children's pain, and second, they were able to acknowledge that their tactics weren't working. In contrast, their parents had been absolutely convinced of the rightness of their way and impervious to their lack of success. Keep those distinctions in mind the next time you are tempted to bludgeon yourself for your parenting errors. We all make mistakes. It is in our willingness to acknowledge our errors and correct them that we remain satisfactory parents.

FEEDING LORE IS NOT RELIABLE

You know about lore. Fishermen trade lore when they tell each other to cast upwind to keep the fish from smelling them. Cooks trade lore when they share a tip like putting a little sugar in too-salty soup to tone down the salt taste. You pass along lore by example and by word of mouth. There is lots of feeding lore around—it has to do with what should go in the bottle or when to start solid foods or when you should stop breastfeeding or how to get your toddler to eat or how to get your school-age child to behave at the table. Parents trade lore when they say kids have to be made to eat vegetables. Or, more likely, parents feed the way they were fed and that, too, was based on lore. Lore gets tested by experience. If you catch the fish or rescue dinner, you know the lore worked—and you tell someone else. Some lore is accurate; feeding lore is not.

To understand why not, let's look at the bit of lore that says that children have to be forced or they won't learn to like vegetables. This is not the usual shrewd advice you get with lore but only a self-fulfilling prophecy. In reality, children won't learn to like anything if they are forced to eat it. Instead, they learn, "If I have to eat this, it must not be so good. So I won't like it." A child who is forced to eat vegetables might continue to eat them when he grows up, but it will be because he should, not because he wants to. On the other hand, the forced child might just quit eating vegetables altogether when parents aren't around to keep up the pressure.

So, why doesn't this bit of lore get thrown away? Probably because feeding is a lot more complicated than fishing or cooking. It takes lots longer to see results with feeding children, and the results may not be what we expect. If a child eats tonight's broccoli, it seems like the forcing tactic worked. And if the parent doesn't push and the child leaves the broccoli, it is further proof, right? Wrong! The proof is not in whether the child eats broccoli tonight; it is in whether the child grows up to enjoy broccoli. To get that proof, we have to turn to research—to careful and systematic observations of how children behave over the long term with their eating.

Many of those observations have been done by L. L. Birch, a psychologist at Penn State University.[2] Over the years, Birch and her students have presented children with one eating challenge after another and observed how they cope. My own observations of children and Birch's research agree. Children are cautious about new food; they don't automatically like new food, and they usually don't eat it the first time it is offered. However, children push themselves along to learn to like new food. They watch their adults eat it, they put it in their mouths and take it out again many times, and eventually they swallow it. Swallowing means they like it, and they start the whole process over again with something else.

Children don't need to be pressured to watch and experiment and do the in-and-out thing in the process of learning to like new food. They just do it. They are in the business of growing up—with respect to eating as with everything else in their lives. If it's on the table, and if nobody puts pressure on them to eat, they assume that one fine day they will eat it too. I will give you more details about what works with children's quirky eating behaviors in chapter 3, "The Feeding Relationship."

EATING ATTITUDES ARE DISTORTED

Distorted attitudes are running—and ruining—our eating. Attitudes are subtle and implied rather than spoken right out loud, and are, in fact, often hard to pin down. But they affect you nonetheless. They can control your behavior, change the way you feel, and get you to make decisions without really thinking through the options. But to raise a healthy eater, you have to deal with destructive attitudes.

Too many people today are unsuccessful

with eating, and unsuccessful with feeding their children. Adults are anxious and ambivalent about their own eating—and these feelings rub off on their parenting. Where does the trouble come from? It comes from prevailing ideas and attitudes about food and about our bodies.

In chapter 2, "You and *Your* Eating," I encourage you to be positive and dependable about feeding yourself. An attitude that has sneaked up on us is that eating isn't important. In some other countries, people take time for meals, and their meals are gratifying for them. In the United States, eating is something you do in a hurry, or when hunger drives you to it, or when children insist on being fed. It isn't something we plan for and invest time and energy in and depend on to provide us with nurturing and companionship.

I complained earlier about events being scheduled at dinnertime. I have other examples of how we have made eating unimportant. Child care centers and schools feed in a hurry and children eat in a hurry to get out on the playground. Families wolf down dinner (or eat in the car on the way home from work) so they can have some fun together or get the chores done. Office workers eat muffins or popcorn at their desks so they can get more work done or run errands at lunchtime.

When we do give attention to our eating, it is negative and rule bound. A particularly destructive example is our obsession with and confusion about body weight. A related example is our attitude that food should be used as medicine.

WEIGHT ATTITUDES ARE DISTORTED

The prevailing attitude is that we weigh more than we should and that we have to be constantly vigilant to keep our weight down. The enthusiasts who have gotten the podium have set arbitrary weight standards, and those standards are so low that over half of us are considered overweight. If we are overweight, what are we to do about it? Why, deprive ourselves, of course. And what does that deprivation do to our trust in our internal processes and our joy in eating? Why, spoils it, of course. In chapter 2, I encourage you to give your body a break. In the appendixes at the end of the book, I address the question of whether or not to diet.

Will you accept your weight and your child's weight and trust yourself? Or will you try to change and control your weight? How you answer will determine whether your eating is positive or negative, whether it is a lifelong struggle or can assume its proper place as only one of life's great issues.

FOOD IS SEEN AS MEDICINE

Attempting to follow current nutritional standards takes the pleasure out of eating and makes us negative, fearful, and controlling. The campaigning about wellness and prevention of heart disease and, to a lesser degree, cancer, implies (or says outright) that these diseases are caused by bad eating habits. The message is everywhere; it comes in the form of press conferences by government agencies, news releases from disease organizations, media features about new studies, and public relations campaigns from the American Heart Association and the American Cancer Society. Food as medicine sells. Food manufacturers see to it that the campaign is everywhere, and their efforts center on finding and marketing the "next oat bran"—the magic bullet that will drastically increase sales.

Most of the advertising and promoting is about the fat content of food. Despite conflicting evidence, current leaders in nutrition policy making are convinced that dietary fat is the culprit causing cancer and heart disease and that restricting fat in the diet can prevent or even cure these degenerative diseases. I call these folks the nutrition enthusiasts. Enthusiasm is all right, but the enthusiasts are often so convinced of the rightness of their point of view that they are judgmental about it. Embedded in nutrition enthusiasm is the attitude "If you get sick it is your own fault."

However, in the barrage of nutrition enthusiasm, there are voices that are not being heard. These are the voices of the nutrition moderates. These are the voices that say, "Wait a minute! There are no guarantees; there is no proof." The one-sided story that reaches the public ignores the substantial disagreement among nutritionists, pediatricians, cardiologists, and other experts about the extent to which dietary fat contributes to disease and about the extent to which modification of dietary fat can prevent disease. The moderates look at the same studies that guide the enthusiasts and conclude that the research does not support making sweeping dietary changes. They point out that available data linking changes in diet to improvements in mortality show modest and variable results.

I consider myself a nutrition moderate. In chapter 4, "Choosing Food for Your Family," I grapple in detail with turning rigid rules into helpful guidelines. My own conviction as a nutrition moderate is that while finding the middle ground is a good idea and while more serious dietary changes may be appropriate for people who have health conditions, the research is not convincing enough to support putting every man, woman, and child in this country on a restrictive modified-fat, low-cholesterol, low-salt diet. Good nutrition is certainly essential for health, and the best way to ward off disease is to be healthy in the first place. I emphasize variety and food seeking rather than avoidance, eating and enjoying food rather than trying to stay away from food-as-poison. A special diet is warranted if someone has heart disease, but if not the benefits from rigid dietary modification are not great enough to justify spoiling the joy of eating. When the joy goes out of eating, nutrition suffers.

As a nutrition moderate, I have set a personal goal in this book of not shaking my finger at you and saying "don't" or "should" or even "ought." I will give you specific advice about how you can be a food seeker rather than a food avoider and find the middle ground between too little and too much. In the process, you can hedge your bets against disease without spoiling your eating. I won't try to motivate you to do anything, because I think you know more about your life than I do, and you are in a better position to make up your own mind about what to do. I assume that you will make decisions that are in your best interests and your child's.

To feel responsible about giving you my blessings to enjoy food and stop worrying so much about making yourself sick, I have had to satisfy myself that my recommendations are safe. I have delved into the heart disease and diet controversy, a deep and murky place if there ever was one. I have carefully read the studies and consulted with nutrition moderates and enthusiasts, and I am satisfied that my recommendations are sound. The appendixes contain most of the pertinent technical and scientific information, which is pretty interesting, but you don't have to read it. You will be able to understand what you need perfectly well without it. The material is there, though, in case you want to go into more depth.

FOOD IS VIEWED AS DANGEROUS

Related to, but not identical with, the food-as-medicine idea is the notion that our food is dangerous. Such convictions label certain foods "bad" and others "good." The idea is that it is more healthful to eat vegetables than animals, and "health," "natural," or "organic" foods are most healthful of all. In reality, both animal and vegetable foods make important contributions to the diet. Any time you avoid entire food groups you run a nutritional risk. Furthermore, foods have the same nutritional value whether or not they are grown organically. The major value of organic foods is ecological—they are grown using methods that are intended to preserve and restore the land they are grown on.

Food scientists agree that the biggest danger associated with food is bacterial contamination. To be safe for consumption, all food needs to be handled appropriately. It must be properly stored: hot food has to be kept hot, cold food cold. All washable food must be carefully washed to get rid of bacteria, pesticides, or fertilizers. This is simply part of safe food-handling practice. In chapter 8, "Planning to Get You Cooking" and in the cooking chapters (chapters 5, 6, and 7), I go into detail about sanitation. The importance of food sanitation is clear; the rest is subjective and political. There are political, ecological, and spiritual reasons why people avoid animal products or grow and buy organic food. To feed your family well, you have to be clean, but you don't have to become vegetarian or buy organic or natural food. Ordinary food from the ordinary grocery store is as nourishing as any other variety.

Summary

As you read this book, it won't escape you that my advice about food selection, eating, and feeding is more liberal than what you usually hear. I think nutrition is important, and I think the way you feed your child is very important. But I don't think you need to be worried or frightened about your food. As I said earlier, I consider myself to be a nutrition moderate, not a nutrition enthusiast. Nutritional enthusiasm has contributed greatly to the conflict and anxiety people feel about their eating and to negative attitudes about food and eating.

I feel strongly that to make a considered decision about how to feed your family you need to get out from under those negative attitudes. In chapter 4, "Choosing Food for Your Family," I'll deal more concretely with public health and medical issues of disease prevention. Here, the issue is attitude. Do your job, expect your child to do his, and settle down.

Throughout this chapter and this book, I emphasize trust: Trust yourself, and trust your child. This message sharply contrasts with today's prevailing attitude, which is "Control your eating and your child's eating." Control makes us ignore our appetite and hunger and makes us impose outside expectations of what and how much to eat. It makes us do the same with our children.

While it is your choice how restrictive you want to be with yourself, it is not wise to be restrictive with your child. Children are a captive audience—they don't have the option of sneaking around to get what they want. Children need enough flexibility in fat intake to let them grow. Adults need to provide them with what they need. Sometimes children grow so fast or are so active that they need a lot of energy. Without flexible access to fat in their diets, they won't be able to get enough energy. (You'll learn how to provide that flexibility in chapter 4, "Choosing Food for Your Family.")

When you try to control what you can't, like heart disease, cancer, and fatness, you try to control your child. In the two stories I told earlier, the parents were trying to control their children and force certain outcomes. In both cases, the parents didn't feel successful, and parents and children were miserable. Eating was being spoiled for everyone, and the children felt bad about themselves.

We must find the middle ground. It is easy to find the extremes, being either too rigid and restrictive or too lax about nutrition and meals. But finding that whole gray area between the two extremes is far more difficult. In *Secrets of Feeding a Healthy Family*, we are after the beautiful and mysterious grays.

Selected References

1. Crawford, P. B., and L. R. Shapiro. 1991. How obesity develops: A new look at nature and nurture. In *Obesity and Health*, ed. F. M. Berg, 40–41. Hettinger, ND: Healthy Living Institute.
2. Satter, E. 1995. Feeding dynamics: Helping children to eat well. *Journal of Pediatric Health Care* 9: 178–184.

How to Feed Yourself

- *Trust* yourself.
- Be positive and dependable about feeding yourself.
- Have food you enjoy.
- Emphasize variety.
- Don't get caught in "being good" and "being bad."
- Give yourself permission to eat.
- Stop being phobic about sugar, fat, and salt.
- Be disciplined but not negative.
- Give your body a break.

CHAPTER
2
YOU AND *YOUR* EATING

Before you can feed a healthy family, you have to feed yourself. To help your child, you have to help yourself. Your child will eat, and feel about eating, the way you do. If that gives you a little thrill of dismay and dread, you have work to do. If you feel conflicted and anxious about eating, it is not surprising, and you are not alone. But most parents don't want their child to feel bad about eating. It feels rotten, for one thing. It isn't a good basis for nutritional health, for another. Today's attitudes about eating are punishing and negative. We feel, surveys find, that eating nutritious food takes all the pleasure out of eating. Eating "properly" comes loaded with overtones of fear, control, and dreariness. Such attitudes are not good motivators. Optimism, pleasure, and self-trust are good motivators.

Celebrate eating. To be consistent and effective in feeding a family, you must build the whole structure of family meals around *enjoyment*. Today, far too much is made of the difficulties of eating: avoiding disease, not getting fat, not *eating* fat. I hope by the time you finish reading this chapter, you will have a more positive vision. Put the emphasis on eating (and feeding) yourself, not on avoiding. Get a satisfying meal on the table, pay attention while you eat it, trust yourself to eat as much or as little as you need, and then forget about eating until it is time to eat again. For your eating fall into place, you have to make it important and gratifying.

Although feeding yourself requires effort and discipline, the discipline need not be negative. Planning and making meals requires sustained effort and may involve considerable learning and change for you. The discipline is positive and achievable, and joyful rewards are built right in, but it is discipline nonetheless. Take it easy on yourself. Don't try to change everything at once. Set your priorities, be realistic about what you can do, and acquire new skills and discipline slowly over time. Eventually you will have put together your own personal, useful, and agreeable way of feeding your family. However, to be free to pleasure yourself with eating, you must first get rid of some interference.

The Trouble with Our Eating

Current eating attitudes and behaviors are negative. The specifics of the advice may vary, but from the latest government directives about the "healthy diet," to articles in the media about nutrition research, to food advertisements everywhere, it seems the official attitude about eating is "don't." Don't eat too much fat, too much sugar, too much salt, too much food, period. Lose weight, eat more fiber. It has gotten to the point where we worry more about *avoiding* than we do about *eating*.

The nutrition enthusiasts have gotten the upper hand. When the principle of medicalized eating was first introduced to the public, many people were very dedicated. Now, it seems we are getting tired of the deprivation. Surveys show that fewer and fewer people are troubling to be really "careful." (To read about those surveys, see appendix A, "What Surveys Say about Our Eating"). Roughly a third of us say we are "already doing it," a generous third of us say "I know I should but . . . ," and nearly half say "Don't bother me." Of course, the gap between what people thought they "should" do and what they were actually *able* to do with their eating was widest for the "I know I should but . . ." people. That gap translates into discomfort and anxiety about eating. The less you are able to live up to your standards, the worse you feel.

Other surveys show that the number one nutritional concern is fat in the diet, with over 50 percent of consumers worrying about avoiding fat and only 10 percent about eating nutritious food. Again, our behavior contradicts our standards. Even while our concern about fat is high, fat intake is going up. We are eating so much full-fat cheese and premium ice cream that we have contributed to a butterfat shortage. Ice cream production is up, but production of low-fat ice cream and frozen yogurt is down. What is the result of this contradiction between our concerns and our behavior? Guilt, of course. We eat it, but we feel guilty about it.

Women in particular feel guilty and anxious about how they eat, especially if they see themselves as overweight (and most do). Some guilt stems from feeling obligated but unable to lose weight, and some stems from feeling obligated but unable to adhere to low-fat eating. I speak and consult with nutrition professionals across the United States, and they report that their clients have considerable difficulty adhering to current dietary standards. These standards are summarized in two government publications, *Dietary Guidelines for Americans* and *The Food Guide Pyramid*. I know some of my readers care deeply about these publications. Others couldn't care less and probably don't even know they exist. The framers of the Guidelines and the Pyramid did what they thought was right, but in my view it was an experiment that failed. If you want to review the set of recommendations that has so many in so much of a tizzy, see the box titled "The Dietary Guidelines" in this chapter and the "Food Guide Pyramid" on page 50. To learn why I have so much trouble with the Guidelines, see my discussion in appendix B,

"The Dietary Guidelines and Why They Are Rule Bound."

THE DIETARY GUIDELINES
- Eat a variety of food.
- Balance food with physical activity-maintain or improve your weight.
- Choose a diet with plenty of grain products, vegetables, and fruits.
- Choose a diet low in fat, saturated fat, and cholesterol.
- Choose a diet moderate in sugars.
- Choose a diet moderate in salt and sodium.
- If you drink alcoholic beverages, do so in moderation.

Even nutritionists who depend on rules acknowledge that the Guidelines are too complex and too confusing for most people to follow. Some of them got together, to form what they called the Dietary Alliance and tried to remedy the problem.* Unfortunately, the solution presented by the alliance was to make more rules. The resulting messages were still externally controlling: "Make small changes over time," and "Balance what you eat with physical activity." The alliance was willing to endorse the concept of enjoyment but couldn't resist throwing in a warning: "Enjoy all foods but *don't overdo it.*" Like most nutrition professionals, the alliance didn't understand that we all have within us natural mechanisms that help us to avoid overdoing it. Clarifying ways to control ourselves doesn't help the basic contradiction of trying to force ourselves to do what we don't feel like doing. Eating goes best when we work *with* our inclinations rather than *against* them.

Dieting Casualties

I work with the casualties, the people for whom the negativity about eating has gotten totally out of hand. I'll tell you about some of the extreme cases because I think we can learn a great deal about run-of-the-mill eating habits

---

*Some of the Dietary Alliance members were professional organizations like the American Dietetic Association and the Food Marketing Institute; federal agencies like the U.S. Departments of Agriculture, U.S. Health and Human Services, and the Food and Drug Administration; and producer organizations like the Dairy Council, Wheat Foods Council, National Cattleman's Beef Association, and Produce Marketing Association.

from their stories. You may glimpse yourself in these cases, and in having that glimpse, you may understand more clearly why you have trouble feeding yourself and your child.

My patients have been so traumatized by weight-reduction dieting or forced eating, often from an early age, that paying attention to their inclinations is out of the question. If the trauma was in the name of weight control, they grew up continually feeling they had to go without, or forcing themselves to eat low-calorie food in order to have a thinner body than the one nature provided. Eventually my patients couldn't stand the deprivation anymore. As one of them recently told me, "If I have to weigh it, count it, or measure it, it makes me crazy."

I have worked with other dieting casualties as well—an eating-phobic woman comes to mind. The only way she could eat was if she distracted herself by reading a book or watching television. Then she got eating over with as fast as she could. She ate rapidly and took in as little food as possible to sustain life. She had been forced to eat when she was little by parents who were vehement about good nutrition. Her parents were downright sadistic in their insistence that she eat the food they deemed wholesome. They often forced her to sit for hours in front of a plate of congealing food— liver was the worst—until she could finally choke it down. The legacy for her was so much internal conflict when she approached eating that she could get food down only by going on automatic pilot. I have seen that unconscious, mindless eating in many people, but she helped me most to understand it. She could only deal with her inner conflict about eating by doing what I have come to call *eating-with-out-eating*.

To help her build a more positive relationship with food, I used desensitization training. I gradually introduced her to food, helped her focus her attention on it, and helped her relax and deal with her upset when she tuned in on her food and her eating. She started with a strawberry, the least threatening food she could think of. It took her three weeks to get to the point that she could put the strawberry in her mouth, and then she couldn't swallow it or even chew it. She had to take it back out again. But finally she was able to chew and swallow the strawberry. Then she learned to enjoy it. From there, she moved on to other foods. By the end of the five months we worked togeth-

er, she was eating and enjoying a variety of food.

My patients, and others like them, are in a bind. They have been so traumatized by dietary restrictions and expectations that they can't go by them anymore. But with all the restricting and forcing, they have lost their sensitivity to their internal sensations of hunger, appetite, and satiety. Because they can't tolerate external regulators, and they can't feel, accept, or trust internal regulators, their eating becomes chaotic.

It takes careful clinical work with dieting casualties to rebuild trust in internal regulation. Because their inclinations toward eating have been so rejected by so many for so long (including themselves), they even feel ashamed that these inclinations *exist*. Children always assume their parents and other adults are right. If the adult says it is wrong to want chocolate cake, then it must be so, and it must be shameful to want it. The child's internal conflict produces so much static that children can't respect—or even know—what they feel inside. The child who grows up in this bind becomes the adult who feels conflicted and distressed about eating.

I teach my adults who have been traumatized with eating how to eat normally. And they have taught me to stay far away from the rules, the shoulds, and the oughts. I will do the same with you. We have all been traumatized at least a little bit with regard to our eating. To eat as well as possible, we have to free ourselves from rule-bound eating.

DISTORTED HEALTH PRIORITIES

Sometimes people become dieting casualties because they are sick and afraid to eat. A 75-year-old woman who was recovering from severe angina and open heart surgery comes to mind. During the critical stage of her disease, she lost 15 pounds and became thin and with depleted body reserves. When she was discharged from the hospital, someone—it is not clear who—casually told her to follow a modified-fat diet and to restrict salt.

Realistically, given her age and condition, it was probably too late for dietary interventions that may or may not have been helpful in the first place. Salt restriction may have been necessary had her heart muscle been weakened by the disease to the extent that it couldn't circulate blood properly to the kidneys. The result is a condition called *congestive heart disease*, in which the body retains fluids, thus forcing the heart to work harder in order to circulate blood throughout the body.

The real problem, however, was that the woman was not given specific enough guidance. It wasn't clear that she was retaining fluids, and given what she had been through with her illness and surgery, the general warning to "restrict fat" and "avoid salt" only terrified her and made her so afraid of food that she didn't eat enough to enable her body to heal. Rigid sodium restriction is not for the casual or uninformed—it is medical nutrition therapy. It carries with it too great a risk of impairing dietary quality overall. Even for people with congestive heart disease, once they get out of the hospital and their diuretic medications have been adjusted, most can keep sodium at about 3,000 to 4,000 milligrams per day—the level I use for the meals suggested in this book.

For our 75-year-old heart patient, as for the rest of us, it was more important to *eat* than to *avoid*. When she lost weight, she didn't just lose fat; she lost muscle and organ tissue. The irony is that she needed to eat to be able to nourish her heart, and she was afraid to do that. She needed a dietitian's help to get a prescription for a specific and realistic level of sodium and to translate that prescription into food.

"Come on back, Ellyn," you may say. "This is a book about young families. Why are you talking about a 75-year-old woman?" Well, I'll tell you why. You may have someone like this is your life, and maybe you can help her get better nutritional care. But, beyond that, much of the panic younger people feel about disease prevention arises because someone they know has heart disease. If she has heart disease and she has to limit salt, we should avoid salt to prevent heart disease, right? Wrong. Bad logic. It doesn't follow at all. When we change our diet to manage a disease, it is because that disease has limited the body's ability to cope with certain nutrients. For instance, people with diabetes can't manage a lot of sugar, so they adjust. However, we can't prevent diabetes by avoiding sugar.

BALANCING THE SHOULDS AND WANTS

Most people aren't dieting casualties, and they aren't ill, but they still have considerable trouble balancing the internals and externals: the *wants* with the *shoulds* and *oughts*. Many just try to find a sensible and livable way through all the mandates about eating and weight. They try to find the middle ground. As in any other area, finding the middle ground is much harder than going to the extremes of "already doing" and "don't bother me."

The enduring middle-ground message about food selection is *variety, moderation, and balance.* Everyone can agree on this message, dietary enthusiasts and moderates alike. It is a good message: Eat a variety of food, do so in moderation, and balance food choices so that together they add up to good nutrition. Unfortunately, people today feel so guilty and negative about eating that even these seemingly neutral guidelines come across as judgmental and withholding. Variety is interpreted as "eat a lot of food you don't like," moderation as "don't eat as much as you are hungry for," and balance as "put together meals you'd rather not eat." It's all very dreary.

The negativity is not working, especially for children. Adults feel that eating nutritious food is a chore, and sometimes they feel like doing the chores, and sometimes they don't. In contrast, children won't make eating a chore—they eat only what tastes good to them. So parents and children come into conflict—parents do what they think is right, and children rebel. Or parents refuse to be bothered, and children don't get the support they need to learn how to eat.

Three Eating-Troubled Children

As far as feeding children is concerned, each of the three survey groups—"already doing it," "I know I should but . . . ," and "don't bother me"—leave something to be desired. To get a better idea of what's happening, let's take a look at three children I have worked with in my practice. Keep in mind as you read that all three sets of parents were doing the best they could for their children and that they sought help because they knew their methods weren't working. Once the parents changed, their children changed right along with them.

ANNIE, WHO ATE ONLY AT THE NEIGHBOR'S

Annie's parents were in the "already doing it" group. They were confident that their food selection and menu planning were above reproach. They served only broiled poultry and fish, vegetables without added fat, bread with a tiny dab of diet margarine, and nonfat milk. But they were exhausted from fighting with their 4-year-old daughter about food. Why, they asked me, was Annie interested in eating only at a neighbor's house, where they weren't nearly as careful about nutrition? Why didn't Annie appreciate what they were doing for her?

I told them, "You have done what you thought was best for Annie. Unfortunately, it has taken all the fun out of eating for her. Children won't eat what they are supposed to—they eat what tastes good. I would guess the neighbors use more fat than you do, and that makes their food taste better to Annie than what you make at home. Extremely low-fat food is not tasty. One way wonderful cooks make good food come alive is to use some fat. Fat makes food taste good. Fat also makes food seem more moist. For children, dry food gets stuck in their mouths."

I encouraged Annie's parents to lighten up on their restrictions. (I will cover disease prevention in more detail in chapter 4.) I also emphasized the division of responsibility in feeding and warned them to stop pressuring Annie to eat. They were loathe to give up their restrictive eating. They were proud of how well they could do with limiting themselves, and truth be told, for them food restriction and avoidance was trendy. But they loved Annie a lot and wanted her back at dinnertime, so they lightened up. As a result, Annie took more of an interest in what they had on the table and stopped reminding them how much better the food was next door. Sometimes Annie ate a little, sometimes a lot.

JOSHUA, WHO COULDN'T WAIT FOR FRIDAY NIGHT

Joshua's parents hailed from the "know I should . . ." group. They *tried* to adhere to what they thought they should eat to prevent disease, but they kept getting ambushed by their fat cravings. Their strategy was to plan for the ambush. They gave themselves weekends off from restrictive dieting. For the parents, this strategy seemed to work. They ate a few preferred foods on the weekend, and then buckled down again on Monday morning. For Joshua, their 8-year-old, this strategy was a problem.

Unlike Annie, Joshua was *too* interested in

food. Joshua ate what his parents prepared—and then some. It seemed that he just couldn't get filled up. During the week, he always seemed hungry and begged for snacks. On the family's Friday trips to the movies, Joshua was up and down all evening—visiting the snack bar to buy nachos, ice cream, buttered popcorn, and all the treats his parents wouldn't let him have any other time. At his grandmother's house, Joshua couldn't get enough fried chicken, mashed potatoes and gravy, and salad with blue cheese dressing.

As with Annie's parents, I encouraged Joshua's parents to lighten up. I taught them some meal-planning strategies and warned against being so restrictive with their food that they had to take a vacation from it. I pointed out that Joshua's energy needs were high and his stomach was still relatively small. He needed some higher-calorie foods throughout the week to have the energy he needed.

After his parents followed my suggestions, Joshua settled down. On Friday nights, they let him have one treat at the movies, and that was all he wanted. After all, now he could get those foods at home. His grandmother worried at first that he didn't like her fried chicken anymore, but he reassured her that now his mom made it sometimes too.

GINNY, WHO ATE FROM A *SHORT* LIST

Ginny's parents were in the "don't bother me" group. When they came to see me, they complained that 4-year-old Ginny was way too finicky. Her short list of acceptable foods included chicken nuggets, French fries, peanut butter on white bread, milk, fruit loops, and orange juice. Ordinarily, they just saw to it that she got what she liked. But Ginny's eating had become a problem recently because she had started going to child care. She wouldn't eat there. She just sat at the table and looked at her food. She might sip her milk, but that was all. She looked so melancholy and ate so little that the child care providers were worried about her.

At home, Ginny's parents continued to prepare what she wanted to eat, but as usual they didn't have meals themselves. They ate at work at their desks or grabbed something on the way home. While Ginny ate dinner, her mother leaned against the kitchen counter and drank a cup of coffee. Usually Ginny's father didn't get home until after Ginny went to bed. He made himself a sandwich, and her mother had cereal during the evening if she got hungry.

Ginny's parents weren't much interested in food. The two of them had a long-standing dispute about who was in charge of cooking. To both of them, meals were negative; they were a big, unrewarding chore that neither wanted to do. Both had grown up in households where meals were intensely important, devotedly nutritious and relentlessly controlling. As children, both of Ginny's parents had to eat certain virtuous (and often drab) food. As a result, *nobody* cooked at Ginny's house.

This time I had to tell the child's parents to shape up rather than lighten up. Their method of eating worked for them—sort of—but it wasn't working for Ginny. Since she hadn't been exposed to a variety of foods, she had learned to like very few. Because she didn't get her parents' social support at mealtime, she frankly wasn't interested in eating, and she didn't know how to behave at the table. Ginny's parents didn't want to be bothered, but they could see that their behavior was creating difficulties for their daughter. We set up a plan to help them get back to the family table.

In that plan, we found appealing, easy-to-prepare food and we negotiated the chores. Perhaps most important, as with my eating-phobic patients, we also did desensitization training to help the parents resolve their negative feelings so they could enjoy eating.

The strategies first employed by these families did not work out well for them. Being overzealous, being inconsistent, not caring—all were causing trouble. To help the children, I had to help the parents. The issue for you is the same as for Annie, Joshua, and Ginny's parents: how to help yourself feel better about food and eating so you can have a pleasant family table. How can you make meals important for yourself and your child without getting caught by the nutrition enthusiasts—or, worse, becoming one yourself? How can you relax with your eating without being neglectful? How can you make nutrition important and be serious about feeding yourself and your child without making it a life's work?

To find the answers, let's see if we can transform those enduring middle-ground messages we talked about earlier—*variety, moderation, and balance*—by looking at them from a more positive perspective. What does it take to neutralize the messages "eat a lot of food you

don't like," "don't eat as much as you are hungry for," and "put together meals you'd rather not eat?" Why, self-trust, of course. Rather than trying to impose a formula—and food—on ourselves, we need to seek out food we like and eat enough of it to get satisfied. To do that, we have to trust our likes and dislikes and our hunger and fullness.

The Key Is Trust

Annie, Joshua, Ginny, and their parents are not the only ones who have a problem. We all do. We can't eat what we think we *should* eat, and we feel bad when we eat what we *like*. Rather than redoubling our efforts to adhere to unrealistic standards, and failing still again, we need to lighten up. I said this before in a slightly different way, and I'll say it again: the secret of feeding a healthy family is to provide yourself with enjoyable food and trust yourself to eat as much as you need. Then do the same for your child. You need to trust and help yourself so you can trust and help your child. Love good food and seek it out. It doesn't matter if your particular definition of good food is different from mine or from that of the nutrition enthusiasts. It is your definition, and you have every right to it. In fact, you are stuck with it.

If you have a joyful attitude about eating, appreciate many different foods, and put the emphasis on having family meals, your diet will be nutritious and healthful and your child will grow up to be a healthy eater. Happy meals are the key, and I don't mean the kind you get from McDonald's. Your child will be curious about food and will want to acquire new eating skills because you show her that eating is a fine thing to do. In the long run, your positive and relaxed attitude and approach will give her the best chance of having a lifelong healthy diet because it will ensure that she eats a variety of food.

To do a good job with your eating, you need support, just as your child does. Earlier we talked about the division of responsibility in feeding. To provide a foundation for your child's eating, you need to provide meals and snacks that are appealing, nutritious, and plentiful, and you need to make eating times pleasant. You need to provide that same foundation for *yourself*. To manage the what, when, and where of your eating—the context—here are some simple guidelines.

Be Dependable about Feeding Yourself

If you want to manage your eating in an orderly and positive fashion, you need to know you are going to be fed. For your child, you take care of the *what, when,* and *where* of feeding. For yourself, you must also provide the *what, when,* and *where.* You must provide yourself with good-tasting food at predictable times in an environment that you enjoy.

Five chapters of this book (chapters 5 through 9) are devoted to helping you manage the what, when, and where of your eating. Those chapters contain suggestions for what to cook and explain specifically how to prepare good food so you leave in—and enhance—the flavor and pleasure.

YOU HAVE TO HAVE MEALS

There is considerable peace and comfort in knowing you are going to be fed. If you have a meal coming, and you know it is going to be something you enjoy, you can forget about eating until it's time. Whether you know it or not, if you wait until hunger drives you to figure out what to eat, you'll scare yourself. If you behave as if every meal is your last, insisting on just the right food, prepared in just the right way, chances are you have been depriving yourself with respect to either the type or amount of food you eat. Getting fed is our most primitive and urgent creature need. Failing to provide for that need in a trustworthy fashion makes it control you. Providing for that need will free you and give you pleasure. When you have a meal and let yourself leave the table feeling satisfied, you know you've been fed. When you eat on the run or graze or munch, there is no beginning, no ending. Without meals, you will find yourself rummaging to get a sense of completion and satisfaction.

Meals have to be satisfying, not just a chore. Plan ahead to make sure you have good food—by that I mean good-*tasting* food. I chose every main-dish recipe in chapters 5 and 6 because I like it, and I like the menus that accompany the recipes. In chapter 8, "Planning to Get You Cooking," I introduce a cycle menu to help you map out several weeks of meals. As you incorporate the suggestions into your own planning, you will find that eating becomes both more and less important. At mealtime, it will be the focus of attention. Between mealtimes, you will be able to forget about it.

Planning or not planning can have a major impact on your food selection as well. If you plan ahead, you'll have a chance to provide yourself with both good and good-for-you food. If you wait until you are hungry to figure out what to eat, you will probably grab something that is not too tasty and also not so good for you. You are also likely to seek out high-calorie food. It's natural to seek out high-calorie food when you are hungry and desperate to eat.

Research shows that hungry children have a marked preference for food they have found by experience to be high in calories and therefore very filling and satisfying. This research has not been done with adults. In fact, it probably wouldn't work, because adults put so much interference between themselves and these natural ways of eating ("I shouldn't have that—it's not good for me—oh, well, just this one time . . ."). So, to find out about natural ways of eating, we have to look at children. Young children don't eat what they *should.* They pick and choose from what is put before them, eating what tastes good and eating as much as they are hungry for.

Watch out for the interference. In planning your meals, beware the overdeveloped conscience that comes from bouts with dieting and concern about health. If you like potato chips with your sandwich, *plan them in.* Don't fall into the trap of avoiding planning as a way of getting around your conscience! Your meal needs to satisfy your *appetite* as well as your hunger, or you'll go rummaging around later, looking for something to give you the pleasure you didn't get at the meal. And don't try to placate yourself with lower-fat potato crackers or baked potato chips. Eat them if you like them, but keep in mind that they are only about 10 percent lower in calories than the real thing. And don't try to trick your body by eating that Olestra stuff. It interferes with the absorption of fat-soluble nutrients, like vitamin A and carotene. The vitamin A is added back in Olestra-fried foods, but carotene is not.

PROVIDE YOURSELF WITH RELIABLE EATING TIMES

For most people, it works best to have meals at regular times, to plan snacks so you can get comfortably through to mealtime without being famished, then to forget about eating between times. If you know you will be fed, and fed well, you won't want to spoil your appetite by grazing on little tidbits here and there. The tidbits are okay, but the lack of attention is not. When you graze, you miss out on good eating because it is hard to tune in and really enjoy your food. Don't force yourself to graze to get the tidbits you want. Include them at meals.

Grazing is rapidly becoming our preferred way of eating. Foods are marketed as commuter foods—the kind you can eat with one hand while you drive. We keep foods on the counter, on our desks, in the break room, even in little dishes on the floor for toddlers to grab as they run by or on low shelves in the refrigerator for children to help themselves when the spirit moves them.

Grazing doesn't work for children. Depending on your food environment and on how your food regulation system is wired, it may or may not work for you. I made a big point about meals in both *Child of Mine and How to Get Your Kid to Eat*. In chapter 3, I emphasize the importance of providing regular planned eating times for children. Children need structure to help them learn to like a variety of foods, consume a nutritionally adequate diet, and eat the right amount to grow well. Adults do too, come to think of it, for many of the same reasons that children do.

If you are willing to follow my recommendations about the importance of structure, enough said. However, grazing is so deeply embedded in our way of eating that you may need to be persuaded. If so, refer to appendix C, "Grazing, Cue Sensitivity, and Your Weight."

STAY IN TOUCH WITH HOW YOU FEEL INSIDE

To make use of your internal regulators of hunger, appetite, and satiety, you must tune in. You need to be able to tolerate your hunger long enough to get to the table, you need to pay attention to how good the food tastes and how your body feels as you eat it, and you need to be aware of what it feels like when you have eaten enough to feel like stopping.

Part of being able to do a good job with your eating is to manage your arousal and to stay in touch with how you feel inside. Being hungry and eager to eat can feel exciting and sometimes distressing, and staying in touch with those feelings can take effort. It is a rewarding effort, though, because tolerating your feelings lets you tune in on eating *sensations*. As you

eat, pay attention to how the food tastes and feels in your mouth, and how your stomach and your whole body feel as you begin to nourish yourself. Over the days and weeks, as you stay in touch with your eating, you will discover a trustworthy sensation of *truly* feeling like stopping. That natural stopping place is quite different from forcing yourself to stop or from quitting because you are so full you can't take another swallow.

When you stay in touch with yourself, you will notice that there are stages in getting enough to eat. First, your hunger goes away. When I train my patients to eat mindfully, they tell me that they feel they *should* stop eating when their hunger goes away. But they are only truly willing to stop when the food stops *tasting* good. As one put it, "I am ready to stop when my mouth is finished as well as my stomach." Another called this extremely subjective point "a feeling of nuffness." I can't improve on that description. It is the point when *appetite* is satisfied.

There are no rules about when to stop eating. You can keep eating beyond the point of satisfying your appetite as well. Next comes the point when you feel quite full. Most people find the too-full sensation generally pleasant and seek it out once in a while. Stopping at this point is okay, too. If you continue to eat beyond the *full* feeling, you will arrive at *stuffed*. For most people, this is an unpleasant feeling. It is the feast-day syndrome, the point at which you would like to make it all go away. There is nothing wrong with eating to this point, either. You need only make a choice about whether it is positive or negative for you and whether you want to seek or avoid it.

The issue is *choice. Awareness brings choice.*

The more you stay in touch with yourself as you eat, the more finely tuned your internal regulators will be. If you don't stay in touch with yourself, your sensitivity to your regulators may be obliterated. My patients who have dieted a great deal and not given themselves permission to eat have been left with only coarsely tuned internal regulators. When they let themselves feel what goes on inside, they can detect only the extremes of *starved* and *stuffed*. Everything else is a blur. They seek my help because they can't recover from this deadening of their awareness on their own. They need guidance to sort it all out. Given all the trauma they have experienced, they have become so distressed and conflicted about eating that their anxiety gets in the way of detecting and trusting their internal regulators.*

DON'T BE SHY ABOUT LOVING TO EAT

I know a little girl who loves eating so much she *moans* when she eats. I know a little boy who gets so excited when it is time to eat that he can hardly sit still in his high chair. Their mothers are mortified. They feel that loving to eat is unwholesome, somehow perverted. And they fear that because their children love to eat that means they are going to be fat.

Not so. Loving to eat is a special sensitivity that offers heightened experience and particular pleasure. People who love to eat are often extremely tuned in to textures and tastes and smells. They are willing to go to some trouble to find food that pleases them. It does not follow that they overeat.

The secret lies in staying connected with the eating experience. To love good food and eat what you need, you need to remain aware of your feelings and responses—and ride them out. Think of the gourmet who seeks the richness of wonderful food and tunes in intensely to eating. The gourmet stops eating when he is satisfied, because at that point food no longer tastes good. Think of the artist who responds deeply to color and form, contains her excitement, and is able to stop painting when the image is captured. Think of the lover who can heighten experience, sustain arousal, and ultimately, gratify.

HAVE PLEASANT MEALTIMES

To stay connected with your experience of eating, you need the support of relaxed and low-key mealtimes. If there is a lot of commotion or tension, it will be hard for you to tune in and eat the amount you need. You may find yourself overeating or undereating. The same holds true for your child.

Pleasant surroundings, good company (if you are eating alone, you can be good company for yourself), good food, and good feelings all have a great deal to do with being able to eat well. Sitting down together for family meals, turning off the television, and having good conversation are hugely important. Taking time to feed yourself is essential. Your eating will work for you if you make mealtimes matter.

---

*I have trained other professionals in my How to Eat method in a workshop called "Treating the Dieting Casualty." Look for these professionals in your area.

Children can make a contribution to the joy of the family table by behaving themselves and taking charge of their own eating. Teach your children how to behave well at the table, excuse them when they finish, and expect them to play quietly while you finish. Children *will* be sloppy, because they are children, but if they are being sloppy just to get your goat, have them leave the table.

Have Food You Enjoy

The shoulds and oughts have gotten in the way of meal planning. Nutrition education today, and the messages that have been picked up by the media, are so rule bound and negative that we have become quite bizarre about eating. To get a grip, you need to make yourself more important than the rules. You need to attend to your hunger and appetite so you can provide yourself with a food environment that keeps you comfortable and safe.

THINK ABOUT WHAT WILL TASTE GOOD

Do you pleasure yourself with food only by cheating? Do you order broiled fish, and then give in to cheesecake when the dessert tray comes around? You aren't alone. Too many people today are being virtuous about their meals, having low-fat, low-salt, low-calorie, low-who-knows-what-else. Then virtue goes out the window and they give in to good-tasting "forbidden" food. In other words, meals are for virtue, desserts and snacks are for fun. This isn't slothful or indulgent. It's just natural.

The flaw in the plan is not the cheesecake but rather the sneaking around and giving in to get it. If you find yourself breaking rules to eat what you like, you are being too strict and withholding. Eating is not a moral issue. It is a necessity, a necessity that is best served by making it one of life's great pleasures. Most of us crave pleasure from eating and will go to some length to achieve it, including "cheating" on our rules. If you can't get pleasure *directly* from eating, you have to be *sneaky* to get it.

The point at which you start to feel deprived is a very individual matter. The nutrition enthusiasts can't tell you when you are being strict and withholding. I can't tell you. I think I am a good model for being lenient and moderate at the same time, and in later chapters I give you lots of examples of what reasonable leniency and moderation might look like for you. However, my permissiveness might seem strict to you—or wildly self-indulgent. The only person who knows what is right for you is you. Be realistic. If you restrict, you will disinhibit—that is, you will go out of control to eat what you want. Eat the foods you like. Use sense in providing for your nutritional welfare. If you have to take a vacation from your menu, you are being too restrictive.

HAVE MEALS THAT ARE BOTH NUTRITIOUS AND DELICIOUS

The baked fish might be fine, if you let yourself have some scalloped potatoes with it, or some sour cream on your potato. In fact, that's exactly what I suggest for the fish menu. Only you know how much sour cream it takes to make the potato taste good. You might, however, prefer fried fish, and that's all right too. It's still nutritious, even if it has some extra fat in it. (You can find instructions on how to fry fish on pages 116-117.) Most people don't enjoy an exclusively high-fat meal, so with fried fish you may find yourself eating relatively low-fat food like a baked potato or rice, salad, vegetables, and bread.

Even if you regularly eat high-fat food, you can still be moderate because your many opportunities to eat allow you to have a *variety*. Sometimes you fry, sometimes you bake or grill. Fried chicken is wonderful now and then. Like the fish, you won't have it every night, but you certainly don't need to give it up forever. It is so good, and broiled chicken is just not the same!

Fat enhances the flavor of food and makes it both more pleasing and more satisfying. Steamed broccoli (if you like broccoli in the first place) will taste better with a dab of butter or margarine. I suggest a teaspoon or two of fat on a serving of vegetables. That amount doesn't drench the vegetables in butter, but it definitely improves the taste. *Some* makes all the difference. Wonderful breads are low in fat (except quick breads), and they benefit from a coating of butter, margarine, or cream cheese. The thickness of the coating depends on you, so experiment. Muffins have more fat, so savor them especially—but don't stop until you have had enough.

Emphasize Variety

Cultivate an attitude of curiosity and anticipation. Seek out a variety of food. Trust yourself to learn to like new food, but reassure yourself that you don't have to eat what you don't enjoy. Know that you have internal processes that you can trust to help you manage your eating. Seek out variety and let the moderation and balance take care of themselves. In a Michigan community, people averaged 16 different foods in 1 day, 31 foods in 3 days, and 64 foods in 15 days.[1] Between day 10 and day 15, the number of different foods increased slowly, indicating that most people exhausted their food repertoire before the end of 2 weeks. People who ate 70 or more different foods during a 15-day period had superior diets to those who had less variety. Subjects who had high variety scores did not necessarily adhere to the Dietary Guidelines. To determine whether your diet has adequate variety, take the test in the box on page 27 titled "Is Your Diet Varied Enough?"

In the cooking chapters (chapters 5 through 7), you may find foods that are unfamiliar to you. I have chosen recipes that make all the foods as appealing as possible, but some may still require some learning. If you give yourself a chance, you *will* learn to like new foods. You mustn't, however, force yourself. Sneak up on unfamiliar foods, just as a child would. When you decide to experiment with a new food, give yourself time and an escape hatch. You may back out at any point. Examine foods at the grocery store without buying them; read recipes without trying them. Prepare food without eating it. Put food in your mouth without swallowing it (keep the paper napkins handy). It is reassuring to children to have familiar foods at the same meal as new ones. One of my bits of advice when feeding children is to always have bread on the table. Bread is easy to like, especially for children. They can eat it when all else fails. The same holds true for you. You'll be braver about trying new foods if you have something familiar to fall back on.

Why do I think variety is so important? Because it is the cornerstone of a nutritionally adequate diet, but more importantly because emphasizing variety has to do with food *seeking* rather than food *avoidance*. And because appetite, respectfully attended to, helps us to have a nutritious diet. Again, let's look at children. Children tire of even favorite foods and seek diversity. We would, too, if we, like children, paid attention to whether the food tastes good. Eating what sounds good and tastes good on any given day encourages you to eat a variety. We can achieve variety and well-balanced eating by attending to *pleasure* rather

IS YOUR DIET VARIED ENOUGH?

Tufts University researcher Katherine Tucker, Ph.D., uses the 37 foods listed below to determine whether people's diets have adequate variety—and therefore an adequate distribution of nutrients. "If you can check off 28 of these foods over the course of 3 days," she says, "you're probably doing pretty well. But if you're eating closer to 14 or 15 foods, you probably should be expanding your food universe."

Tucker notes that a variety of foods in each cat-egory makes the diet that much better. In the citrus category, for example, it is better to eat a tangerine, an orange, and half a grapefruit over 3 days than to eat 3 tangerines.

Note that there are 5 vegetable groups and 5 fruit groups but only 1 group for sweet baked goods and desserts. In other words, a Twinkie, a doughnut, and a brownie are not the kind of variety health experts are talking about when they recommend eating many different types of foods.

1. ☐ milk
2. ☐ yogurt
3. ☐ cheese
4. ☐ ice cream/milk-based desserts
5. ☐ other dairy
6. ☐ eggs
7. ☐ poultry
8. ☐ beef
9. ☐ pork
10. ☐ lamb, veal, game
11. ☐ fish
12. ☐ liver/organ meats
13. ☐ processed meats
14. ☐ beans and legumes
15. ☐ nuts and seeds
16. ☐ green leafy vegetables
17. ☐ orange and yellow vegetables
18. ☐ tomatoes and tomato products
19. ☐ potatoes and other root crops
20. ☐ other vegetables
21. ☐ citrus fruits
22. ☐ berries
23. ☐ melons
24. ☐ other fruit
25. ☐ fruit juices
26. ☐ white bread
27. ☐ whole wheat bread
28. ☐ cold breakfast cereals
29. ☐ hot breakfast cereals
30. ☐ rice
31. ☐ pasta
32. ☐ other grains
33. ☐ margarine, butter, and oils
34. ☐ sweet baked goods and desserts
35. ☐ salty snacks
36. ☐ soft drinks
37. ☐ candy

Tufts University Health and Nutrition Letter, August 1997. Reprinted with permission.

than by getting caught up in *obligation*.

Emphasizing variety is the best way to hedge your bets against disease. Our understanding of the connections between nutrition and disease is far from complete and is always changing. Emerging research questions what we did in response to earlier research. For example, we emphasized all-vegetable shortenings; then we were told the trans fatty acids they contain are bad for us. We emphasized polyunsaturated fat; now we are told that monounsaturates are better. Emphasizing variety rather than jumping on the latest bandwagon increases the chances that you are doing something *right* and decreases the negative effects if you are doing something *wrong*. Researchers from Michigan examined variety and applied their studies to the so-called French paradox.[2] The paradox is that the French break what we in the United States consider to be the rules of healthy eating by consuming a relatively high-fat diet. Nevertheless, they have a relatively low incidence of heart disease. Why? We have heard many theories, including the highly appealing idea that drinking wine somehow protects against heart disease. But another answer may have to do with variety. The French eat a considerably greater variety of food than we do. They take their eating seriously, celebrate good food, and use fat to make it appealing. They set aside time for meals and expect their meals to be tasty and filling. When checked for *variety*, the French scored high. But when it came to adherence to the U.S. Dietary Guidelines, the French got failing grades. Those who scored well on the Dietary Guidelines, however, scored poorly on variety.*

What is the point? Well, a number of points emerge, really: For one, all the answers aren't in. For another, the way we behave in this

---

*In nutrition circles, adherence to the Dietary Guidelines is scored using *The Healthy Eating Index*, put out by the U.S. Department of Agriculture.

country is not necessarily the right way. Furthermore, we must consider many possible explanations, some that we may not yet know, for why some people get heart disease and others don't. Finally, and most important, it's possible for healthy eating to be positive and permissive.

Alarming words, you may say. Like the nutrition enthusiasts, you may fear that, given permission to eat what you like, you will simply throw away all controls and eat like there is no tomorrow. Not so. It only seems that way because we are so restrictive about our eating. And we sometimes behave in bizarre ways because of the restriction.

Don't Get Caught Up in "Being Good" and "Being Bad"

Rather than talking about "being good" and "being bad," I prefer to talk about restraint and disinhibition because that sets aside value judgments. However, since none of my reviewers knew what *disinhibition* meant, I had to find different words. Restraint and disinhibition are jargon thrown about by eating disorder specialists, myself included. Restraint means eating less and different food than we really want. We do it because we think we *should*, for whatever reason, possibly because of health or weight concerns, or as a result of some fuzzy idea about proper eating, or in response to what we learned at our mother's table. Disinhibition means setting aside the restraints and eating as if we could make up for lost time.

Restraint and disinhibition go hand-in-hand. If we restrict ourselves, sooner or later we come to the point of disinhibition, when we throw off the restraints, often chaotically. When we disinhibit, we don't just stop restricting, we jump way over the line, often feeling that we are careening out of control. We might do it at a given meal, when we try to be stern and find out it doesn't work. We might do it once a week, as Joshua's parents did. Or we might do it over a much longer cycle as we lose and regain weight. We respond this way because our fundamental need is to be nourished and satisfied, and the rules say we can't do that. To get around the rules, we periodically throw them away. We are being restrained if we feel deprived. We are disinhibiting when

we sneak off to eat.

The rules are unrealistic. Joshua's parents, whose theme was "I know I should but . . . ," were restraining and then disinhibiting by taking vacations from low-fat eating. It is restraining and disinhibiting when we impulsively do the fish/cheesecake thing.

This issue is so difficult for so many of us, let me clarify. There is nothing wrong with eating fish for dinner, then savoring cheesecake for dessert. In fact, the combination is good menu planning because the high-fat, high-calorie cheesecake balances off the low-fat, low-calorie fish (more about this in chapter 5, "How to Get Cooking.") The problem is in attitude, and in the process by which we arrive at the menu— and eat it. Good menu planning becomes restraint and disinhibition when we judge cheesecake to be bad or forbidden, try to avoid it, then throw away restraint by eating it anyway. Often the throwing-away-restraint eating is rapid and guilty eating that involves very little savoring. Such unsatisfying, out-of-control eating may lead to another piece of cheesecake, then another after that, since we may feel that having broken restraint we might as well eat a lot. Such eating leaves many people feeling ashamed and out of control.

The problem is not you, but the rules. If we have to take vacations from the rules, they are unrealistic. Rules are unrealistic when they say we have to go without, either in amount or type of food, and we have to do it forever. Restraint is profoundly unrealistic. Going without is painful. Going without forever in the name of weight management or disease avoidance is unthinkable. But that is what we expect of ourselves, so we find ways to cheat.

Give Yourself Permission to Eat

"But," say the nutrition enthusiasts, "what we are recommending isn't going without—it is moderate and realistic." Well, maybe to them. People in the "already doing" group didn't feel they were going without. They *liked* eating that way. But I *don't*. I don't like low-fat or fat-free versions of my favorite foods, I don't like reading nutrition labels and cross-examining the waiter to make sure everything balances out, I don't like worrying about whatever I put in my mouth, and I don't like going without salt. I don't consider myself slothful and careless. I do a good job of feeding myself, and I did a good job of feeding my family. I still do, when my grown children will let me.

If you don't like being restrictive, whatever restrictive means to you, admit it to yourself and take a more realistic approach. Contrary to the fears of the food police in all of us, being more realistic and relaxed about what and how much to eat doesn't mean going out of control. You can trust your body. Your body *does* regulate. It *forces* you to regulate. It does this with two basic, very powerful drives: hunger and appetite. Hunger is a great mobilizer. Hunger tells you your body needs energy and moves you to seek food to fill you up. Appetite is a mobilizer too. Appetite tells you your body needs variety and your soul needs pleasure. Appetite moves you to seek out food you enjoy and encourages you to eat a variety of food.

Rather than fighting against these drives, you will be better off working *with* them. Give yourself permission to eat. Have meals, and know that you can go to the table hungry and that you can eat until you are satisfied. Have foods at those meals that you enjoy, not just foods that you serve because you *should*. Reassure yourself that there will be enough and that you can eat another time, rather than scaring yourself by trying to be restrictive.

It seems like a contradiction, and it is, but out of this permission will come control. Forbidden foods won't be so enticing when you can have them any time. Virtuous foods will be more appealing if you don't *have* to eat them. Eat the *real* version of your favorite foods, rather than the pale imitations. You'll be better off in the long run because you will be more satisfied, and you will probably consume fewer calories. Many low-fat copies of our favorite foods, like frozen yogurt that serves as a substitute for ice cream, are so high in sugar that they have more calories than the high-fat versions. If you disinhibit when you eat them, eating low-fat foods can make you eat more than you need.

Stop Being Phobic about Sugar, Fat, and Salt

My son-in-law, Glenn Herlinger, was astonished when I told him, "celebrate the cookie." Glenn's discriminating tastes become particu-

larly apparent when he considers the important matter of chocolate chip cookies. I encourage him to honor his passion rather than apologizing for it. I am happy to say he learned quickly.

Alison Lockridge, one of my assistants, told me she was surprised that my menus included potato chips, ice cream, cookies, and other salty foods and sweets. To her, said Alison, such eatables had not been real foods. They were just something to do—almost a hobby, like watching television. As Alison put it, "I realized when I included the potato chips, ice cream, or cookies in my meals that I enjoy them more and quit eating them because I get enough. The other way, I stop because I feel full and uncomfortable or I detach from my body and stop when they are gone."

Sugar, fat, and salt are such nutritional bugaboos that most people don't realize that fatty, salty, and sugary foods can make a nutritional contribution. And even if they don't, it isn't going to kill you to eat them. If you have meals and feed yourself regularly with pretty good food, it won't hurt you to include some fatty and sugary food. If you don't, no amount of avoiding fatty and sugary food will help you.

Sugar is getting a slight vacation from scrutiny, and some people even emphasize eating sugar as a way of avoiding fat. But, as I said earlier, over 50 percent of consumers are more concerned about avoiding fat than they are about eating well. Many people have come to regard eating less fat as a nutritional magic bullet, feeling that if they choose something low in fat they have improved their health. Salt avoidance is not far behind, gathering 25 percent of consumer concern. How many rank nutrition as a primary concern? Only 10 percent. The emphasis on avoiding fat, sugar, and salt is backward.. To consistently feed yourself well and be a positive role model for your children, you must reverse these priorities. Love good food. Emphasize meals. Seek diversity. Use sugar, fat, and salt to make food taste good. Healthy eating will fall into place. In chapter 4, "Choosing Food for Your Family," we will talk more about these issues. For now—settle down!

Be Disciplined, but Not Negative

There is positive discipline in feeding yourself well. It takes discipline to set up regular and predictable mealtimes, to plan the shopping list, to get the food in the house, to do the cooking and cleanup, to set aside the time to tune in on the meal—the list goes on. In later chapters, you will learn ways to harness the chores to decrease time and preserve satisfaction. But even if you become really efficient, you still need discipline to follow principles of menu planning and keep food clean and wholesome. Without discipline, we would have chaos, and like Ginny's parents (who didn't want to bother), children (and adults) won't get the support they need to eat well. But if you become negative or too heavy-handed on the discipline, you, like Joshua's parents, will have to take vacations from it. Not a good idea.

Give Your Body a Break

Take good care of yourself with your eating, take good care of yourself with your activity, and let your body be healthy and weigh what it will in response. You do not have to be thin to be healthy. To understand in more detail why I say this, read appendix D, "To Diet or Not to Diet—That Is the Question."

Your weight is not optional. Your body has a preferred weight, and you have the food-regulation mechanism, inclinations to move, and metabolism to support that preferred weight. You can help your body regulate by getting some activity and feeding yourself reliably, but you can't shift too much from your preferred weight. You can starve to force your weight down, but you will become preoccupied with food and prone to the restraint-disinhibition cycle. You can stuff yourself to force your weight up, but eventually you will tire of the bloated, turned-off-to-food feelings that go along with overeating, and you will give up the effort. Your weight will return to what it was before you started trying to change it. If you are lucky.

If you are *not* lucky, and many people—children and adults alike—are not, you will experience a rebound effect. Over my professional career, I have worked with hundreds of people who have become fatter because of their dieting. Despite the casual way many people jump on and off diets, weight-reduction dieting is serious business with the potential for considerable negative consequence. It can screw up your homeostasis, that is, the mechanisms that keep your weight pretty stable without you having to think too much about it. Once homeostasis

is corrupted, it is beastly difficult to restore it to order.

Your dieting is not helpful for your child. Parents who diet have children who diet at an early age. Parents who diet have trouble trusting their children's ability to regulate their eating and develop the body that is right for them. Parents who diet tend to be cranky and tired, and they make less interesting meals than people who take good care of themselves with eating.

Again, the Key Is Trust

You know how much you need to eat. Your internal signals of hunger, appetite, and satisfaction can guide you. You get that guidance by emphasizing positive, orderly, tuned-in eating. Go to the table hungry, tune in to your food, eat what you enjoy, and continue to eat until you are truly ready to quit. Then you can stop, knowing that another meal or snack is coming later and you can eat again then. If you eat until you have *genuinely* had enough (until your mouth says enough, not just your stomach), eating will take its place as only one of life's great pleasures.

If you help yourself by having reliable meals, you can even trust your body to make up for variations in your eating. You might eat a lot today (just because it feels good, or by accident), and tomorrow or the next day you won't be as hungry. You might eat a lot of some food because it tastes really good to you or because you don't have it very often. Another time, you will eat less. You might not eat very much at a meal or for a whole day, and you will make up for it another time. You don't have to count calories to keep the balance—your body will do it for you.

Summary

In summary, being a role model lets you both teach and learn from your child. Give your child a joyful, trusting model of eating. Let your child teach you, in return, what normal eating is like. Imitate the way your child eats. Children trust what goes on inside of them. They pay attention to their sensations of hunger and appetite. They automatically tune in to their sensations of satisfaction to know when they have had enough to eat. Children don't stop when the rules dictate but when they *feel* like stopping. And they stop because they know adults will give them another good meal or snack before too long and they can do it all over again.

Children don't eat all of what is put before them but only what tastes good on a given day. That's because, unlike most adults, they still pay attention. If you start paying attention again, you may be surprised to find out that even though you may have planned and even cooked the meal, when you get to the table some foods taste better than others. Emphasize what tastes good to you at any meal. Don't worry about nutritional imbalance—if you continue preparing nutritious meals, your appetite will vary and you'll eat different foods different days.

Children eat as much as they are hungry for on any given day. Some days they are hungry, some days they are not. The same holds true for you. The amount you need to eat will vary from one day to the next.

Trust.

Selected References

1. Drewnowski, A., S. Ahlstrom Henderson, A. Discoll, and B. J. Rolls. 1997. The dietary variety score: Assessing diet quality in healthy young and older adults. *Journal of the American Dietetic Association* 97: 266-271.

2. Drewnowski, A., S. Ahlstrom Henderson, A. B. Shore, C. Fischler, P. Preziosi, and S. Hercberg. 1996. Diet quality and dietary diversity in France: Implications for the French paradox. *Journal of the American Dietetic Association* 96: 663-669.

The Division of Responsibility

In infancy, the division of responsibility is very simple:
- The parent is responsible for *what* the infant is fed.
- The child is responsible for *how much* he eats, as well as how often, how much, how fast, and at what skill level he eats.

However, toddlers and older children need structure. Thus, the division of responsibility becomes more detailed:
- The parent is responsible for *what, when,* and *where* the child is fed.
- The child is responsible for *how much* and *whether* he eats.

THE PARENTS' FEEDING TASKS
- Choose and prepare food.
- Provide regularly scheduled meals and snacks.
- Make eating times pleasant.
- Provide mastery expectations.

THE CHILD'S EATING CAPABILITIES
- Children will eat.
- Children know how much to eat.
- Children will eat a variety of food.
- Children will grow predictably.
- Children will mature with regard to eating.

CHAPTER
3
THE FEEDING RELATIONSHIP

To feed a healthy family, you need to understand children's eating behaviors. You need to know how to feed so your child can do a good job with eating. The rewards are enormous. If you set up your feeding relationship in a wise and positive way, your mealtimes will be pleasant and you will have the satisfaction of knowing you are doing a good job.

Children want to eat. They can't help it. They are in the business of growing up, and they watch the adults and older children around them to find out how to do it. They see others eating, and they assume, on whatever level they are able to assume it, that one fine day they will do the same thing. Sometimes, however, it starts to look like children *don't* want to eat. They turn away from the spoon, or refuse to try a new vegetable unless they are made to, or get hysterical when they are asked to come to the table. Parents plead and reward and force and, in the most alarming cases, start to fear that without all the pressure, their child simply won't survive.

Parents ask me, "Why won't this child eat?" I ask a different question.[1] Since I have such a basic trust that *children will eat*, I wonder, "What is going on in this child's world that makes it *appear* that he won't eat?" What makes the difference between a child who takes an interest in food and one who does not? One who sits up to the table without a fuss and participates in family meals and one who creates such a fuss that the meal is spoiled for everyone?

At the other extreme, sometimes children

seem to take *too much* interest in food. "He is always hungry," his parents observe. "I feel if I let him eat as much as he wanted, he would get terribly fat. Why does he eat so much?" Again, if we assume that children know how much they need to eat, the question becomes, "What makes this child behave like he can't get filled up?" What makes the difference between a child who eats a lot and one who eats more moderate amounts? One who knows when to stop eating and one who does not?

The answer to all these questions is the *feeding relationship*. The feeding relationship can support stable, competent eating behavior, or it can create distortions in eating behavior in which the child shows too much or too little interest in food. The feeding relationship consists of all interactions between parents or other important adults and children as they deal with choosing food, eating it, and deciding how much to eat. The child asks for food, with more or less clarity and civility, and the parent responds, with more or less promptness, skill, and willingness. The child reacts to the parent's attempts at feeding with more or less capability and tolerance. And the parent reacts to the child's behavior with more or less acceptance and flexibility.

And so it goes, with each reacting to the other and initiating still more responses until they move into a dance where it isn't at all clear who is leading and who is following. Like any dance, if the partners become more expert, the rhythm gets smoother and more pleasant for both. However, if partners can't get their steps to mesh, the dance becomes choppy and unpleasant. The child reacts poorly to what the parent does, and the parent feels so upset and frustrated that the next move is awkward—and it makes things worse. They step on each other's toes over and over again, and neither feels successful; neither has any fun. It's nobody's fault. Sometimes the partners just need some help to work out a better way of being together.

How can we get the dance to be smooth and stay smooth? The answer lies in the division of responsibility in feeding.

The Division of Responsibility

You are no doubt aware by now that feeding requires a division of responsibility between you and your child. Now we will examine this central issue in more depth. Initially, when your child is an infant, the division of responsibility is very simple:

- The parent is responsible for *what* the infant is fed.
- The infant is responsible for *how much* he eats (and how often, how fast, and so on).

During most of the first six months of your child's life, your choices are limited. You get to decide whether to breastfeed or bottle-feed, and you get to pick out what goes into the bottle. Your child gets to decide everything else: How often, how much, how fast, and at what skill level he eats . Your job during the early months is to devote yourself to understanding what your baby is saying to you about feeding, sleeping, and comforting; you follow his lead and do what is necessary to make him comfortable and happy.*

However, if you do the same when your child is a *toddler* (somewhere between 8 and 36 months of age) and completely follow his lead to try to keep him comfortable and happy, you will fail him utterly. As a toddler, your child's needs are radically different from what they were when he was an infant. When he was a baby, he was learning to get settled and adjust to his new world. He was learning to love you and to know that you love him. Your toddler has those achievements under his belt, and he's ready to find out that he is his own person. He is ready to expand on the close, one-on-one relationship with you and start trying himself out in the larger world around him—the family, the neighborhood, or the child care setting. The toddler is driven to explore the world and to make up his own mind about what he wants to do. However, he has absolutely no judgment about what is safe or appropriate for him.

To do well at this stage, the toddler needs room to explore, and he also needs structure and limits. Thus, for the toddler, the division of responsibility shifts to the pattern we've observed before: The parent is responsible for *what, when,* and *where* the child is fed. The child is responsible for *how much* he eats and *whether* he eats.

You, the parent, are still responsible for choosing and offering nutritious food that your child can safely chew and swallow. But toward the end of the first year and into the second, rather than continuing to feed on demand, you will move toward structure. You will learn to make use of snacks to allow your toddler to come to the family table hungry but not famished and ready to explore the food that is served there. But it will continue to be up to your child to decide how much and even whether to eat the *food you have made available.*

THE CHRONICLE OF THE DIVISION OF RESPONSIBILITY

The idea of the division of responsibility came to me about 20 years ago, back in my dietitian-in-a-medical-clinic days. It was one of those sessions that taught me to keep deodorant in my desk drawer. A chubby little boy and his disgusted mother had been referred to me to find out what should be done about his eating and weight. As we talked, the boy slumped in the corner of his chair, his feet dangling, looking absolutely miserable. I felt the best thing I could do for this humiliated child was leave him alone. So I talked with the

---

*Alarmingly, control and scheduling are making a resurgence among young parents. Many of these parents are reading *On Becoming Babywise*, a book by the Gary and Anne Marie Ezzo based on their parenting classes for churches, *Preparation for Parenting*. The Ezzos have established Growing Families International (GPI), which advocates an authoritarian parenting style from birth, including rigid scheduling of feeding for infants. I vigorously *do not* recommend using the methods recommended by GFI. The authors are not trained child care professionals in any sense; their medical claims are untrue, misleading, or unsubstantiated; and infants raised using these methods have too high an incidence of dehydration and slow growth.

mother. I asked her about how she cooked and what she planned for meals, and it sounded pretty good to me—regular meals, tasty food, plenty of choices. I suggested a few ways to tweak her menus to make them more balanced, but for the most part she was doing very well.

My suggestions only made her feel more angry and frustrated because she was already trying hard and felt she was doing all the right things. But she wasn't getting the desired results. And here she was in my office, taking the rap for what she saw as her son's poor willpower. She had reminded him, as she put it, "time and time again not to eat so much. But look at him," she sputtered. "He is still too fat."

Clearly, this child was in pain. His mother made it abundantly clear she would be happy with him only if he were thin. But the mother was in pain, too. She had been made to feel responsible for her son's weight. She felt her mothering would be labeled substandard as long as she had raised a fat child. I wasn't too happy, either, come to think about it. I was supposed to give them the solution, and I didn't have one. So I kept talking. I talked about menu planning and having planned snacks and not letting him graze for food or beverages between times. I thought then, and I think now, that dieting is bad for anybody, and that for children it is brutal.

Finally, the mother had had enough. "I am already doing all that!" she exploded. "What am I supposed to do?" she demanded. "I have one at home who is too thin, and this one is too fat. How am I supposed to get that one to eat more and this one to eat less?"

Well, she had me there. What in the world could I say? After a pause that seemed to go on forever, I blurted, "You don't have to worry about how much either one of them eats." The mother looked startled, and I rushed on. "That's not your job. Your job is to put the meals on the table. After that, they are the ones to decide how much to eat."

The mother glared. The little boy smiled and straightened up in his chair. I gulped. "Holy smokes," I thought. "Where did that come from? That is pretty revolutionary. Is it really true?" But it was better than anything else I had said that day, so I let it stand.

I don't think I helped that mother and child as much as they helped me. The part I *didn't* say, the part that would have made it come

together, was "You don't have to take responsibility for how your sons' bodies turn out. That is up to them and nature. You need to do your job with feeding; the rest is up to them." (That session, and others like it, also taught me to do a careful evaluation before I start giving advice. See the box below titled "Evaluating Feeding Problems.")

Since then, I have tested the division of responsibility with all kinds of families with children of all ages and applied it to many different feeding problems. I have written about it in two books and heard from lots of parents who say that applying it has completely changed their relationship with their child around food. I have taught the concept of the

---

EVALUATING FEEDING PROBLEMS

I don't know what factors contributed to the problems experienced by the boy whose difficulties led to my first insights regarding the division of responsibility with feeding. I don't really know if his fatness was normal or abnormal for him. It seemed he was in a real struggle with his mother about eating, and often those struggles make children fatter than nature intended. He might have regularly eaten more than he wanted to defy her or because he was afraid he would have to go hungry later.

I have learned since then to make recommendations only after I have carefully evaluated the child's medical history, food intake, growth patterns, and parent-child feeding dynamics. So many factors can affect eating and growth that it is impossible to responsibly identify and treat the problem without looking at the situation in detail. When I met with the little boy and his mother, I didn't do a complete evaluation, so I didn't know whether his size was normal or abnormal for him. He may have been a normally large child who was growing consistently. Or he may have gained weight in a way that was abnormal for him. If his growth was inconsistent, I didn't know why: Was there some medical problem that interfered with his activity? Was there a greater problem with the family menu than the mother was willing to let on? Were food restrictions causing him to be preoccupied with food and more likely to overeat? Had he been small or ill when he was a baby and been overfed because of it? Had the family had some crisis that made him overeat and gain weight?

With a more-detailed understanding, I could have advised the mother about how to solve the *real* problem rather than just guessing that the problem was food selection and focusing on that.

division of responsibility to lots of professionals who work with children and their eating in lots of settings. I have held my breath while I read the careful research that people in universities have done with children and their eating—and seen my beliefs confirmed. And I have seen this concept enter the public consciousness. "It is a traditional principle of feeding well-known in the child development world," said one government publication, "to observe a division of responsibility in feeding." It is one of those understandings that is so right that it becomes generic.

The division of responsibility in feeding is based on some basic assumptions, both about the tasks of the parent and about the capabilities of the child. To take charge of their eating and do well, children depend on parents and other adults to provide them with both love and limits. They need a positive framework. The division of responsibility in feeding provides just such a framework.

The Parents' Feeding Tasks

For children to do a good job with eating, parents and other adults have to do certain things to support them. Those tasks include providing food, making eating times pleasant and predictable, and showing your child what it means to grow up with regard to eating.

CHOOSE AND PREPARE FOOD

You are the gatekeeper when it comes to the food that is in your home and on your table. You need to know enough about your child's physical ability to eat, and enough about nutrition, to offer him food that is both developmentally and nutritionally appropriate. By *developmentally* I mean that food has to be the right texture and consistency to match his mouth and hand skills. By *nutritionally* I mean choosing foods that combine to give a well-balanced diet. In chapter 4, "Choosing Food for Your Family," we will go into more detail about how to attend to nutrition.

During your child's first 6 months, when he can only suckle and cuddle, you feed him with a nipple—either breast or bottle. You provide breastmilk or a formula that is specially adapted to be nutritious and digestible for the young infant. Then, when he is ready to sit up and open his mouth for the spoon, you offer

soft baby cereal. Because he still depends on breastmilk or formula for nutrition, there is no rush about his eating cereal. It may take several weeks before your baby learns to tolerate the spoon in his mouth and discovers that the cereal is *food*. Nutritionally, these early solid-food meals are most important as sessions that build eating skills. The same holds true as he gets better at swallowing and gumming food and you introduce him to thicker and lumpier food. Often by 8 to 10 months, children are ready to eat soft pieces of food and are ready to join in at the family table. At that point he will start to depend nutritionally more on solid food and less on breastmilk or formula. Throughout the period of rapid transition from nipple-feeding to table food, your child develops capabilities, and you offer the food so he can learn to eat.

Part of choosing and preparing food for your child is understanding the way his mouth and hands develop so you can provide textures he can manage. You also need to know about his nutritional requirements and choose accordingly, and you need to be aware of his social development so you'll know when to include him at the family table. I cover these issues in detail in *Child of Mine* (see appendix K for how to obtain a copy). But one important aspect of choosing food for toddlers and older children that most often gets overlooked is offering a variety—even when your child doesn't eat a variety.

DON'T CATER TO CHILDREN

It doesn't work—for parents or for children—to limit the menu to what children readily accept, or to short-order cook for them. You know how that goes: "Aargh, I don't like that!"

"Well, what do you like?"

"Peanut butter. Macaroni and cheese. Hot dogs."

So the parent gets up and makes hot dogs, and the child may or may not eat them.

Letting children dictate the menu is not a good idea. Your child finds out from you what is next on the list of skills he needs to learn and foods he needs to master. If you cater to him, he will learn that you don't expect much of him. Your child learns to like a variety of foods by being exposed to them. He is growing up to join the family table—the family table is not limited and adapted to suit him. Your child will learn to eat and enjoy what you eat. Give your child the same consideration in menu planning as you do other family members—sometimes he gets lucky, sometimes somebody else does.

On the other hand, don't do sadistic menu planning. A sadistic meal would be something like liver, boiled potatoes, and cooked cabbage: all challenging foods, nothing that really offers your child an "out." A menu that would give him a better chance of succeeding would include some bread. Children can usually eat bread when all else fails. A child-friendly menu might include corn instead of cabbage, because cabbage-family vegetables (like cauliflower and broccoli) often taste bitter to children. Mashing the potatoes with milk and butter would help, because children can generally manage soft and creamy foods better than dry, hard foods. And it *certainly* would help to not insist that your child eat the liver—or anything else that is on the table. He may learn to like it eventually, but only if you don't force it on him. Liver is such a strong-smelling, strong-flavored, and strange-textured food that your child might not learn to like it. In that case, liver will give your child an opportunity to learn to politely say, "no, thank you." He need not say "Oh, yuck!" or "How can you eat that stuff?" If he does, check yourself to be sure you are not putting pressure on him to eat it. If you're not being pushy, let him know, in no uncertain terms, that you expect him to cut it out.

Plan meals with familiar foods as well as challenging ones. That is not short-order cooking or limiting the menu to what your child can manage, but simply giving him some help. Your child wants to be successful with eating the food on the family table. You can help him by having some familiar foods, some that are less familiar, and at least one food that he can eat if all else fails—like bread. At mealtimes, put a variety of food on the table: a main dish, fruit and/or vegetable, two carbohydrates (always bread—or what you have that serves as bread, like tortillas or chapatis—and one other) and milk. Offer them all at the same time, and let your toddler pick and choose. Otherwise he will play the nifty game of turning foods down one at a time and watching you get frustrated.

PROVIDE REGULARLY SCHEDULED MEALS AND SNACKS

For your child to join you at the table, you have to have a table for him to join. Get in the habit of cooking for yourself before you need to cook for your child. That way, you will be clear that you are cooking for a family and your child is learning to join in by eating family food (adapted, of course, to make it safe for him to chew and swallow). Most children are ready to eat from the family table before they are a year old.

Toward the end of the first year and into the beginning of the second, your child will go longer between feedings and will become more regular in his eating times. To make his hunger coincide with family mealtime, you can make strategic use of snacks. Eventually, he will come to depend on his meals and snacks for nourishment, and you will no longer feed on demand. In fact, for toddlers and older children, on-demand feeding is known as panhandling, and panhandling children do poorly with eating. They fill up on food handouts and don't learn to eat nutritious food at meals and snacks.

In all ways, once children get past the on-demand feeding of infancy, they benefit from structure and predictability. With feeding, it is especially important. Structure lets your child know you will take care of feeding him so he doesn't have to worry about it or make it happen. Offer three meals at reasonably reliable times, and offer enough snacks so he gets the opportunity to eat every 2 1/2 or 3 hours. Plan the snacks and keep control of where and when they are served—don't just give food handouts in response to panhandling.

That goes for beverage handouts as well. Letting your child have even nutritious beverages, like juice or milk (or even breastfeeding him), will spoil his appetite for meals and he won't eat as well. Giving in to his random begging for food and beverages puts him in charge of the menu (your job) and keeps him from working up enough of an appetite to take an interest in meals (his job).

MAKE EATING TIMES PLEASANT

Children (and the rest of us) need a positive emotional climate to do the best job with eating. The most important way to make eating times pleasant is to be there yourself. Keep your child company, make easygoing conversation, enjoy your own meal, help him get served, then let him take care of the rest. Don't nag or push him to eat. Even when your child is a older and seems independent, he benefits from having you there at mealtime. When parents don't take an interest in eating with them, children lose heart, lose interest themselves, and eat poorly. Your child will always do more and dare more with eating if you are there. Your presence provides the reassurance he needs to try new foods and move himself along.

Children need to be included in mealtime conversation, but they don't need to be the center of attention. Talk with your child a bit, then talk with others at the table. If your child knows he will be included in the conversation, he will enjoy listening and will learn from it.

An absolute key to making mealtimes pleasant is to let your child decide what and how much to eat *from what you have made available.* Notice that this is *from what you have made available.* I am not recommending throwing away control. I am emphasizing planning and serving the meal, then letting your child take it from there.

Although your presence is important, you must be careful not to take over. If you are having trouble in this respect, you are not alone. Parents of preschoolers who were observed in the Western Massachusetts Growth Study did a good job of providing structured meals and snacks.[2] However, they did a poor job of letting their children manage their own eating. At mealtimes, parents dictated food choices and portion sizes. However, between meals, children were allowed to graze for snacks. They helped themselves freely to the cupboard and the refrigerator, eating what and how much they wanted.

The implications of this method of feeding are grave, and they go beyond eating. Preschoolers love their parents and are more comfortable and willing to experiment with eating when parents are around. But in this study, when parents were around they spoiled eating for their children by being controlling. The only way the children were able to eat what they wanted was to go off by themselves and eat, when parents were not around. The message to the child? The only way you can be your own person is to get away from your parents. If you are careful to observe a division of responsibility with feeding, your child can be with you and be his own person too.

PROVIDE MASTERY EXPECTATIONS

Cultivate the attitude that your child will progress with his eating. As I said earlier, your child wants to eat, and he wants to learn to eat

more and more grown-up food in more and more grown-up ways. However, he looks to you to find out what being grown up is all about. You show him, with the food and the feeding situations you offer. For instance, when they are offered the nipple, most babies instinctively know how to suck. Some babies have some learning to do before they get a good suck-swallow going, and they learn by eating. You time introduction of solid foods by looking for the signs that your baby is ready to learn to eat from the spoon. Is he sitting up in his high chair, possibly with a couple of pillows to support him? Is he opening his mouth when you hold the spoon in front of him? Can he close his lips over a spoon? Sitting up gives him more control with spoon feeding, and he will do and dare more if he feels he has control. He can lean forward to eat, and lean back or turn away to stop eating.

Even when he is ready, it will take him some time to learn to tolerate the spoon in his mouth, to scrape the food from the spoon, and to swallow. Your child might learn to eat from a spoon so fast it looks automatic. Or, if he is more cautious, he might react, make a face, turn away. Then you need to stop and give him another chance another day. Keep offering the spoon, but stop *right away* when he says to stop, and he will learn.

And so it goes—with learning to eat pieces of food and joining others at the family table— you are the one to give your child the occasion to learn; he does the learning. You respect your child when you let him take charge of his own eating. You give him mastery expectations when you put food on the table, give him the support he needs to get served, and then leave him to his own devices. The message is, "I know you can do this."

YOUR FEEDING BEHAVIOR MAKES A DIFFERENCE

Whether your child takes charge of his own eating depends almost exclusively on the way you treat him with regard to feeding. More and more, I hear complaints about finicky children. When I have an opportunity to evaluate children who eat only a limited variety of food, I generally find the problem to be in the feeding relationship.

Often parents give children little opportunity to learn. They expect children to eat and like something the first time it is presented to them. If the child refuses, that food disappears from the menu. Finicky children often eat a lot of high-fat, high-sugar foods, like candy and French fries, because these tasty, easy-to-like foods are easy for them to master. A child can learn to like a new candy bar the first time he eats it. Learning to like a new vegetable takes longer—lots longer.

Finicky children often behave poorly at the table. Poor mealtime behavior comes both from pressure to eat and from a lack of limits around eating. One usually accompanies the other. Parents often go to a lot of trouble to get a child to eat: they short-order cook or limit the family menu to foods the child will readily accept. But even the most indulgent parents, the ones who cater to the child's every whim, get fed up after a while. Then they put pressure on the child to eat. And the child fights back. Often, the child provokes the fight. Children know when they are behaving poorly, and they look for limits. So they mess. Or whine. Or refuse to be pleased by even the most special food. Parents who have an investment in getting their child to eat let them get away with it. Parents who protect their own rights don't get into the struggles in the first place. When children behave badly, these parents excuse them from the table.

Your Child's Eating Capabilities

If you do your job with feeding—and no more—your child will do his. He will take charge of his own eating. It seems simple, but it involves finding the middle ground between offering too much support and too little. If you become controlling and try to do your child's job as well as your own, he will feel overwhelmed and put off and probably won't eat well. If you are not supportive enough and fail to remain present with your child while he learns how to eat, he won't eat well either.

It is hard to play the supportive role. It means you have to slow down and tone down what you do and offer your child the opportunity to learn. He will pick up the food and drop it, pat some of it into his mouth (and on his cheeks), sample the same foods over and over, spit foods out and gag them up. In the midst of all that struggle and commotion, your job is the hardest of all—it is to wait and watch. He will love doing it, but you may have

to sit on your hands. To give him the chance to learn, you have to be able to trust that your child will eat. And, despite all the awkwardness, he really wants to do it himself. In fact, he cares deeply about doing it himself.

YOUR CHILD WANTS TO EAT

Children are born with the will to survive and the drive to eat. Even the sickest baby has the drive to eat. That drive can be blunted, but it never goes away—and it takes a lot to blunt it. Children want to eat because they see people around them eating, and because that is just the way they are—the desire is inborn.

If your child looks like he doesn't want to eat, the question to ask is "Why not?" What is going on that makes it appear that your child won't eat? Often the reason is that an adult is being too pushy, insisting that the child eat certain amounts or types of food. Parents are most likely to be pushy if a child has been ill or grows slowly. Sometimes a child appears not to want to eat because he doesn't get enough support: the food isn't right for him, or his parents don't give him the kind of company he needs to do a good job with eating.

Occasionally, a child seems like he doesn't want to eat because he *can't* eat. Something is going on inside of him that he can't overcome on his own. Babies who were born prematurely often have trouble learning to eat. Tube feeding and the many procedures done to their mouths make it hard for them to realize what eating is and how to do it. Some children have a birth problem that interferes with eating early on. For instance, a problem with a child's stomach or esophagus may need to be corrected surgically before he can eat. Other children have problems with nerves or muscles that first become apparent in feeding. All these children *want* to eat. They just need some extra help so they can *do* it. Some of the issues to think about in considering approaches to teaching children how to eat are outlined in the box on the next page titled "Helping Children Learn How to Eat."

YOUR CHILD KNOWS HOW MUCH TO EAT

Your child was born with an internal regulator adapted to his own physical requirements. He will be hungry, and eat, and get filled up, and stop eating (even in the middle of a bowl of ice cream). He may be a relatively hungry child with a high energy need. Or he may have

HELPING CHILDREN LEARN HOW TO EAT

Helping a child who appears unwilling to eat requires professional help. Before such a child can do well with eating, we need to be sure that he can chew and swallow properly. We need to know there is a way of supporting him nutritionally while he learns to eat. And we need to know that parents are in a position to follow through with the intervention.

Schools of thought about teaching such a child to eat break down into the same trust and control issues we considered with other children. The trust school assumes that at least on some level the child wants to eat. Feeders and parents build on that assumption by giving the child mastery expectations and opportunities. An occupational therapist from the trust school waits to get the child's permission before trying to put something in his mouth. A feeding therapist from the trust school finds a way for parents to give the child the messages: "It's time for you to learn to eat," "You can do it," and "Here's how to do it." Then the therapist supports the parents and child while the child gets a grip on himself and puts food in his mouth. They teach parents to off-handedly say, "Good for you." Approval that is too enthusiastic makes eating the feeder's business, not the child's.

The control school assumes that the child's eating is the feeder's idea and that the child has to be enticed, rewarded, or manipulated into eating. Feeding therapists are usually the ones to intervene rather than parents. An occupational therapist from the control school finds often-ingenious ways to ignore or bypass the child's refusal to put something in his mouth. A feeding therapist from the control school applauds enthusiastically or rewards the child with a favorite toy for putting something in his mouth.

While I don't have to tell you that I prefer the *trust* approach, both methods work if they are well planned and constructed and followed through to the point where the child takes charge of his own eating—and finds it rewarding. The assumption that the child is in charge of his eating is built in from the first with the trust model. With the control model, a final step in treatment needs to be that of phasing out enticement and maneuvering and turning over eating to the child.

Even with the best treatment, however, sometimes a child's ability to control his nerves and muscles is so limited that he can't eat as much as he needs to supply his nutritional needs. In those cases, parents and child can enjoy the sociability and accomplishment of his eating *part* of what he needs. Then, when everybody's energy and interest run out, his food intake can be supplemented by tube feeding.

a relatively small appetite and not require so much food to keep him going. Whether he needs a lot or a little, he knows instinctively how much he needs. If you do your job—no more and no less—he will automatically eat the right amount of food to grow and be as active as is right for him.

Provided you don't try to control him, your child can even make mistakes in eating and then make up for his mistakes later. He can eat a lot today and make up for it by eating less tomorrow—or the next day. He doesn't have to think about it or use his willpower. His instinctive regulators of hunger and fullness do it for him.

Some children are naturally large, and some naturally small; some eat a lot, and some don't eat so much. But when children eat and grow at the extremes, parents often worry about how much their children eat and try to control it. In our weight-obsessed culture, a robust child with a hearty appetite may make parents hesitate to feed him all he wants for fear he will get fat. A small, thin child with a small appetite may make parents push food. Neither approach works. Children who don't get enough to eat—or fear they won't—become preoccupied with food and are prone to overeat when they get a chance. Children who have food pushed on them become turned off by eating and are likely to undereat when they get the chance.

The large child and the small child, the big eater and the picky eater, all know how much to eat. All grow in the often-surprising way nature intended. Children face a whole lifetime of having to regulate their food intake in order to maintain a stable body weight. To do well with food regulation, they need to be allowed to preserve their sensitivity to their internal sensations of hunger, appetite, and satiety. For more on this topic, see appendix E, "Children and Food Regulation."

YOUR CHILD WILL EAT A VARIETY OF FOOD

If you offer your child a variety of food, over time he will eat a variety. At a given meal or snack, he probably won't eat some of everything that is put before him. Only adults eat some of everything. We know we paid for it or that it is good for us, so we eat. That reason means nothing to children. Your child will eat what tastes good to him on a given day, and what tastes good today will be different from what tastes good tomorrow. That is where the variety comes in.

Studies show that children tire of even a favorite food and will eat something else at another meal or on another day. We tire of foods too, and we have the same inclination to seek diversity in what we eat. However, unlike children, we often don't pay attention to our internal cues. If we think we should eat something, we eat it whether it tastes good or not.

The positive benefit of children seeking a variety of food is that over time they tend to have a nutritionally adequate diet. The negative effect is that it worries parents. Children's erratic eating fools and alarms many parents to the point that they feel they have to take charge to even things out. Try to stick to doing your job, and let your child do his.

If you look at only one day, it may appear that your child eats poorly. He may go on a fruit kick one day, breads and grains another, meat another. This kind of day-to-day shift in food choices is fine. When I analyze children's diets, I always ask for at least a week of menus. (On my better days, I also ask the parent to tell me what they are *offering*, as well as what the child is eating.) It generally looks pretty strange: a bite of this, a cup of that, no vegetables, lots of vegetables. However, I consistently find that the week's intake adds up to a nutritionally adequate diet.

I also find that what is on the table, and the emotional climate at the table, has more to do with a child getting the nutrients he needs than what he actually eats on any given day. If the table is a pleasant place to be and the food is nutritious and well balanced, a child gets the nutrients he needs. For background on children and food acceptance see appendix F, "Children and Food Acceptance."

YOUR CHILD WILL GROW PREDICTABLY

Your child was born with a blueprint for growth. If he gets enough to eat, he will grow according to that blueprint. If you let him eat as much or as little as he wants to eat, he will grow in a consistent and predictable fashion—you don't have to worry about it.

Look at yourself and then look at your child's other parent. Visualize what an average between the two of you would look like, in height and weight, and that is what your child's height and weight are likely to be. For instance, if one of you is tall, one short, one fat, and one thin, your child will probably be medium in both height and weight by the time he is 7 or 8 years old. Of course, there are exceptions, but for the most part, that is how the genetics of size and shape play themselves out.

Each age has a large range of heights and weights that are considered "normal." Your child's height and weight are mostly determined by genetics. Most people know that height is inherited, but not everyone realizes the extent to which weight is inherited as well. The law of averages as it applies to genetics says that it is normal for some children to be relatively light and some to be relatively heavy. Unfortunately, even many health professionals don't realize that the child who is at the outside extremes for growth, and still growing predictably, is doing just fine. Many times professionals and parents react negatively to normal growth and try to get the small child to eat more and grow more or pressure the large child to eat less and grow less. Almost without exception, putting this kind of pressure on a child leads to struggles with eating, and that, in the long run, can undermine the natural balance of the child's energy regulation and growth. Even if a child is relatively large or relatively small, if he grows predictably according to the growth charts, that natural balance is working for him. His growth is likely to be normal.

Your job is to feed your child and let him grow. That is not an easy job, because it also means that you have to keep your nerve. Sometimes children grow fast, sometimes slowly. Some children grow up to be tall, others short, some thin, others fat. You don't get to choose, and neither does your child. What you do get to do is help your child to have the healthiest body possible, to feel good about that body, and to learn how to use that body in the way it works well. Your small, thin child might not turn out to be a Green Bay Packer; your large, fat child might not become an Olympic gymnast. But strange turnarounds happen as children grow up. So there's no telling what might happen. But if you try to make something happen, you will do damage. There are plenty of opportunities besides professional football and championship gymnastics. One part of growing up is for your child and you to come to terms with what he can and can't do.

YOUR CHILD WILL MATURE WITH REGARD TO EATING

I have already said this, but I will say it again because it is so important. *Your child has within him the drive and the desire to grow up with regard to eating.* He will acquire new skills, learn to eat new food, and will come to enjoy eating in a healthy, positive way. If you think your child will eat only if you make it happen, you are working too hard and holding him back. *Your child will eat.* But you might never know it to watch him.

Your child will not automatically like new food. When he sees a new food, he may not even allow it on his plate, let alone near his lips. But he will learn to like it using a laborious process of trial and error. As he becomes more familiar with a food—as he sees it on the table and sees you eat it—he will get over some of the feeling of newness. Eventually, he will get around to putting a bite in his mouth—and taking it out again. To us, this looks like food refusal, but it is actually a child's way of becoming accustomed to the taste and texture of the food and ready to swallow it. (If this seems strange to you, remember the last time you tried to swallow a bite of "mystery meat.") Research shows that it takes 10, 15, or 20 tastes, in as many meals, before a child will like something.

Your child will likely be erratic about eating. He may eat a lot one day and hardly anything the next. He may *love* a food one day and eat a lot of it. Another time you will make extra, and he will turn it down cold. He will hardly ever eat what we think of as a full meal. Instead, he will eat the one or two foods that taste good to him at that meal.

By now, I hope you have figured out that it doesn't pay to hold your breath waiting for your child to eat. You can also see why I warned earlier not to limit the menu to foods your child readily accepts. You would go berserk trying to outguess him. Your child needs exposure to a variety of food to do his learning. You need to manage meals so you can be casual about his experimentation. If you cook especially for him and are invested in getting him to eat, you won't be casual. You will watch him with an eagle eye and try to get him to eat. Any self-respecting kid can only react to that catering and hovering by refusing to eat.

How to Apply This Information

If your child is an infant, you can start off on the right foot. You can establish and maintain a division of responsibility from the first, and your child will grow up with the eating capabilities we have talked about in this chapter. If, however, your child is older and you have been crossing the lines of division of responsibility and getting into some struggles about feeding, you have some repair work to do.

Since you are reading this book, it is likely you feel the need of some improvement in your child's eating habits. My message, which not all parents are pleased to hear, is that the way you feed determines to a large degree the way your child eats. Children have a regrettable habit of behaving exactly as we teach them to! If you have been controlling the *how much* and *whether* of your child's eating (or trying to), your child will let you (or let you try) and then find ways of getting around you. If you have had an open kitchen policy, then your child will likely be a grazer and grabber, eating only the most appealing food and not taking much interest in meals or in learning to like more challenging food. If you have been limiting your child's food intake, your child will behave as though he can't get filled up.

But not to worry. We all make mistakes—the name of the game with raising children is to give it your best try, find out if it works, and then tinker with it. Children have a wonderful way of changing if their parents change—provided their parents really mean to change and follow through. The younger children are, the more quickly they change.

If your child is a preschooler or older, you need to tell him there is a change coming, why, and what that change is going to be. You may say, "You know, I have been trying to get you to _____ (eat your vegetables, eat less, use your silverware all the time, *put your feeding error here*). It seems like it hasn't worked. You don't like it, and I don't like fighting with you about it. So, from now on, here is what I am going to do. I am going to put the food on the table, and I am going to leave it up to you to decide what to eat from what's on the table. What do you think of that?"

Now, chances are your child will like the sound of this quite a lot. "Does that mean I can have all the dessert I want?" he will ask. "No."

(The answer is no.) "But I will put your serving of dessert by your plate and you may eat it when you want to."

Wow! Cool! What kid wouldn't like that? Well, wait, there's more. So you go on.

"Now, part of the reason I nag you about eating is so you don't keep snacking all the time. So the snacks are going to change, too. From now on, instead of letting you eat whenever you want to the way I do now, we will have special snack times. We'll talk about foods you like and foods I am comfortable giving you. I'll put the snacks on the table for you just like it's a meal. And just like at mealtime, you can eat what you like and as much or as little as you like. What do you think of that?"

Younger children may not have much to offer at this point. They may think of a few things they want for snacks, and you can negotiate about that. Keep in mind that "snack" doesn't mean "treat"; it means "little meal." If your child has been grazing to get treats, simply incorporate those treats into your planned meals and snacks. Otherwise, the changes you are making will be more negative than positive, and you will get a lot of unnecessary resistance.

Older children may have thoughtful contributions to the planning. A 12-year-old I worked with balked when his parents talked about set snack times. They all agreed on what foods were acceptable, and since he was older, he was getting his snack himself. But they objected to the way he loaded up on food just before dinner and asked him to get his snack out of the way by 4 P.M. He objected to that, so we asked why. "Well," he responded, "the reason I eat so much before dinner is because we always have something I don't like at dinner, like roast beef, and then you make me eat it." His parents saw his point. They agreed to lay off the strong-arm feeding, and he agreed to save his appetite for dinner. And the next time they had roast beef he surprised them by trying a little. It is impressive what kids will do if they feel their parents respect how they feel and what they have to say.

Just because you and your child have agreed on a plan of action doesn't mean instituting it will be trouble free. Like grown-ups, children can be very enthusiastic about setting up the rules, but acting on them becomes another story. Your child will want to bend the rules. Reasoning with him and reminding him he helped make them won't help. You still have to take the lead in implementing the rules you agreed on.

Clearly with younger children these discussions and negotiations are mostly nonverbal. Do tell your toddler in simple words about meals and snacks—he is likely to understand more than you think. But the real communication will come with your acting it out. You will "tell" your toddler about the division of responsibility by having more-or-less set times for meals and snacks and by limiting his between-time food (and juice) begging. Your toddler may "tell" you about his displeasure by having tantrums. You answer back that you are undeterred by his theatrics by working around him while he rages. The good thing about making these changes with toddlers is that toddlers change quickly. If you can weather the storm for 3 or 4 days and are consistent with setting limits, he will come around. If you can manage to continue to be consistent for another month or two, you will have changed the way you do things. Older children take longer. I figure it takes a preschooler or a school-age child on average about 3 months before he really trusts that his parents mean what they say and won't go back to the way things used to be. Then the child will learn to behave in the new way. If you waffle and slip and give in sometimes, it will take even longer.

One mother, a dietitian, told me that after she decided to stop forcing her kids to eat their vegetables (and having fights about eating) it took over 6 months before the children started experimenting with a variety of food. At first, all they ate was meat and bread. As you can imagine, having her children not eat vegetables or drink milk made that dietitian mother pretty nervous. In fact, it may have taken her kids longer than usual to start experimenting because they felt her nervousness. Kids are perceptive—her sons probably knew how important it was to her that they eat well, so they gave her plenty of time before they really believed she wouldn't go back to pressuring them.

The keys are *realistic expectations* and *consistency*. If the struggle goes on and on, someone is being controlling or giving the child the message that they don't really mean it. Two of my small patients continued to whine and behave badly at mealtime, even though their parents insisted they weren't pressuring the children to eat. After very careful questioning, it emerged that the father was hounding his 3- and 5-year-old sons about table manners. He insisted they neatly use their silverware and napkins. Were the boys fighting back, or were they simply overwhelmed? Probably both. Their father's rigid expectations were keeping them from growing up with regard to eating.

If you decide to change the way you handle feeding, be advised that before your child's eating gets better, it will get worse. You need to weather the storms, to keep your courage, and not revert to old habits. You may need to consult with a feeding specialist to plan your strategy and then get help maintaining your courage and commitment. You may need outside help to catch yourself when you go back to your old ways. You will benefit from help dealing with your feelings while you make the changes. You may feel so sorry for your child or so angry at him that you can't be steady and consistent with feeding. You may have been so worried for so long about your ill child that you fear he won't survive. You may be so afraid your child will be fat that you can't let go of control. In such instances well-informed help for a few weeks while you make your changes can be a very good investment. In *How to Get Your Kid to Eat* I go into more detail about how to solve childhood feeding problems. (See appendix K for how to obtain a copy.)

OLDER CHILDREN STILL NEED SUPPORT

As your child gets older, he will become more independent. He may seem so independent, in fact, that you may forget how important you as parent continue to be. An 11- or 13-year-old child can make his own sandwich or even warm up his own food. In many families, older children get home first and even eat before parents arrive. Food companies capitalize on this trend with "meals for children" or "cooking classes for kids." They want to convince you that feeding is a do-it-yourself business so you'll buy their products. It's not. Your children still need you to feed them.

Do-it-yourself feeding is *not* good for children, even older children. Children do benefit from learning to cook. But for children cooking is best done *with* parents, not *instead* of them. In chapters 5, 6, and 7 I give lots of ideas for how children can contribute to meal preparation. But the *really* important thing that happens in the kitchen is spending time with you. Through their teen years children continue to benefit from your time and involvement and

from the nurturing and structure of family meals. It is not easy to hold the line with preserving the mealtime ritual, but it is so important. Cooking and eating together gives your busy family a way to connect. Food gives pleasure that you can enjoy together.

Where You Can Get Support

It is relatively easy for parents to get advice about what to feed children. Most nutrition advice nowadays, however, starts out with what to avoid. If you skip over those parts, chances are that the rest can be helpful. In *Child of Mine: Feeding with Love and Good Sense,* I cover nutrition in detail and give age-by-age advice about feeding your child. Many young parents have told me they keep *Child of Mine* on their bedside table.

But it is more difficult to get good advice about *how* to feed your child. Even parenting professionals give feeding advice based on how *they* were fed, and those methods are more likely to be controlling or forcing than really helpful. I have made it my mission to change that. To provide parents with loving and effective advice about feeding, in my second book, *How to Get Your Kid to Eat,* I focus on the feeding relationship. There I go into more depth about feeding dynamics and parenting with food. (See appendix K for how to obtain a copy.)

I make it my business to provide other professionals with training and teaching materials so they can effectively help parents with feeding. I have written and published two packages that I market to health professionals: *ELLYN SATTER'S NUTRITION AND FEEDING FOR INFANTS AND CHILDREN: Handout Masters* and *ELLYN SATTER'S FEEDING WITH LOVE AND GOOD SENSE: Video and Teacher's Guide.* The *Handout Masters* are a set of reproducible masters that give routine nutritional guidance for the first 5 years and answer questions most often asked by parents about feeding. The *Video and Teacher's Guide* shows children as parents feed them—sometimes successfully, sometimes not—and gives lessons and handouts to help you make sense of it all. Many clinics use these materials and find them tremendously helpful. You can be instrumental in seeing that your clinic provides them, as well. Let your health professional or clinic know that you would like to have access to these materials. (See my Web site—*www.ellynsatter.com*—and appendix K for more information.)

PRIVATE HEALTH CLINICS

Your private health clinic may or may not offer nutrition and feeding education and support. Many health clinics have dietitians on staff who provide clinical nutrition counseling. A few are in a position to give routine guidance on nutritional care for children. If your health clinic is like a lot of others, it depends on free handouts from drug, formula, or baby food companies for nutrition education. Those materials may be good, but they are often too brief and general to be much help. Furthermore, they are written to promote a product.

On the other hand, the powers that be in these clinics do recognize the need for health education, and they do respond if a committed person makes it their business to see that materials and programs are provided. Consider the success of Edie Applegate, a registered dietitian in the Rockford Health System in Rockford, Illinois. Thanks to Edie's vision and leadership, copies of *ELLYN SATTER'S NUTRITION AND FEEDING FOR INFANTS AND CHILDREN: Handout Masters* were placed in the offices of all physicians who are responsible for routine health care of infants and young children in the system. At Rockford Health System, classes in feeding from infancy through the preschool years are regularly offered and are based on *ELLYN SATTER'S FEEDING WITH LOVE AND GOOD SENSE: Video and Teacher's Guide*. Dietitians and other health professionals are trained in feeding dynamics so they can teach and solve problems.

When you take your newborn to the Rockford Clinic, your doctor gives you a packet of handouts about scheduling, breastfeeding, and bottle-feeding. At 1 month you'll get another packet, at 3 months, still another. And if you want more specific help, you will be referred to a dietitian who knows how to help with feeding and food selection. Parents love the program and feel more successful with feeding their children; doctors find there are fewer feeding problems.

Pediatric nurse practitioners (PNPs), who are taking on an increasing role in private health clinics, want to know how to intervene more effectively with feeding dynamics.* Consider

that over 20 PNPs have gone to considerable trouble and expense to take my class *Feeding with Love and Good Sense*, an intensive course on nutrition and feeding of young children. Periodically, the National Association of Pediatric Nurse Associates and Practitioners (NAPNAP) invites me to speak for their annual meeting. They recognize the importance of the feeding relationship and the need for expert help in this area. If you are lucky enough to work with a pediatric nurse practitioner, you know that PNPs are wonderfully committed, expert, and helpful professionals who can guide you caringly through the mysteries of being a parent.

If you feel strongly about nutrition and feeding, and about helping other parents get accurate information about the feeding relationship, you may want to become an advocate with your health clinic. Approach your health provider about instituting programs and materials. Approach the administration. Talk with other parents and get a movement going. Check out my Web site and investigate my materials (see appendix K). They are produced for just this purpose.

In today's health care world, the parent is increasingly being made responsible for the child's health maintenance. Given that assumption, it seems that your health care provider's responsibility is to make an investment in up-to-date, accurate, authoritative educational materials. Do what you can to request that those materials be made available at your clinic.

LOW-INCOME PROGRAMS

Ironically, it will be easier for you to find feeding help if your income is low. Many excellent federally sponsored programs, such as the Special Supplemental Nutrition Program for Women, Infants, and Children (WIC), provide nutrition and feeding education and consultation to families. (WIC also provides vouchers for foods high in the nutrients that are likely to be low during pregnancy and early childhood.) The Expanded Food and Nutrition Education Program (EFNEP) is sponsored by university extension services to take an active role in teaching low-income families nutrition and food management skills.

---

*PNPs get master's degrees in patient care so they can be health providers. They work under the supervision of physicians and do examinations, routine health care, and diagnosis. However, they don't prescribe drugs, and they don't do surgery.

University extension services also provide nutrition education to food stamp recipients through the Food Stamp Nutrition Education Program (FSNEP). Not every area has EFNEP and FSNEP, but extension offices and programs are available everywhere, and they can help you not only with *what* to feed but also with *how* to feed.

If you are eligible, I urge you to participate in these programs. They are education and public health programs, not welfare programs. Our society offers little enough help for young families, so why not accept what help is offered? Most participants are working parents who need help for a time during the particularly challenging early childhood years. Recipients benefit greatly from help in managing money and food. You will be treated with respect, offered materials and training, and supported with your job of parenting your child nutritionally.

CHILD CARE AND HEAD START

The Child Care Food Program (CCFP) is a fine program that offers child care providers advice, standards, and financial support with their meal planning. Increasingly, CCFP consultants are gaining expertise with feeding dynamics as well, and they help providers solve feeding problems with their young charges.

Head Start takes feeding seriously and provides a good model for feeding in child care. The program considers teaching children eating and mealtime skills to be part of their educational responsibility. Head Start nutrition programs feed children family style, teach them to serve themselves, to pass food, to say "yes, please" and "no, thank you," and to clear away dishes after the meal. Despite the richness and availability of the Head Start program, only 2 of every 5 eligible 4-year-olds are enrolled.

A good child care food program or Head Start program that observes and maintains a division of responsibility in feeding can help your child grow up with regard to eating. Look for a child care provider who makes meals an important part of the program day by helping children to settle down for eating and by taking plenty of time for meals. Look for a provider who enjoys eating, who sits down with the children at mealtimes, who serves family style, and who neither pressures children to eat nor deprives them of food.

SCHOOL NUTRITION

Although it is a fine nutrition program, the National School Lunch Program (NSLP) will be more helpful to you and your child with food than with feeding (read more about NSLP on pages 196-198). While that represents considerable help, eating attitudes and behaviors that your child takes to school are likely to be the ones he uses in the school lunchroom. You can, however, expect that nothing will happen at school to interfere with your child's ability to do a good job with eating. He needs to be given time to eat, and he must not be forced to eat anything that he doesn't want to.

Summary

Feeding goes best when you do your jobs with feeding and trust your child to do his. Your child wants to grow up with respect to eating, the same as with everything else in his life. You are the one who knows what growing up is and can help by understanding your child's growing ability to eat and offering food he can manage. He is the one with the eating capabilities, and he will retain those capabilities if you maintain the division of responsibility with feeding. When he is little, he needs you to keep his food world to the size he can handle. You help him to feel secure when you maintain the structure of regular meals and snacks rather than by throwing open the kitchen or turning him loose in the supermarket. You support his independence by letting him pick and choose from what you have made available. As he gets older and gains experience and mastery with food, he will start to do some food selection himself at school and at friends' houses. However, through high school, maintaining the structure of the family meals is important, both for nutrition and for nurturing.

Selected References

1. Satter, E. M. 1990. The feeding relationship: Problems and interventions. *Journal of Pediatrics* 117: S181–S189.
2. Anliker, J. A., M. J. Laus, K. W. Samonds, and V. A. Beal. 1992. Mothers' reports of their three-year-old children's control over foods and involvement in food-related activities. *Journal of Nutrition Education* 24(6): 285–291.

Choices and Attitudes

- Avoid trying to follow dietary formulas. Not only is doing so generally unhelpful and unrealistic, but it can also be discouraging and even harmful.
- Place more importance on *yourself and your family* than on *rules*. Emphasize self-trust rather than self-control.
- Give yourself and your family opportunities to learn and explore. Optimism, self-trust, and adventure are good motivators.
- Make the effort to have family meals and focus your energy on meal planning.
- Choose food that tastes good, but don't try to please every family member all the time. Choose some foods that are familiar and easy to like and some that are more challenging.
- Avoid common pitfalls in feeding children: don't cater to your child at the dinner table; be realistic about your child's mealtime behavior; schedule meals and snacks so that children are hungry when it's time to eat, but not too hungry.
- Seek a wide variety of food.

CHAPTER
4
CHOOSING
FOOD FOR YOUR
FAMILY

We turn in this chapter to the issue of what to eat, and more important, the issue of *attitude*. You can be thoughtful about selecting food without being negative and rule bound. Following the recommendations in this chapter can free you from the fears and anxieties about eating that are so prevalent today. You and your family are more important than your diet. Your positive feelings about food and eating—and those of your children—will do more for you in terms of your physical and nutritional health than adhering to a set of rules about what to eat and what not to eat. Feeling positive and comfortable about food and eating puts you in a position to do a good and thoughtful job of feeding yourself and your family. Emphasize meals; nutrition will fall into place.

If you are like most people, you have difficulty doing your job of putting food on the table. More and more young families are strapped for time and money. The economy is booming for those in higher income brackets, who tend to be older, more-established people, not young families. More and more parents must work long hours. Then when they get home, they try to parent and cook and get the chores done. If it seems hard, it's because it is hard. This book is intended to make it a little easier for you to do a good job. Here, you'll learn realistic and manageable principles of nutrition and food selection. In the next few chapters, you'll learn how to apply those principles to your cooking, planning, and shopping.

Nutrition Rules Are Negative

The nutrition rules are making us anxious. As I said in chapter 2, some people have become so fearful and upset about health and weight they are dietary cripples. But most people are just moderately irrational about food. Take, for example, Darlene, whom I bumped into recently in the grocery store. "I am here on a junk food run," she announced, shielding the soda and potato chips in her shopping cart. "I shouldn't let a dietitian see this."

I do not enjoy being made into the nutrition police. "Come on, Darlene," I objected, "don't put that on me. I like that stuff as well as the next person, and I buy it. I wouldn't have gotten the low-fat potato chips, though. I like the regular ones better." It's a matter of proportion: I don't eat potato chips and drink soda all day every day, and I expect Darlene and her family don't either. What ever happened to enjoying food? Food will nourish you and make you strong and give you joy. Instead, choosing food has become a truly negative and puritanical business. No wonder people are so anxious. They have gotten the message that food will kill them, and I am afraid that current national nutrition and health policy has contributed to this notion. In my view, that policy was an experiment that failed. Certainly, it was a well-considered experiment launched by well-intended people based on their interpretation of an incredibly complex set of data. But it failed, nonetheless.

WHERE THE NUTRITION RULES COME FROM

Nutrition messages have always been a tad rigid and proper, but starting in 1977 with the McGovern Committee on Dietary Goals, nutrition advice took a distinctively morbid turn. Now, I grew up in South Dakota and have always been loyal to former Senator George McGovern. I even voted for him when he ran for president. However, I don't think he did us any nutritional favors. Because the priority was disease avoidance rather than nutritional enhancement, the committee's goals were negative, and they stayed negative when they were jointly reviewed and presented for the public in the first set of Dietary Guidelines issued by two U.S. government agencies: the Department of Agriculture and the Department of Health and Human Services.

The Dietary Guidelines are reissued every five years by the same two government agencies. The priority continues to be disease avoidance, and the emphasis is still on laying out a formula for managing our food selection. In 1992 the Food Guide Pyramid was issued, by the same two agencies, to give concrete guidance in food selection based on the Dietary Guidelines. (See the box titled "The Food Guide Pyramid.") The framers have tried to make the language more positive to reduce food anxiety, but the root of the problem, the formula, remains. In fact, the formula got even more prescriptive with the conservative weight guidelines that were included in the most recent version of the Dietary Guidelines. One of the biggest sources of worry about our eating comes from unrelenting pressure to lose weight.

With the institution of the Food Guide Pyramid, the emphasis in nutrition advice for the public drastically shifted. Before that, we were told the minimum we needed to eat to consume a healthful diet. Nutrition guidelines were easily satisfied and allowed for a big fudge factor. (The fudge factor is the margin between the calories we need to spend on nutritious food and our total energy requirement; it gives flexibility.) The Food Guide Pyramid is a closely defined food selection formula with little or no fudge factor that was constructed not only to support health but also to prevent chronic and degenerative disease.

Rather than just putting a floor under our food selection, the creators of the Pyramid put

THE FOOD GUIDE PYRAMID

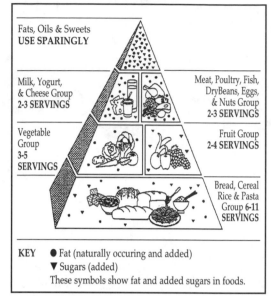

Fats, Oils & Sweets
USE SPARINGLY

Milk, Yogurt, & Cheese Group
2-3 SERVINGS

Meat, Poultry, Fish, DryBeans, Eggs, & Nuts Group
2-3 SERVINGS

Vegetable Group
3-5 SERVINGS

Fruit Group
2-4 SERVINGS

Bread, Cereal Rice & Pasta Group **6-11 SERVINGS**

KEY   ● Fat (naturally occuring and added)
       ▼ Sugars (added)
These symbols show fat and added sugars in foods.

up the walls and roof as well. In fact, the framers did a brilliant job of defining a total diet integrating the nutritional principles of variety, moderation, and proportionality. Unfortunately, the Pyramid ended up being so meticulous that the overall message to the public became rigidity and avoidance. The supporters of the Food Guide Pyramid maintain that it is flexible, and I can see that. However, those supporters are nutrition professionals and so am I. We love our formulas for managing food selection, and we know so much about food composition that we can manipulate the formula to allow us to eat anything we want. That doesn't mean that other people can do the same. Other people are simply overwhelmed.

DIETARY FORMULAS DON'T WORK

Of course, hindsight is always twenty-twenty, but I could have told the committee that formulas for managing eating don't work, and other experienced clinical dietitians could have done the same. During my many years of doing nutrition counseling, it gradually dawned on me that my beloved formulas were not helping; in fact, they were making my patients miserable. My patients would try to comply with the formula, then fail, then try again, then fail again, always blaming themselves rather than me or my formula. They let me off easy, but I didn't. Whether the problem was excess weight, diabetes, heart disease, or some other malady, it was clear that extremes in their eating were caused by my diet, and those extremes weren't helping. On the other hand, when I made the *person* more important than the *diet* and began by respecting his or her usual ways of eating, we could collaborate in doing the least we could to get the results we wanted. Their eating patterns became more positive and stable, and medical indicators improved as well.

It comes down to the same theme we have grappled with before: control versus trust. Formulas are controlling. Honoring people and their relationships with food is trusting. Most of us can't get our eating to conform to closely defined formulas, and it isn't necessary or even wise to try. Any time we try to follow a dietary formula to control weight, prevent disease, or control any other outcome, we distort our eating attitudes and behaviors. In the long run, the impact is negative, not positive. Following the rules with children is even more unrealistic, because no child ever ate according to a formula. Eating is a complex brew of habit, attitude, intuitive capability, and physical processes. When expected to control it deliberately, we become as overwhelmed and confused as the centipede:

> A centipede was quite content,
>   Until a frog in fun
> Said, "Please, which leg comes after which?"
> This worried her to such a pitch,
> She lay distracted in a ditch,
>   Considering how to run.
>   —Anonymous

The frog has become a part of our everyday lives. Read the paper or watch the news: Almost every day some new bit of research scares us about what we eat or sends us off on another tangent in search of a magic potion to keep us healthy. (Read the box on the next page titled "Protect Yourself against the News.") Advertisers for food, clothing, exercise businesses, weight loss businesses, and others have picked up the message, "Do right or you will die and so will your children." That's bad. It's bad because it is so pessimistic and alarming. It's also bad because it takes away self-trust and makes us controlling with our eating.

What Is the Alternative?

In decrying the current rigidity in nutritional guidance, I am not encouraging you to throw away your efforts to eat well. I am saying to lighten up and take a more positive approach. The Food Guide Pyramid is the only nutrition guideline we have, so instead of ignoring it, I will do my best to interpret it for you in a way it doesn't spoil your eating.

We'll start out with *attitude*. As I have said repeatedly, negativity, fear, and avoidance are not good motivators. Optimism, self-trust, and adventure are good motivators. How can we restore these qualities to our eating? Perhaps we can learn something from our children. Unless we spoil it for them, children are curious about food and expect to like it, just as they are with everything else in their lives. Children don't eat food because they feel they *should* or because it is *good for them*. They eat it because it *tastes* good. If you do your job of presenting your child with a variety of nutritious food, she'll do her job of learning to like it. She'll also do her job of getting it all to add up to a nutritionally adequate diet. She doesn't need a formula to do that—she will automatically and intuitively eat different foods one day than she will the next, and over time she will get what she needs. So will you, if you stop trying to impose the formula and go back to trusting what goes on inside of you.

How can we restore to ourselves a child's curiosity about food and the expectation that we will like it? How can we learn to trust our hunger and appetite and satiety to guide us in our eating? By giving ourselves opportunities to learn and encouragement to explore, just as we do for our children. To be helpful to ourselves and our children, we must be positive rather than negative.

I have done my level best in this book to approach nutrition in such a way that it can introduce you to the possibilities of delicious foods that contribute to your health and well-being. You will learn to prepare food for yourself and your family so it is beautiful, tasty, and wholesome and so the nutritional value is preserved (usually each supports the other). I offer strategies for putting together meals that are likely to be satisfying for everybody. It is my conviction that good nutrition information is freeing, not limiting.

YOU HAVE TO MAKE VALUE JUDGMENTS

Our children depend on us to make value judgments about food. Up to about age 12 or 13—the scope of this book—it's better if your child doesn't have to worry about choosing

PROTECT YOURSELF AGAINST THE NEWS

The media feature scary messages about nutrition and health because they sell, and they sell because we are concerned and want to do the right thing. Because health and nutrition are such popular topics, many issues that used to be argued only in professional meetings are now being argued in the media. We hear about somebody's ideas before scientific colleagues get a chance to examine them and determine whether they are valid or even reasonable. A lot of the stories we hear in the media are, at best, *preliminary results*—somebody's statement of what they think they found, before other scientists have been able to grill them about it.

To keep yourself steady with eating, you have to be able to take these media releases, as they say, with a grain of salt. An article in the *Tufts University Health and Nutrition Letter* of September 1998 helps you to do just that. "Yet Another Study—Should You Pay Attention?" gives questions you can ask yourself as you hear about study results. I summarize and paraphrase them for you as follows, and as usual I put in my own two cents worth.

1. What are the *actual* numbers as opposed to the *relative* numbers? Three of the early studies about diet and heart disease claimed a 50 percent reduction in heart attacks with dietary modification (see appendix G, "Dietary Fat and Heart Disease: It's Not as Bad as You Think"). However, a look at the actual numbers showed a reduction of from 1.4 to 0.7 deaths per 1,000 men per year, a modest reduction and certainly a far less alarming figure. If the release doesn't give you actual numbers, ignore it.

2. What type of study was it? Many media releases are based on epidemiological evidence: observations of large groups of people. The nature of epidemiological studies is to give preliminary results—an educated guess. From epidemiological studies, scientists make educated guesses about cause and effect. The guesses must, in turn, be tested in animal studies and then clinical trials with humans before they can be accepted as accurate. Unless the evidence has been well tested, it is speculative and doesn't give you grounds for making changes in your diet.

3. Does the study stand alone, or are its results corroborated by other research? Before a conclusion can be accepted, it has to be supported with evidence from a variety of approaches. A study that stands alone must be regarded as giving preliminary results and, again, doesn't provide grounds for making dietary changes. Responsible nutritional and medical change take place slowly. If the information is startling and revolutionary and calls into question accepted scientific fact, it probably stands alone.

4. Was the study published in a peer-reviewed journal? (You can find out by asking a medical librarian at your local hospital.) Peer review sets out to poke holes in a study's design or conclusions. This acid test helps to ensure that authors haven't distorted data or conclusions. In some nonreviewed journals, authors can make poorly substantiated claims and without having them challenged.

5. Are the conclusions of the article supported by the data presented? For example, given current mind-sets about heart disease and weight, authors of even peer-reviewed articles draw subjective conclusions that contradict their own data. For instance, that study that showed reductions in heart disease from 1.4 to 0.7 deaths per 1,000 (again, see appendix G) described results as "striking" and "highly significant." For another instance, in the Iowa Women's Study on weight and mortality, the data confirmed the observations of other studies that women whose weight varied or went down significantly showed higher mortality than women whose weight remained stable.* The conclusions of the authors? That the question needed more study.

*Folsom, A. R., S. A. French, W. Zheng, J. E. Baxter, and R. W. Jeffrey. 1996. Weight variability and mortality: The Iowa Women's Health Study. *International Journal of Obesity* 10: 704–709

food. That is your job. (To learn about teaching children food selection, see chapter 10, "Raising a Healthy Eater in Your Community.") We have to make value judgments about food for children, and we have to make them for ourselves. We have to weigh the positives and negatives of a food, put it in the context of the overall diet, and decide whether a particular food makes a contribution.

So what information can help you feed your family? How can you learn about nutrition without putting the whole family on a guilt trip? Our job, in this chapter, and in this book, is to find balance, to help you settle down—to reduce your anxiety about nutrition and health so you can use good judgment with regard to your eating. The goal is not to teach you a whole new set of rules but to free you to find out what works for *you and your family*. Choosing delicious, wholesome food is important when it comes to caring for body and soul, but it is not a life-or-death matter. Being thoughtful about food selection doesn't mean you have to give up your potato chips and soda. (Horrors! What a terrible thought!) It simply means that you need to pay attention to what you want and need.

Have Meals

For feeding a healthy family, meals are absolutely essential. I realize it is not easy to have family meals. There is so much interference. Workdays and commutes are long. Events get scheduled at family dinnertimes. To make matters worse, advertising makes it seem that family meals are unimportant. Instead of breakfast, children on television are handed a high-energy bar on the way out of the house. Frozen, microwavable "meals for kids" with pictures of children doing the preparation assure us that children can cook for themselves. Prepackaged food and fast foods are readily available. Children can take some money and buy dinner for themselves. It all makes it seem that family meals are a thing of the past.

They are not. A Food Marketing Institute–Better Homes and Gardens survey indicates that our commitment to dinner is strong and that we eat dinner together on an average of five times per week. When asked why they believed family dinners to be important, survey respondents said they felt strongly that eating meals together strengthens family ties and unity and that children who have family dinners eat a more healthful diet. They felt that eating together gave important opportunities for family communication and promoted a better family atmosphere, including giving a sense of stability and togetherness. The parents in the survey appear to be right. A survey of Cincinnati teens showed that those who more frequently ate dinner with family members were more likely to do well in school, had better relationships with their friends, and were less likely to fall victim to depression and drugs than teens who had fewer family meals.

Despite the evidence, I often get resistance when I press for meals. People say they don't have time to shop and cook. I can sympathize with that, but it's a matter of priorities. To eat well and to keep eating in perspective as only one of life's important issues, you have to be willing to devote time and energy to it. In chapters 5, 6, and 7 I have outlined strategies that will cut that time and energy to a mini-

mum. However, it still takes time.

When I talk about meals with some parents, they argue with me. "It's unnatural to be so structured," they say. Or, "making children wait for meals is not the way we do it in our family." Well, maybe—or maybe not. Before the advent of the corner store or convenience foods, someone in every household had to cook. There had to be a pot somewhere, and to get food from that pot, children needed the help of an adult. The realities of cooking from scratch meant that there were likely to be some predictable times for eating. Preparing food took time, and the busy adult was not in a position to be a short-order cook.

Focus on Meal Planning

You will get the nutrition and food satisfaction you need if, one meal at a time, you follow the rituals of good meal planning. Here is where you go back to what you learned at your mother's table—what I call the *Mother Principle*. A meal needs to have some protein, it needs a starch (different cultures have different starches, like grits or potatoes or plantain or rice), a vegetable (or fruit, or both), bread (or tortillas or biscuits), some good source of calcium, like milk, and some fat. At breakfast, milk may do double duty as both protein and calcium source and the fruit/vegetable may be orange juice.

Now, like any good guideline, at times you will disregard it. You will miss something. Occasionally you will have what you think is a nutritionally worthless meal. Like many families, you may enjoy having popcorn and cocoa in front of the television for Sunday supper (which is really pretty good nutritionally). Or when you go to the fast-food joint, you and your kids may miss your vegetables. As you can see by both of my examples, coming up with a truly worthless meal is pretty hard. And even if you do, it will happen only occasionally. It's your everyday meal planning that has the real impact on your family's nutrition.

The foods you choose for your meals, and how you prepare them, will depend on your location, your nationality, your preferences, your feelings about cooking, and lots of other factors. You might consider a meal without tortillas or without grits to be incomplete, or you might be convinced that a meal without potatoes isn't a meal at all. You might depend on baked beans to be your protein, or you might think baked beans are a vegetable you have along with your hot dogs. You may be in the habit of putting the protein and vegetables together in a stir-fry or a curry, or you may add the starch as well and have a one-dish meal like lasagna or enchiladas. On the other hand, you may feel that mixing the meat with something else just doesn't do at all.

I tend to make up Midwestern menus, because I live in the Midwest. I have tried to be somewhat universal, but I expect you will need to adjust the suggested menus and recipes for your own food traditions. Use my ideas to learn the principles of menu planning and cooking and to spark your own ideas. Whatever your mealtime tradition, or the tradition you borrow from another culture, it is likely to be trustworthy. Based on the available foods, every society has, through trial and error, put together a nutritious diet and tested that diet over the centuries. If the diet worked, people survived at least long enough to reproduce. It is as simple as that. The diet wasn't just based on a whole bunch of rules that dictated what people *should* eat. It was based on what tasted good and what was available and satisfying. Cooks went to real trouble to make the available foods taste good because they knew that, unless food tasted good, the family would not eat. Which brings us to our next guideline—*taste*.

Choose Food That Tastes Good

Cook foods that you and your family (generally) enjoy. Go to some trouble to make food taste good. Use fat in your cooking. Once your child has been introduced one by one to a variety of foods and textures, don't be afraid to experiment with spices, mixtures, and sauces. Children like interesting food, even if it is a little challenging at first. So-called ethnic food, after all, is somebody's else's standard fare, and *their* children learn to like it.

Everyone is entitled to food likes and dislikes, and some foods won't appeal to your child or you. It appears that to some people, for example, cauliflower and broccoli taste bitter. Children in general are more sensitive to tastes and textures than adults are, and some

tastes and textures may make your child gag. You have to accept your child's reluctance to eat certain foods—and your own. All you can do is trust that you and she would eat it if you could. You both, however, can be polite about saying "no, thank you." You cooked it and others enjoy eating it—people's feelings must be respected. But you don't have to eat it.

In the matter of eating what tastes good, you might benefit from imitating your child. *Your* food needs to taste good to you, too, in order to be satisfying. If you are the cook, you do have the advantage, like most cooks, of preparing only what you like. But even if you plan the meal and cook it, you can't know what will taste good to you until you put it in your mouth. Choosing to eat your vegetables even if they taste only so-so, just to get the nutrition, is all right. But try to include something else that is really tasty so you can get up from the table feeling satisfied.

Avoid Common Pitfalls in Feeding Children

Before we can get down to choosing food, however, we have to adjust some attitudes about feeding children. From my clinical work, and from my consulting and public speaking, I have found that certain traps capture parents again and again. These traps can discourage them from making meals and may leave them feeling like angry, worn-out failures.

STAY AWAY FROM CATERING
One of the biggest obstacles to family meals is the cook's feeling of having to please every eater with every food on the table. "I don't even want to cook any more," one frustrated parent complained. "Somebody always complains about something. If the meat is okay, the vegetable isn't. The bread is wrong, or somebody won't eat the dessert."

Don't drive yourself crazy trying to cook everybody's favorite food. Do give some thought to what family members like. Some parents feel they have to find food that their kids will like so they will eat. Don't do that—it's taking over your child's responsibility. Instead, plan menus that combine liked and familiar foods with less popular foods, and make sure that there is at least one food on the table that each person *usually* eats. I say *usually* because even if someone likes something, he or she won't eat it every time you serve it. With children particularly, it just doesn't pay to try to outguess their fickle appetites on any one day. Sometimes your child will get lucky; sometimes someone else will. What she doesn't eat this meal, she will another.

Planning menus that help your child to be successful with the meal is all right and is different from catering to her whims or short-order cooking for her. Your child wants to eat, but there is a lot of food that looks pretty challenging to young eyes. Your child is encouraged when she sees familiar food like bread on the table. If she can be successful eating bread, she will be more likely to experiment with a new vegetable. It helps to always put bread on the table—most children can eat bread if all else fails. Having another source of carbohydrate is also a good idea. A child who isn't ready to tackle the stir-fry can still eat the rice.

Use these meal-planning guidelines to be considerate, not to offer your child the easy way out. Offering the easy way out would be to always have a jar of peanut butter on the table or to let her have cereal if she isn't interested in eating what you have prepared. The family meal provides your child the opportunity to learn to cope with family food and tells her you assume she will develop new eating skills and learn to enjoy a variety of food. Making other foods readily available tells her you don't expect her to learn and grow.

What about the adults at your table? If you are the cook, remember that you don't have to please your partner (or yourself) with everything you prepare. Give him or her the same consideration you do the children (or a little more). In return, you can expect your partner to say "yes, please" and "no, thank you" and make do with the available food without making a big issue of it. If you and your partner can't be flexible and reasonable about food, you might as well stop reading this book right now, because in that case things aren't going to get any better with your children and their eating. If the adults at the table are narrow and rigid about what they eat, the children will be, too.

DON'T TRY TO GET FOOD INTO YOUR CHILD

I know a mother—good, dedicated, thoughtful—who is being jerked around by her son. This appealing and charming little boy has figured out that his mother is concerned about what and how much he eats. Very concerned.

His mother tries not to let on, but the little boy knows. Ordinarily he eats very little. His mother looks the other way and doesn't say anything. Once in a while he eats quite a lot. "See how much I ate!" he announces to his mother.

"Oh, you really did! That is just great! Good for you!" his mother enthuses. And the little boy smiles to himself because he knows that his mother wants him to eat. Because his mother wants him to eat, the little boy can jerk her around whenever he feels like it, and that has become more important to him than eating. So he might eat. Or he might not.

The mother feels her job isn't done until her child eats. In reality, the job is done when the meal goes on the table and the mealtime environment is established. Eating is the little boy's job, not the mother's, and the son won't take charge of his eating until the mother expects him to.

Like this mother, you can't pin your feelings of success on getting food into your child. You have no control over that. But you do have control over getting a meal on the table. About *that* you can feel successful. As I said in chapter 3, as long as you hold steady with your *feeding*, your child may be erratic and inconsistent with eating, but she will still be all right nutritionally.

You do have to hold steady. You have to keep planning your meals according to the *Mother Principle* and letting your child pick and choose from what you have made available. Don't try to anticipate what your child will eat. It will drive you crazy. All you can do is put it on the table and let your child take care of the rest.

BE REALISTIC ABOUT YOUR CHILD'S MEALTIME BEHAVIOR

To be successful at mealtimes, your child needs to come to the table, be pleasant to be around, say "yes, please," and "no, thank you," and act her age with regard to eating. A toddler eats with her fingers almost exclusively. A preschooler picks up a fork and spoon and uses it a lot of the time—along with her fingers. The older child almost always eats the way you do. If you use utensils, she'll depend mostly on utensils. But she'll still use her fingers from time to time, so don't get too concerned about it.

Your child wants to learn to eat like you do. However, her little fingers can master only so much at one time, and the muscles in her mouth won't develop grown-up chewing patterns until she's about 8 years old. For a long time she won't be too neat or skillful at the table. Be tolerant of spills and childlike eating.

Your child wants to please you. If she is regularly behaving badly at the table, take a look at what is making it seem like she doesn't care about pleasing you. It could be that she's feeling too much pressure. Begin by examining your division of responsibility. If you are trying to do your child's job—or failing to do your own—she will be confused and may feel she has no choice but to rebel.

For your child to do well with eating, the table has to be a pleasant place to be. You make it pleasant by being there yourself, by keeping the conversation light and positive, and by not badgering her about eating. Your child needs to help make it pleasant, too. Teach her how to do her part. Manners don't have to be exquisite, but they do have to help keep other people comfortable. Your child can help make meals enjoyable by not whining or criticizing the food choices or begging for alternatives.

If your child is hungry and can find something on the table that she likes to eat, she will pay attention to her eating. When she starts to get full, her attention will begin to wander. When she is full, she will lose all interest in food and will want to get down. If you keep her there after she is full, she will misbehave.

Many times parents keep children at the table after they are finished in hopes that they will eat a few more bites. Children behave badly, parents wheedle them to eat (and are upset when they don't), and nobody has any fun. When I ask them why they don't just let their child run off and play, parents say, "If she doesn't eat, she will be right back, begging for snacks."

"Ah," I say, "that is a separate problem. The solution to *that* is the *planned snack*."

AVOID TOO MUCH OR TOO LITTLE HUNGER

To do well with meals, children (and the rest of us) need to come to the table hungry and interested in the food there but not so famished that they are distraught and can't settle down to eat. To eat well and to be willing to learn to like new food, children need to come to the table hungry but not starved. Enter the planned snack.

Children need snacks. Their stomachs are small, and their energy needs are high. To keep from getting overly hungry and cranky, they need something nutritious to fill up on every 2 to 3 hours. Keep snacks from spoiling meals by keeping them soon enough before meals so that children have time to get hungry again. Keep snacks from spoiling nutrition by making them like little meals: protein, starch, some fat, and some fruit or a vegetable. A good snack might be cookies and milk; apples and peanut butter; crackers, cheese, and fruit juice; or cereal and milk. Snacks help make up for what is missing the rest of the day—if you had lunch at a fast-food place, include fruit or vegetables in the snack.

Giving snacks is not the same thing as throwing open the refrigerator door and letting your child go on a raid. Snacks are like meals—*you* need to be in control of the menu. And you need to be in control of the timing. Let's say your child has hardly eaten her meal and wants to leave the table. You know full well that in 5 minutes she will be back looking for a cookie. What do you do? You say no. You say (in whatever language your child understands), "Snack time will be in a while. You can have your cookie then." If your child is a toddler, the bottom line is "no." Tell her in words, but the language she really understands is your not giving her a cookie. Don't try to reason with her or explain—she won't understand or accept the explanation. She will only understand "no."

If she is like most toddlers when they are learning that no means no, she will pitch a fit. The best thing to do is to step over her. When she gets done yelling and kicking the floor, the answer will still be "no." And it will be "no" until it is time for her snack. She will learn, little by little, to tend to business when it is time to eat.

"Isn't that a little harsh?" parents ask me. "After all, she is so little and it *is* only one little cookie. Why make such a big deal over it? What if I offered her some whole-wheat crackers instead?" Sorry, it *is* a big deal. Your child depends on you to set a limit. This is not a power trip on your part. If she is allowed to graze for food and beg for handouts, the nutritional quality of her diet will suffer. She won't do as well with her eating, and she will be frightened.

When she begs, she doesn't beg for broccoli. She begs for crackers and cookies and candy and potato chips and all the easy-to-like stuff she has already mastered. Children push themselves along to learn, but they also take the easy way out if it is offered. If you give in to food begging you offer her the easy way out. You buy yourself some peace in the short run—but in the long run, you pay for it. When children are allowed to beg for food handouts, the list of foods they like becomes shorter and shorter, and their behavior at meals gets worse and worse.

Why does your child find a lack of limits frightening? To feel safe, your child needs to know you are able to stand up to her. When you set a limit, it is possible she will throw a tantrum. When she first starts having tantrums, it is because she is frustrated. But if you give in, she will learn that tantrums are effective in getting you to back down. Your giving in also tells her that she is stronger than you are, and that is frightening for her. Whenever you set a limit, you are conceivably picking a battle, so be prepared to stand your ground. Don't set limits casually, and do follow through. The structure of meals and snacks is an important limit, so don't hesitate to enforce the rule—just be sure to follow through.

Stay Positive in Choosing Food

Now that you have a better fix on your child's behavior, the stage is set. Let's get down to the business of food selection. How do you plan those meals we have talked about? I will loosely follow the Food Guide Pyramid for recommending *what goes on the table*, not for dictating what goes into your child—or into you. I will tell you the minimums you need from each food group to have a nutritionally adequate diet, but, unlike the Food Guide Pyramid, I won't try to oversee the total amount of food you eat from each food group. It is up to you if you want to exert control over the proportions of food you eat. However, if you begin to break your rules and show extremes in your eating, keep in mind that trying to follow a formula could be causing it.

Put another way, I will give you the floor to put under your eating, but I trust you to put up the walls and the roof. The walls and the roof are what and how much you are hungry for. The floor is the minimum for nutritional

adequacy you need to get from each of the groups in the Food Guide Pyramid (see page 50). To keep the confusion to a minimum, see the section on pages 67-68, "Don't be Enslaved by Serving Sizes." For now, see the box for the floor for each of the food groups:

> **NUTRITIONAL MINIMUMS**
> **Bread, cereal, rice, and pasta group:**
>   6 servings
> **Fruit group:** 2 servings
> **Vegetable group:** 3 servings
> **Fruit and vegetable groups put together:**
>   5 servings
> **Meat, poultry, fish, dry beans, eggs, and nuts group:** 2 to 3 servings or 5 to 7 ounces
> **Milk, yogurt, and cheese group:**
>   2 to 3 servings

To help you trust yourself, remember that your body knows how much to eat and that you will automatically seek a variety. And remember the fudge factor. Most of us could squander a third or more of our calories on nutritionally worthless food and still get the nutrients we need. For children, the fudge factor is even higher. It's unlikely that you or your child would actually need that much of a fudge factor. As I have said elsewhere, it is hard to find nutritionally worthless food. Most good-tasting food contains some nutrients, so if you eat what you like to make up your fudge factor, you will automatically nourish yourself as well.

Enjoy Bread, Cereal, Rice, and Pasta

Starting from the bottom, the Pyramid suggests we emphasize enriched and whole grain bread, cereal, rice, and pasta. For each meal include bread and one other complex carbohydrate, like rice or pasta. I think potatoes can count as the starch, as well. In fact, I count them on whichever list I need them. However, my nutritionist friends remind me that potatoes are not on the *bread* list but on the *vegetable* list and that they are not as rich in iron or B vitamins as bread.

The Pyramid says to eat 6 to 11 servings of bread or bread equivalents per day, which nutritionally is more than we need. Six servings is enough to get the B vitamins and iron we depend on this group to give us. The Pyramid recommends *more* than we need to get us to eat more of these low-fat, relatively low-calorie foods and less of higher-fat, higher-calorie foods. And, of course, the thinking is that these foods will help you keep your weight down and avoid disease. I am not sure I buy that thinking, but I won't quibble. I will point out, though, that that kind of encouragement turns these foods into *medicine*; instead of being fun it makes eating them a chore. We are going to have to do something to counteract that negativity.

Generally, children have no trouble eating what they need from this group. They eat starchy foods because they like them. You may feel the same way, but enough is enough. Don't eat any more of the starchy stuff than tastes good, even if it is supposed to be healthful. Pay attention to your appetite. Seek out good-tasting breads; eat rice and noodles if you like them. Use butter or a sauce to make starchy foods more interesting.

Again, *if they taste good to you*, you can emphasize the complex carbohydrates in your diet by making those the foods you and your family fill up on. With all the restrictiveness and external control we use with eating, the idea of "foods to fill up on" has gotten lost. We eat sparingly and try not to fill up on anything (not a good idea). Fill-up food is a concept worth bringing back. The traditional strategy for stretching food dollars is to fill up on starch. People who do hard physical labor need to go away from the table feeling fully satisfied in order to have energy for their active lives. Many times they have extra servings of rice or potatoes. A few years back, we thought meat was the food to fill up on. Now starches are the fill-up food of choice.

Serve whole grains about half the time, but again, only if you like them. Eating all whole grain is not necessary and isn't even good for children. All the fiber and other components in whole grain can interfere with iron and zinc nutrition.

Enjoy Fruits and Vegetables

Fruits and vegetables are on separate lists on the Food Guide Pyramid, but they give many of the same nutrients. Surveys show that adults eat, on the average, 1 to 1 1/2 servings of fruits and 2 1/2 to 3 1/3 vegetables a day. That's remarkably good. I suppose there's room for improvement, particularly because white potatoes (in French fries and chips) and tomatoes (in spaghetti sauce and salsa) make up most of the vegetable choices. The low fruit consumption is a particular surprise. Most people say they like fruit and find vegetables more challenging. Most children find fruit easier to like than vegetables. They *certainly* like juice. The Department of Agriculture's nationwide food consumption survey—*What We Eat in America*—showed that two to three times more children and teens drank apple juice, grape juice, or a noncitrus juice blend on a given day in 1994 than they did in 1977.

The Pyramid says eat 3 to 5 servings of vegetables and 2 to 4 servings of fruit a day. These daunting recommendations are intended to get us to eat more of these and fewer high-fat foods. A total of five servings of fruits and vegetables is enough. That number gives the vitamins A and C, B vitamins, fiber, phytochemicals (and other mysterious, possibly protective ingredients) we need from this group.

Including more fruits and vegetables is a good idea. The more we learn about nutrition, the more we realize that fruits and vegetables contribute to health and vitality. But we don't want to turn our food into medicine. Instead, we must entice ourselves and our families with fruits and vegetables. How can we do that? First, make them more interesting. In chapters 5, 6, and 7 I have dressed up vegetables with butter and sauces. I have given you tasty recipes for casseroles and soups that have vegetables in them. I have included recipes for fruit cobblers and crisps, and I have reminded you to consider including dried fruit in your menus.

Then, even though the fruit or vegetable will be as delicious as it can possibly be, give yourself an out. For both yourself and your children, keep hold of the distinction between *serving* and *eating*. That keeps you in touch with appetite: how the food tastes at the time. If the food is new to everyone, allow time for it to catch on. Remember, research with children shows that they need 10 or 15 or 20 tastes, in as many meals, before they like a new food. You are likely to need the same. Experiment the way a child does, and always give yourself an out: Look but don't taste; taste but don't swallow; swallow but don't force yourself to take another bite. If you pay attention to whether you really enjoy the food, you—like your child—will be more interested in eating it the next time you have the opportunity.

Use canned and frozen vegetables and fruit to cut down on preparation time and to vary the taste. Fruits and vegetables don't have to be fresh to be nutritious. Keep cans of fruit and vegetable juice around, reach for those rather than soda and use them for a late-afternoon pickup. Apricot and peach nectar are wonderfully tasty and nutritious and are simply fruits in a different form. Raisins and dried apricots or prunes give vitamin A and iron and make a nutritious sweet snack.

Don't forget about breakfast as a place to include fruit and vegetables: An omelet with spinach or a dish of peaches can add to the day's offerings. Depending on how big it is, the daily glass of orange juice can add up to one or two servings. Snacks also may include a fruit or vegetable: A banana, a few slices of dried apple, raw vegetables with a dip, a pear with some peanut butter, frozen peas eaten frozen like little ice cubes—all can add to the day's offerings. You notice I said *offerings*. I really mean it: Your job is done when you put it on the table. Increase your vegetable and fruit use slowly—don't shoot for the whole five a day at one time. Start, for instance, by trying to offer two fruits a day. When you are consistent about that, nudge it up one more. You will still be doing very well.

Lumping the fruit and vegetable lists together and trying for five servings altogether helps when planning meals for children. Sometimes children eat fruits, sometimes vegetables, and there is no predicting which it will be! When you get so you regularly include fruits and vegetables in your menus, try to offer two at each of your main meals to increase the chances your child (and you) will find one of them appealing enough to eat. This might be a fruit and a vegetable, like corn and peaches; two fruits, like a big fruit salad; or two vegetables, like tomatoes in the lasagna and a vegetable salad.

You can use all your ingenuity to come up with a variety of fruits and vegetables to put on the table, but once again beware: You mustn't try to force your child—or yourself—to eat them. Take it slowly and trust your child—and yourself—to learn to enjoy them. Best intentions aside, you will keep eating fruits and vegetables only if they give you pleasure. Forcing them down out of duty will work for a while, but eventually you will give it up.

Enjoy Meat, Poultry, Fish, Dry Beans, Eggs, and Nuts

The Pyramid suggests 2 to 3 servings from the protein group each day, with the total being the equivalent of 5 to 7 ounces of cooked lean meat, poultry, or fish. (See chapter 6, page 120, for what counts as an ounce.) Politically correct protein foods right now, in order of the virtue attributed to them, are dried beans and peas (especially soybeans), nuts, fish, and poultry. In last place, in fact, and generally considered *not* to be virtuous at all, is red meat.

ENJOY RED MEAT

Meat's sad fate is based on urban rumor. You know the urban rumor—it is the story that gets passed around and told for the gospel truth and attributed to a friend of a friend. The story about Mao Tse Tung condemning mosquitoes, instructing every man, woman, and child in China to kill 20 a day and upsetting the balance of nature is an urban rumor. It seems logical; it could be true, but it isn't. The same goes for red meat. The urban rumor is that meat is bad for you. It is not. Even the Food Guide Pyramid, that guidepost of cautious eating, says to eat 2 to 3 servings a day from the meat group, and it assigns lean meat equal importance and virtue with other foods in the group. It does recommend using trimmed, lean meats. It does not say to stop eating red meat.

Here is how the urban rumor got started. Unlike the grains and fruit/vegetable groups, the Pyramid tells us to limit our consumption in this category to 5 to 7 ounces of meat, poultry, or fish a day. While that is certainly enough for nutritional adequacy, the problem is that most people took that recommendation to mean that meat is bad for you. That interpretation is as factually based as Mao Tse Tung's mosquito shortage. On the contrary, red meat is good for you. National statistics indicate that from beef alone, which accounts for only about 7 percent of the calories we consume, we get 18 percent of our protein; over 25 percent of our vitamin B_{12} and zinc; 10 percent of our vitamin B_6, iron, and niacin; and significant amounts of thiamin.[1] Moreover, red meat (and to a lesser extent poultry and fish) contains meat factor (the substance that helps the body to absorb iron). In other words, meat carries more than its nutritional weight.

Even though the enthusiasts who wrote the Dietary Guidelines and the Food Guide Pyramid didn't say to give up red meat, they urged caution based on its saturated fat content. Instead of being cautious, we have begun avoiding red meat altogether. I don't think we are stupid or reactionary; I just think the warning turns meat into something we have to measure and limit instead of something to eat until we feel satisfied. Eating red meat has become a *control* issue rather than a *trust* issue.

In my view, the caution is misplaced. Compared with the 18 percent of protein and all the other nutrients it gives, beef contributes only 11 percent of the saturated fat we eat. Moreover, about a fourth of the saturated fat in red meat is stearic acid, which has been shown by newer research (and older research revisited) to neither raise nor lower blood cholesterol.[2] Not only that, but beef contributes 13 percent of our monounsaturated fat intake and 2 percent of polyunsaturated fat, both considered "good" fats by the enthusiasts.

Some people avoid meat for religious reasons, or out of concern for animal welfare. Those reasons are personal, and I won't quibble with them. It is not my choice, but it can be yours. However, avoiding any category of foods, like animal protein sources, increases the difficulty of getting a nutritionally adequate diet. As a consequence, to ensure that you follow a healthful vegetarian diet, understand the principles of vegetarian menu planning. See the box "Vegetarian Menu Planning" in chapter 8, page 152.) Others avoid meat out of concern for the environment, and with that argument, I will quibble. The objection I hear most often is that meat is high on the food chain—supposedly meat animals compete with humans for the same food. Presumably, growing animals is inefficient use of land—it requires several times the amount of acreage to grow grain to feed the animals than it would if we just ate the grain in the first place. Well, that would be true if meat animals ate only grain. But usually, meat animals are raised by grazing on grassland pastures—they are fed grain only in the last few weeks before they are slaughtered.

Sixty percent of the earth's cropland is grassland; without grazing animals, that land could not be responsibly or efficiently used for agri-

culture. Because of the way pastureland is managed, grazing does not deplete or destroy the land. Most animals are grazed in a way that sustains the grasses growing in the pastures. If the land is used destructively—if it is overgrazed—it wrecks fragile pastureland for decades and destroys its usefulness. The majority of ranchers know to avoid overgrazing and are responsible environmentalists who manage their grasslands well.

ENJOY EGGS

The Food Guide Pyramid says "Go easy on egg yolks; use one egg yolk per person in egg dishes and make larger portions by adding egg whites." Not only do I think that that limit is too restrictive, but I have observed that people in general have exaggerated the advice to be even *more* restrictive about eggs. Many people feel they shouldn't eat eggs at all. The American Heart Association won't like my saying this, but I think eating an egg a day or 10 a week is moderate, especially for children. Eggs are an important source of protein; vitamins E, A, and D; and B vitamins. Children like eggs and generally eat them well. When cooking for a family, eggs are a mainstay.

So why would I encourage you to eat eggs? Egg yolks, as you undoubtedly know, are a rich source of cholesterol, so it stands to reason that they should be avoided. Not so. Cholesterol plays an essential part in the makeup of the walls of all the cells in the body and is a major component of brain and nerve tissue. Your body uses cholesterol to manufacture essential hormones like estrogen, testosterone, and adrenal hormones. Your body has to have cholesterol, and if you don't eat it, your body makes its own.

If you cut down on your cholesterol intake, your body manufactures more to make up for it. If you eat more, your body cuts down on production. As a consequence, varying the amount of cholesterol you eat doesn't have much impact on your blood cholesterol. Most agencies that make dietary recommendations recognize this phenomenon. Many countries have dietary guidelines that are similar to our own, but the United States is the only country that recommends restricting cholesterol intake.

A certain small percentage of people lack the biological feedback loop that enables them to make less cholesterol when they eat more of it. For them, a low-cholesterol diet is important. Their blood cholesterol falls if they cut down on dietary cholesterol. If you have high blood cholesterol, it is worth a try to lower your intake of cholesterol to see if you are one of these few "cholesterol responders." If you aren't, go ahead and eat eggs. In my view, we don't all have to go without eggs just because some people are cholesterol responders.

ENJOY POULTRY AND FISH

In defending the inclusion of meat and eggs in your menus, I do not mean to slight poultry and fish. They, too, provide protein, vitamins, minerals, and some meat factor. Eat poultry the way you like it. It really isn't necessary to be slavish about removing the skin. True, most of the fat is in or just under the skin. True, you get rid of that fat if you strip the skin away. True, even if you add a marinade it doesn't equal the amount in the skin. *But*, if you like the skin and enjoy eating it, why deprive yourself? If you check the box titled "Fat in Meat" on page 170, you will see that leaving the skin on poultry changes it from a lean meat to a not-quite-so-lean meat. Is the added pleasure worth it to you? Only you can decide.

ENJOY DRY BEANS AND NUTS

Cooked dried beans are on the meat list as well. Beans offer fiber, minerals, and B vitamins, and they are filling, economical, and delicious. An offshoot of meat phobia is that people have discovered an assortment of wonderful beans. Tofu is making its way onto our tables from time to time, and we are beginning to use seeds and nuts as a source of protein. All that is well and good. However, you do not have to forsake meat to embrace beans and nuts. Include them all, and your diet will be the better for it. The greater your variety, the better your diet. Have beans as a main dish (see the recipe for **Savory Black Beans and Rice** on pages 110-111), or combine them with meat (see the recipe for **Minestrone Soup** on pages 108-109, or have them as a side dish, as in wieners and beans. For ideas about using seeds and nuts in main dishes, see the "Complementary Plant Proteins" box. Do keep in mind, however, that you need to wait to give children whole nuts until they are about 3 years old and are able to chew and swallow well.

PEANUT BUTTER

Let me share a special word about peanut butter. This mainstay of children's diets has gotten some bad press recently because some people experience life-threatening reactions to it. Children most likely to be seriously allergic to peanuts are those with strong family histories of allergies. Whether from food or environmental agents such as house dust, pollen, or animal dander, allergies make themselves

---

COMPLEMENTARY PLANT PROTEINS

Plant proteins, in contrast to animal proteins, are incomplete: They don't have all the components (amino acids) needed to build and repair muscle and body tissue. Since plants vary in the amino acid limitations, a plant from one food group can combine with a plant from another food group to make a complete protein. We used to think we had to have these combinations at the same meal. Newer research shows that we have a day or more to consume the combinations. That means you can be more casual about combining plant proteins: If you prepare a variety of legumes and grains, and if you use some eggs and milk, chances are you are balancing things out.

It seems to me, however, that half the fun of cooking vegetarian is making use of complementary proteins and cooking traditional vegetarian dishes. Centuries of eating—and surviving—have demonstrated the nutritional utility—and the taste appeal—of these dishes. Here are some combinations of plant protein that add up to make a complete protein.

Legumes + Grains:
- split pea soup and crackers
- peanut butter on wheat bread
- black beans and rice
- corn tortillas and refried beans
- tofu and bulgur (wheat)

Legumes + Seeds:
- hummus (chickpea and sesame seed dip)
- sunflower seeds sprinkled on navy bean soup
- falafel patties with tahini (sesame butter)
- snack mix of roasted soy beans and seeds
Don't give seeds and nuts to young children.

Grains + Milk:
- macaroni and cheese
- cheese and crackers
- rice pudding
- cereal and milk

Grains + Egg:
- fried egg sandwich
- French toast

Legumes + Milk or Eggs:
- cheese sauce over kidney beans
- bean frittata
- lentil-yogurt salad
- peanut butter milk shake

apparent through skin rashes, breathing problems, stomachaches, or indigestion. If someone in your family has allergic reactions, keep your child away from peanuts and peanut butter until she is 2 years old.

Peanuts and peanut butter, however, are not such a concern for children without histories of allergies. Your 1-year-old can have peanut butter on bread or toast, if you spread it thinly to keep down the risk of choking. By age 12 months, her immune system will have matured and her intestine will be less likely to take in the whole protein molecules that cause allergic reactions.

Enjoy Milk, Yogurt, and Cheese

Milk is good for children. A few children are allergic to milk or can't digest the sugar that milk contains (lactose), but most children benefit from drinking milk. So do grown-ups. The Pyramid recommends the minimum: 2 to 3 servings per day. It won't hurt you or your children to drink more unless you drink milk instead of eating something else you need.

Milk and milk products contribute important amounts of protein to most children's diets and are a primary source of calcium and vitamin D. In 1997 the National Academy of Sciences announced new guidelines for recommended calcium intake: Children between 1 and 3 years old need 500 milligrams of calcium per day, between 4 and 8 years they need 800 milligrams, and between 9 and 18 years 1,300 milligrams. A cup of milk or yogurt or 1 1/2 ounces of cheese give about 300 milligrams of calcium. See the box titled "Sources of Calcium" for some other good sources of calcium.

Unfortunately, children's milk consumption appears to be dropping markedly across the board. Instead, kids are drinking more juice and soft drinks. The *What We Eat in America* survey found that preschoolers drank four times more juice (mostly apple juice) in 1994 than they did in 1977. Many toddlers drink so much apple juice, and drink it so often, that they spoil their meals, and some even rot their teeth. Teenage boys tripled their soft drink consumption during the same period. Although it would be hard to spoil a teenage boy's appetite, that requirement of 1,300 milligrams of calcium is hard to meet if kids routinely choose soda instead of milk.

The rumors (and even press conferences by seeming authorities) ballyhooed every so often that milk is bad for people in general and for children in particular are simply wrong. Such ideas are based on flimsy evidence by people on crusades. Charges against milk do not hold up to careful examination. Pasteurized milk sold in regular grocery stores is safe and wholesome for your child. It is subject to strict regulation.

Give your baby breastmilk or iron-fortified formula until she is at least a year old and is eating a variety of other food. Then switch to pasteurized whole milk. Why is it all right to give pasteurized milk at age 1 year but not before? Because by that time, the other foods your baby eats makes up for the nutrients lacking in milk, such as iron and vitamin C, and because other food mixes with the milk in your child's stomach to make milk easier to digest. Don't feed unpasteurized milk of any type at any age.

Why whole milk? Because fat is an important source of energy. Younger children, especially, depend on milk to provide them with fat. After age 2, whole milk is still okay. So is 2 percent, 1 percent, or skim milk, *if* your child likes it and drinks it well (many children don't) and *if* she has other good sources of fat in her diet. *But be careful!* Pennsylvania State researchers found that it was all too easy to overdo fat restriction, especially for toddlers (see also chapter 10, "Raising a Healthy Eater in Your Community"). Do *not* use low-fat milk if you use mostly lean meats *or* use low-fat food preparation techniques or limit the butter or salad dressing your child uses at the table. If you are in doubt about whether your child is eating enough fat, give her whole milk.

If you can, make milk the mealtime beverage. Drink it yourself. Don't push it, or you will turn it into something your child wants to avoid. Just make it available and wait. I realize that some cultural traditions don't support milk as a mealtime beverage. In that case, be careful about making the alternatives too appealing. Water is best. For some reason I do not understand, many young children would rather drink than eat their meals. If you make juice, Kool-Aid, or soda readily available, your child may eat poorly.

It's okay to occasionally put flavorings in milk. But be careful of your attitude. If *you* are

SOURCES OF CALCIUM

Food	Amount	Calcium (mg)
Dairy Products		
Milk, fluid	1 cup	300
Milk, powdered	1 Tbsp	60
Cheese, natural or processed	1 oz	200
Cottage cheese	1/4 cup	40
Yogurt	1 cup	300
Ice cream	1/2 cup	110
Cream cheese	1 Tbsp	10
Meat and Other Protein Sources		
Meat, poultry, fish	3 oz	10–20
Canned fish with bones	3 oz	250
Egg	1	30
Cooked dried beans	1/2 cup	45
Nuts and seeds	2 Tbsp	20–40
Peanut butter	2 Tbsp	20
Tofu with calcium lactate (brands vary—check label)	4 oz	50–250
Bread, Cereal, Pasta		
Bread	1 slice	25
Biscuits, rolls	1	25
Corn tortillas	1	60
Cooked and dry cereals, unfortified	1 serving	15
Noodles, macaroni, rice	1/2 cup	15
Vegetables and Fruits		
Vegetables, average	1/2 cup	20–40
Green leafy vegetables, average	1/2 cup	100
Fruits, average	1/2 cup	20–40
Calcium-fortified orange juice	1/2 cup	150

so invested in getting your child to drink milk that *you* are willing to go to a lot of trouble to make it happen, your child will know that. She will make drinking milk *your* thing, not hers, and she will use it to manipulate you. Even the child who drinks milk will go through periods when she doesn't drink much milk, especially right after she is weaned. Don't make a fuss about it; don't try to push milk. Just wait. And drink *your* milk. She will go back to drinking milk when she's ready. After all, if you drink it, it must be the thing to do.

Enjoy Sweets

Although people generally think of sugar as bad and sugary foods as forbidden, children benefit from eating some sugar. Their energy needs are high, and their stomachs are small, and sugar gives them concentrated energy. But, to state the obvious, it's not a good idea for either you or your child to fill up on sweets.

Sugar doesn't have to be a nutritional no-no. Some of the calories in the fudge factor I mentioned earlier—the margin between the calories we need to spend on nutritious food and our total energy requirement—can go for sugary foods. You can also use sugar to help make nutritious foods more interesting, like the spoonful of sugar we put in the **Herbed Peas** (recipe on page 140) to make them taste fresher, or the brown sugar we put in Applesauce (recipe on page 144) to make it chunkier. Sugar can carry nutrition if you make most sweets nutritious, like pudding or oatmeal cookies. Candy and Kool-Aid are okay, but offer them only occasionally.

The only disease caused by sugar is tooth decay. Sugar of all kinds nourishes the acid-producing bacteria in the mouth. Mouth bacteria can learn to live on the sugar in milk (lactose) and fruit (fructose) as well as the sugar in candy and soda (sucrose) as well as on sugar broken down from starch. The primary considerations with food and tooth decay are frequency and duration—how often bacteria-supporting nutrients are in the mouth and for how long. Munching all day on raisins can decay your child's teeth as surely as chewing on caramels; both are sticky and sugary and stay in contact with teeth. Because it keeps sugar in contact with the teeth, drinking fruit juice all the time can cause tooth decay as surely as drinking Kool-Aid. For up-to-date information about nutrition and oral health, talk with your dentist. Dental professionals care about nutrition and go to some trouble to support their patients' nutritional health.

There is no reliable evidence that eating sugar causes children to have behavior problems. However, *hungry* children have behavior problems. Eating sweets instead of something more substantial can soon leave a child empty—and cranky. To keep your child from having that post-sugar emptiness and crankiness, reserve the sweets for meal and snack times and offer other foods at the same time. The other food will stay with her longer and keep her comfortable until the next feeding time.

Enjoy Salt

If you want to know what I recommend for your salt use, read on. If you want to know why I recommend it, see appendix I, "Sodium in Your Diet." It is more important to eat—and enjoy—a variety of nutritious food than it is to rigidly restrict salt (or anything else, for that matter). Use the salt you need to make your food taste good. Don't drive yourself to eating out so you can let someone else do the salting. As with the rest of your eating, finding the moderate middle ground is the trick. Getting enough salt is important, particularly during pregnancy and when doing hard physical labor. It is not necessary to be enslaved or afraid to use salt, nor is it a good idea to throw caution to the winds and eat an unrelieved

diet of high-salt foods.

I show you the middle ground with my cooking strategies. I use moderate amounts of salt in cooking, include canned vegetables, sauces, mixes, and even soups in cooking and occasionally use bacon and other high-salt foods in cooking. Cooking—and eating—in that way gives you about 3,000 to 4,000 milligrams of sodium per day—a reasonable and moderate amount. More important, it will allow you to be *consistent* in your sodium intake.

With sodium, as with the rest of your eating, think about sustainability. Find a way of eating that you can maintain without the extremes of restraint and disinhibition. If you want to restrict salt and can be consistent about it, you have my blessings (unless you are pregnant, sweat a lot, or take certain medications). Be aware, however, that if you, like most people, can't consistently maintain that level of restriction, you'd better lighten up. If you restrain and disinhibit, you will lead your body's sodium-processing system a merry chase, and it won't be good for you.

Enjoy Fats and Oils

Now we come to the crunch: What to do about fat? The standard advice about fat is so negative and restrictive that it's difficult to talk about fat and still stay out of the food-as-medicine trap. While many consumers avoid fat in the name of weight control, in the nutrition community the big debate is about dietary fat and heart disease and the avoid-fat advice is in the name of heart disease. If you want to know only what I recommend, I will tell you now. I am satisfied that my recommendations are safe and realistic because I have thought carefully about them and done more reading on the topic than I care to think about. If you want to know why I tell you that you don't have to be so scared about diet and heart disease and so restrictive with fat, see appendix G, "Dietary Fat and Heart Disease: It's Not as Bad as You Think."

Lighten up on fat restriction. You must have fat. Fat provides essential fatty acids and carries fat-soluble vitamins. Fat conveys flavor in food, tastes good on its own, and gives food appealing color, texture, and moistness. Fat gives food "staying power" because eating fat with a meal retards the emptying time of the stomach and makes energy available to your body more slowly and for a longer time.

We act as if fat were poison. Many consumers, especially those in the "I'm already doing it" group, set their goals at eating no fat at *all*. Fifty percent of consumers put fat avoidance at the top of their list of nutritional concerns. It is unclear whether they avoid fat for weight control or for disease avoidance, but the principle is the same either way. Avoiding fat is dangerous. You can't be healthy without eating fat.

My best recommendation is that you lighten up and hedge your bets. Eating fat doesn't make you fat, unless you get into the restraint/disinhibition cycle. In my carefully considered view, unless you have a strong family history of heart disease, you can safely relax about your own fat consumption and your child's. Be moderate in your use of fat, but not restrictive. Do use butter on vegetables or sauces on foods (if you enjoy them). Most of my recipes have 1 or 2 teaspoons of fat per serving, and they are still moderate in fat. Using a tasty sauce or some butter (I endorse butter, but by *butter* I mean *butter or margarine*) in food preparation will make you and your children feel more like eating. Fat carries the flavor in food and makes it more interesting.

Put butter and salad dressing on the table, and use them to make food taste good. Notice that while you eat and enjoy some fatty foods, a steady diet of them is not pleasant. Internal mechanisms that seek variety provide guidance with low- and high-fat food, as well as with other foods. If you pay attention, you will observe that you get enough of even luscious, fried food and will look around for alternatives. For specific guidelines on making your cooking moderate in fat, see the chapters 5, 6, and 7.

Use a variety of fats (see appendix J, "A Primer on Dietary Fat"). Emphasize monounsaturated fats—like olive, canola, and peanut oils—in your cooking, frying, and salad dressings. It is okay to include polyunsaturated fats as well—like corn, sunflower, and soybean oils—just don't emphasize them as much as the monounsaturated ones. If you use margarine, make sure it adds to the quality and variety of oils in your diet. Ideally, the first ingredient of a margarine is a liquid form of one of the monounsaturated fats. Hardened, or hydrogenated, oils in vegetable shortenings don't have the nutritional advantages of liquid oils. They work great for baking cakes, but for

frying and cooking, the oils are better for you.

Don't feel you have to give up butter. Its wonderful taste adds greatly to good food flavor, and because it tastes so good, you may end up using less than if you try to settle for margarine. The same holds true for more "traditional" shortenings like lard. Lard "shortens" more—you need less of it than hydrogenated vegetable shortenings. It browns beautifully. For some dishes, like authentic, south-of-the-border refried beans, lard is an essential ingredient. Like other animal fats, butter and lard are not all saturated fat. Both have gotten an undeserved bad name by being put on oversimplified "bad" lists. Recent research, in fact, indicates that lard is a better choice than the solid vegetable shortenings we have all been using.

All foods have a place in a wholesome and varied diet. I use moderation as my guideline in the recipes in chapters 5, 6, and 7. I have defined moderate fat levels in recipes as roughly 1 to 2 teaspoons of fat per serving, and I have ensured that the recipes call for a variety of dietary fats.

TREAT LOW-FAT FOOD WITH RESPECT

Eating low-fat can make you fat. Research shows that over the last few years, as the percentage of fat in our diets has gone down, our weight has gone up. What does this mean? The nutrition enthusiasts say that we have to be more disciplined about watching our portion sizes, even for low-fat food. But that is a *control* message. The *trust* message is that your body knows how much to eat and that adhering to a low-fat diet could be undermining that ability to regulate.

Why would that be? Because for most people, eating a low-fat diet involves restriction. People tire of restriction, take a vacation from it, and overeat. In fact, periodic overeating is built into the restrictive low-fat lifestyle through the erroneous idea that "if it is low-fat, I can eat a lot of it." Low-fat food gives an escape from restriction and essentially is used as license for disinhibition.

When women in a Pennsylvania research study thought they were eating low-fat yogurt, they ate far more than when they ate unlabeled yogurt. Presumably they tuned in on internal controls for the unlabeled yogurt and ignored them for the low-fat yogurt. They are typical. Why is it necessary for us to overeat on low-fat foods? Why don't we just eat until we are satisfied? Because we feel deprived. Being comfortably satisfied is not part of the restraint/disinhibition cycle. The irony is that the throwing-away-control, eating-a-lot type of eating isn't really tuned-in and is therefore unsatisfying. It is often just excessive.

RELAX ABOUT CHILDREN AND DIETARY FAT

You may think my advice is too wildly liberal, and you may choose to be more restrictive with your fat intake. If you can be cautious and *consistent*, then carry on. (If you are going without and then making up for lost satisfaction, you are not being consistent.) However, it is not wise to be restrictive with your child. Children depend on fat to get the calories they need, and they depend on fat to make food appealing to them. Children's energy needs are high, and their stomachs are small. A low-fat diet may be too bulky for a child to be physically able to consume enough to get the energy she needs. In many cases, when children's fat intake is restricted, they eat sugary foods to get the high-energy food they need. The fat is more desirable, though, because it is more likely to be hooked onto high-nutrient foods like main dishes and vegetables. To find out *what* I recommend for children and fat, keep reading. To find out *why*, see appendix H, "Children, Dietary Fat, and Heart Disease: You Don't Have to Panic."

Since children are so tuned in to their hunger and appetites, and since children's energy needs vary so much from time to time, you need to choose foods for meals and snacks that vary in fat and calories. Have some that are high in fat, some that are moderate, and some that are low. Then let children choose what they will. When they are hungry because they are active or growing fast, they will likely eat more high-fat, high-calorie foods.

Let children use regular salad dressing and table spreads like butter and/or margarine to make their food taste good. Children may not want butter, or they may put on a lot. Typically, children experiment and learn. Unless butter becomes something you and she struggle about, if your child eats a lot of butter it is because she needs the calories.

The cooking methods you will learn in this book are moderate in fat. When your child is active or growing fast, she needs more fat than she'll get from those main dishes or vegetable recipes. Let her eat as much butter, margarine,

or salad dressing as she wants. She knows what she is doing. Children choose high-fat foods partly because they need the extra calories and partly because fat enhances the food's flavor. One mother worried when her daughter piled on the butter and doubted me when I said her daughter would find her own moderation. "You were right," she announced recently. "The other night we had cornbread and Julia put on a lot of butter. Then she said, 'you know, I put on so much butter I can't taste my cornbread.' " We are so concerned about fatty foods that we make butter, margarine, and salad dressing forbidden fruit. Like other forbidden fruit, children find those foods especially appealing precisely because they are forbidden. When parents restrict foods, children want them all the more, and they don't have the opportunity to discover, like Julia did, that some is good but too much isn't.

Offer and use a variety of fats and fat sources, including saturated, monounsaturated, and polyunsaturated fats from both animal and vegetable sources. Children benefit from learning to like a variety of fats, just as they do with other foods in their diets.

A Postscript about Fat, Sodium, and Even Weight

You need to know that since I have taken my moderate stance about fat, sodium, and weight, I have been advised by my enthusiast colleagues that I am too negative and extreme—apparently I am well on my way to being a rogue dietitian. "Why don't you just recommend being sensible and quit being so critical?" they ask. I have a little difficulty wrapping my brain around the challenge. Let me see if I have this right: I am being negative and extreme about negativity and extremism. I won't even dignify that contradictory question with an answer.

However, I will speak to the matter of being "critical." If being critical means being picky and faultfinding, I don't agree. I am bluntly identifying the issues and letting you decide about them for yourself. However, if being critical means being analytical, I will own up to it. I am questioning and challenging the current nutrition policy, and there is no doubt that it would be safer for me not to. To me, recommending sensible use of fat, for instance, without dealing with the basic issues of fat and disease would amount to a bland message, and I don't think a bland message would break through the panic. Without addressing the basic issues, recommending moderation just seems like more of the same.

We are too worried to be sensible. To become more sensible, we have to reduce our anxiety to the point that we can learn and change. Some of my colleagues are alarmed when I say "lighten up," and they fear that I am saying "don't be concerned." I'm not. I am saying, "don't be terrified," as well as "do no harm." As I point out in appendix G, my assessment is that for most of us, the wolf we fear is at the door is not a wolf at all—it is an irritable pussycat.

Furthermore, I feel I am on the firm middle ground because I encourage normal eating. Normal eating is what you do when you pay attention to what you want and need and are accustomed to eating. As you pay attention, you will find ways of eating that work for you. I do think the way you eat is important and needs to be attended to, but I don't think the way you eat is so bad or so irresponsible that you have to be scared into making drastic changes. Wherever today's dietary disapproval, fear mongering, and rigid formulas come from, they are spoiling our eating.

Don't Be Enslaved by Serving Sizes

If you make yourself more important than the rules, a serving is how much you eat. Too often, a discussion of servings becomes a dis-cussion of how much you *should* eat for a serving, and *BAM!* eating becomes controlling and negative. Just like that. You don't need it. Your eating will always be worse if you are controlling and negative. You will be oh, so good, and then you will make up for lost time by being oh, so bad.

Serving sizes are nothing more or less than a unit of measurement, like a gallon of gas. A gallon of gas costs a certain amount, a cup of milk gives certain amounts of nutrients. When I fill up my car, I buy 14 gallons of gas or more. When I fill up on milk, I drink a cup or more. Simply because the label on a container of milk says a portion is 1 cup, that doesn't mean I have to stop at a cup. That would be as silly as going to the gas station every time I need a gallon of gas. With eating, as with buying gas, a *portion* and a *fill-up* are two different things.

You can use serving sizes to get a feeling for how you are doing nutritionally (if you drink 12 ounces of milk you get credit for one and a half of your two to three servings). When I assess the nutritional quality of a child's diet, I use serving sizes as a basis for my nutrient calculations. The guidelines I have been giving you are for numbers of servings a day needed to have a *nutritionally adequate* diet, not a *filling* diet. In general, for adults, those servings are as follows:

- 1/2 cup of cooked rice, noodles, or grits
- 3/4 cup of juice, vegetables, or fruit
- An average piece as commonly served (a banana, an apple)
- 2 to 3 ounces of cooked meat, fish, or poultry
- 1 to 2 ounces of cheese; 2 to 3 eggs
- 8 ounces of milk

For children, check the box titled "Serving Sizes for Children." Keep in mind that a child

SERVING SIZES FOR CHILDREN				
	Age 1–3	**Age 3–5**	**Age 6–8**	**Age 8+**
Meat, poultry, fish	1–2 Tbsp	1 oz	1–2 oz	2 oz
Eggs	1/4	1/2	3/4	1 egg
Cooked dried beans	1–2 Tbsp	3–5 Tbsp	5–8 Tbsp	1/2 cup
Pasta, rice, potatoes	1–2 Tbsp	3–5 Tbsp	5–8 Tbsp	1/2 cup
Bread	1/4 slice	1/2 slice	1 slice	1 slice
Vegetables	1–2 Tbsp	3–5 Tbsp	5–8 Tbsp	1/2 cup
Fruit	1–2 Tbsp or 1/4 piece	3–5 Tbsp or 1/3 piece	5–8 Tbsp or 1/2 piece	1/2 cup or 1 piece
Milk	1/4 to 1/3 cup	1/3 to 1/2 cup	1/2 to 2/3 cup	1 cup
Note: Children may eat more or less, but this is how much you can serve them to start with.				

might eat more or less—the recommendations are just a place to start. Remember, the serving size doesn't dictate the amount that you—or your child—need to eat. It simply gives you a way of knowing how you are doing nutritionally. You can trust internal processes of hunger, appetite, and satiety to arrive at how much to eat. Use the "Serving Sizes for Children" box as a guide for how much to put on your child's plate. Children eat better when parents offer them child-sized helpings.

I don't give portion sizes for fat because foods vary so much in the amount of fat they contain. When you emphasize variety and use fat moderately to make food taste good (you will learn how in the chapters 5, 6, and 7), you and your family will get the right amount of fat.

Summary

We have covered a lot of information in this chapter, and it is pretty detailed. Here is the bottom line:
• Focus on meal planning.
• Seek variety.

As Grandpa Eddie says: "A little of everything will keep you alive. Too much of anything will kill you." You don't know Grandpa Eddie, but like other sages, he makes a good point. Maybe you can think of him the next

time you read one of the news releases about a new miracle food that will ward off disease or when you hear one of those alarming statements that tells us we are killing ourselves with our knives and forks.

Meals make variety possible. Variety increases your chances of doing the right thing and decreases the negatives if you are doing the wrong thing. Striving for variety allows you to be positive in exploring food and keeps you in touch with the joy of eating. It lets you expose your child to the wonderful world of food and helps her grow up with the joy of good eating. Each food has something to offer. You can help your family be comfortable in the world of food as well as hedge their bets against disease if you help them learn to like a *variety*.

Selected References

1. Subar, A. F., S. M. Krebs–Smith, A. Cook, and L. L. Kahle. 1998. Dietary sources of nutrients among U.S. adults, 1989 to 1991. *Journal of the American Dietetic Association* 98: 537–547.
2. Grundy, S. M. 1994. Influence of stearic acid on cholesterol metabolism relative to other long-chain fatty acids. *American Journal of Clinical Nutrition* 60 (6 suppl.): 986S–990S

Getting Started

- Build a foundation for good, fast, and wholesome cooking.
- Don't be a food snob—food does not need to be sophisticated, trendy, or complicated to be delicious.
- Don't be afraid to use salt and fat to make food taste good.
- Increase your efficiency by thinking ahead about your cooking, preferably the night before.
- Increase your efficiency by cooking pre-prepared meals.
- Your children will grow up to be comfortable with cooking if you let them help with meal preparation.
- You can adapt dishes and menus to help your children eat well without catering to them.

CHAPTER

5

HOW TO GET
COOKING

In previous chapters I have encouraged you to celebrate eating and take good care of yourself with food. Now we move on to extending and supporting that celebration with cooking. Our task is to translate these principles into food preparation. Unless you have unlimited resources, to celebrate eating and take good care of yourself with food, you have to cook—and keep on cooking. For you to keep it up, it has to be rewarding, and you need to feel successful at it. How do you manage that in the everydayness of time constraints and competing priorities?

Approach your cooking with the anticipation of pleasure, respect for the food, a clean kitchen, an organized mind, and flexible expectations. Cooking can be intensely rewarding, but it can also be a chore that has to be attended to day in and day out. You may love cooking and find it relaxing and energizing. You may put up with cooking for the reward of eating good food. You feel the way you feel.

In the next five chapters, I approach cooking and food management with the assumption that you don't know much about it. My young adult friends tell me, "My generation doesn't cook." Cooking magazines say that their readers long for home-cooked food, want to get back to the family table, but feel they don't know how. Women's magazines say that food preparation articles are the most popular with readers. This chapter, together with chapters 6 and 7, will help you build a foundation for being a good, fast, efficient, and wholesome

cook. I am serious about building a foundation. I hope my ideas will give you ideas of your own and help you to become comfortable creating your own ways in the kitchen. Because building a foundation requires bricks and mortar, to be successful with cooking you need to orchestrate your equipment and supplies. You will learn about those issues in chapter 8, "Planning to Get You Cooking," and chapter 9, "Shopping to Get You Cooking."

I have chosen recipes that will help you learn food skills and strategies so you can be successful with the everyday challenge—and reward—of getting meals on the table. I find food fascinating, and the science of food even more so. Knowing the basic principles of cooking and why certain things work and others don't can give you the satisfaction of knowing what to do and, more than that, why you're doing it.

I chose every one of the recipes in this book to teach you something about food, nutrition, or cooking. I take it back. I chose every recipe because I like to eat it, and most other people do, too. Many of them are recipes I used when I was raising my own family, and my children still make them. These recipes make good tools for teaching because they use a variety of foods and cooking methods. They are easy, use familiar foods, and can be assembled in 20 to 30 minutes. Because some are cooked in the oven, others in the slow cooker (Crock-Pot), and still others simmered on the stove, they may take longer to cook in some cases, but your actual *production* time is low. I hope that

71

the recipes spark your own ideas and that you'll feel comfortable expanding on them.

We will start with success and build on it. There is much to learn, and developing cooking intuition takes time. On the principle that you will benefit from learning to walk before you can enjoy running, this chapter starts out easiest and ends up easy. The next chapter, "How to Continue Cooking," has recipes that are equally timesaving, have a few more steps, and may be a bit more interesting. Wait to prepare those recipes until you have had some success with the simpler ones in this chapter.

I hope that dealing with food and cooking so concretely will help you settle down and stop worrying so much about fat, nutrition, food safety, the environment, and who-knows-what-else that you can't get a meal on the table. To help you relax about those worries, I will help you find the middle ground. For food to taste good, you have to use some salt and fat in preparing it. You don't, however, have to throw away all controls and let the sky be the limit. You will discover an in-between, where you use fat and salt but don't overload your food—or yourself—with it. We will be moderate, but we will *not* filter out the essence of good taste by trying to cut out all the fat and salt. These recipes will help you know what is moderate—not too high and not too low.

These are dinner recipes. Because I want this cooking lesson to be brief and accessible, I haven't tried to give you guidelines for breakfast or lunch. However, you can provide very well for your lunches by eating leftovers or even doubling recipes and having the extra for lunch. Breakfast is often a simple meal, and that's fine—the important thing is *having* it. Children will eat breakfast well if you do. In chapter 9 I make some suggestions for breakfast cereals, and in chapter 7 I suggest using pumpkin or apple custard for breakfast. To help you with longer-term planning, the recipes in all three chapters have been combined into a cycle menu in the planning chapter. For now, we are going to have fun learning how to cook!

Don't Be a Food Snob

We are starting with tuna noodle casserole. Do not sneer or scoff! If you are a gourmet cook, turn your head away. For many of us,

this was the very first meal that we ever cooked, and proud of it we were! This dish tastes great, it is easy to make, and it uses ingredients you can easily keep on hand. As a matter of fact, three of the first four recipes use concentrated soup, including the ever-versatile cream of mushroom soup, a commodity that Garrison Keillor on *A Prairie Home Companion* calls "the everyday sacrament of Lutherans." Of course, he is poking fun at the eating habits of Minnesotans. Always quick to pick up on social trends, Keillor capitalizes on the current fashion of ridiculing unsophisticated eating habits. In addition to being just too-too ordinary, cooking with canned soup has fallen into disfavor because of the high salt and presumed high fat content. However, diluted in the recipes we use here, the amount of sodium or fat per serving is reasonable.

Scorning or being afraid of everyday food is one obstacle that can get in the way of your feeding a healthy family. Another obstacle is being daunted by cooking because your mother was such a good cook. Let me tell you a smutty secret about her and others of my generation: we started out cooking with canned soup. I had a recipe book called *Take a Can of Soup . . . ,* and I learned that you could mix canned soup with almost anything and turn it into dinner. You could even get it to turn into a cake, as the famous tomato soup chocolate cake testified. No, I haven't given you the recipe. It wasn't that good. It was just something odd and wonderful to do with food, like the apple pie you make with Ritz crackers and fool your friends into thinking really is apple pie.

In choosing these recipes, I have attempted to cater to many food preferences and offer food that is interesting and good-tasting but not overly challenging to prepare or to eat. Most people will be able to find at least some recipes and menu suggestions that suit them. If you find, however, that there is very little that you feel you can eat or that pleases you, you might take a look at your own eating attitudes and behaviors. You may be following a list of dietary rules that is just *too* restrictive. You may need to work on food acceptance—your ability to learn to like variety of food. Finally, you may be laboring under the "last meal" mentality that many too-cautious eaters experience, where every morsel of food has to be just right.

Use Salt and Fat

The amount of salt and fat called for in these recipes is moderate; it makes the food taste good. Cooking without salt and fat will make food unappealing to you and your family, and will make you feel unsuccessful as a cook.

AMOUNT OF SALT

In preparing these recipes and menus, I have figured an average of 3,000 to 4,000 milligrams of sodium per day. That is higher than the target level of 2,400 milligrams recommended by the enthusiasts, but it's still a moderate level for children and healthy adults. I have used as my standard 1/4 teaspoon of salt per cup of food. Each of these recipes gives about 500 to 600 milligrams of sodium per cup, an amount that tastes good to most of us. Broth that tastes good to most of us contains about 1/4 teaspoon of salt per cup, or around 525 milligrams of sodium. To salt water for cooking noodles, rice, and vegetables, I recommend adding 1 teaspoon of salt per quart to the water, which again is pretty standard. (A quart contains 4 cups, so each cup has 1/4 teaspoon of salt.) Many recipes tell you to salt to taste, and your taste is likely to come out at around 1/4 teaspoon per cup of food. To avoid oversalting and spoiling the dish, add a little salt at a time and taste after each addition. When you read labels, you can tell if a main dish, soup, or vegetable is relatively high or low in sodium from going by the 500-milligrams-per-cup guideline. For instance, canned chicken broth is high in sodium: it contains 1,000 milligrams per 1-cup serving.

Canned, concentrated soups, like cream of mushroom and cream of potato, are good ingredients for jump-starting your cooking, and you will find them in the recipes that follow. The salt and fat in the canned soup can be high: diluted with water according to the directions on the can, canned soups generally give 750 to 1,000 milligrams of sodium per cup. However, when canned soup is used in cooking, the recipe dilutes the sodium to moderate levels by letting soup provide the salt for the recipe.

If you choose to keep your daily sodium usage down to 2,500 milligrams or less, leave out the salt in recipes, choose "no salt added" soups, avoid cured meats, and use frozen or fresh vegetables rather than canned. If you have congestive heart disease or high blood pressure that needs to be treated with diet, see a registered dietitian. For sodium restriction to make a difference in blood pressure, you have to cut your daily intake even less than 2,500 milligrams, and that takes very careful planning.

AMOUNT OF FAT

For the most part, each of my recipes has 1 to 2 teaspoons of fat per helping, and usually I use low- to medium-fat cuts of meat (see the "Fat in Meat" box on page 170). My menus contain liberal amounts of fruits and vegetables and starchy foods. Put together, that adds up to a moderate-fat diet. If you use modest amounts of salad dressings and table fats (butter, margarine, cream cheese, and sour cream), drink 2 percent or skim milk, and hit the fast-food joints only once or twice a week, you will end up with a moderate-fat diet. It won't be high and it won't be low. That is good for grown-ups, but it may or may not so good for children, young children especially.

Because children don't eat so much meat, casserole, or vegetables, the menus I recommend may not give them enough fat. Foods higher in fat that help as fat sources include desserts, crackers, cookies, ice cream, hot dogs, and high-fat casseroles like macaroni and cheese. If children eat too little fat, they may not get enough calories to grow properly. Only your child knows how many calories he needs, and he automatically eats more high-calorie foods when he is hungry from being active or growing fast. To give him the flexibility he needs, my menus specify bread and *butter*, meaning a table spread like *butter* or *margarine*. In addition, use at least 2 percent milk *and* let your children use as much salad dressing, butter or margarine, and other table spreads (cream cheese, sour cream) as they want.

TYPE OF FAT

With respect to fat selection, I have gone by the principle that it won't hurt you to eat a variety of fats and oils and even to emphasize those recommended by the enthusiasts. It might even help. When I say "cooking oil" in these recipes, I mean liquid vegetable oils. Consider using oils that contain predominantly monounsaturated fatty acids like canola, peanut, or olive oil. If you want more detail about fat chemistry and selection, see appendix J, "A Primer on Dietary Fat."

I diverge from the enthusiasts, however,

with respect to butter. I use butter because it tastes better and browns better. In my view, even the enthusiasts need not be concerned about butter. It contains about 30 percent monounsaturated fat and carries so much flavor that you can get by on less butter than if you try to make do with margarine. If you prefer margarine, be my guest. Do, however, read the list of ingredients and find one that lists a liquid monounsaturated oil, like canola oil, as the first ingredient. If the label says the oil is "hydrogenated" or "partially hydrogenated" (hydrogenation is a chemical process that hardens liquid fat), it won't do you any good and may even do harm. Fatty acids in hydrogenated oils are in the *trans* form, which has been shown to raise blood cholesterol as much as saturated fat.

When I think a recipe needs the flavor of olive oil, I say so. Use one of the virgin oils for dressings and sautéing and a refined oil for frying. Olive oils are graded informally according to the method of extraction and the free fatty acid composition. The grade determines the flavor and smoke point of the oil—the temperature at which it can smoke and, eventually, burst into flames. Smoking oils impart bad flavor and are dangerous. In order of decreasing free fatty acid content, *virgin, fine. superfine*, and *extra virgin* olive oils all come from the first pressing of the olives and are unrefined. The virgin oils have a relatively low smoke point and taste good in salads or in recipes that aren't heated too much. Subsequent pressings extract substances that give a harsh flavor to the oil and further lower the smoke point. Olive oil labeled *pure* is generally a combination of first and second pressings and has a higher content of less-good-tasting free fatty acids than the ones I listed earlier. In contrast to *pure*, olive oil labeled *refined* has been treated to remove the flavor components and raise the smoke point. Use refined olive oil for frying.

For sautéing use butter, margarine, virgin olive oil, or one of the monounsaturated oils. I like butter for sautéing because it browns well—food develops a lovely golden color with relatively little heat and cooking time. By the same token, butter does burn easily, so you have to watch carefully when food is browning. For frying, use one of the vegetable oils or refined olive oil. Butter, margarine, and virgin olive oil have low smoke points and can't take high frying temperatures. For solid shorten-ings, use butter, margarine, or lard. Unless you are baking a cake and want it to have a perfect, fine texture, avoid partially hydrogenated vegetable fats like solid vegetable shortenings.

If you have a favorite fat I haven't named, don't give up on it until you have a dietitian analyze it for you. People who love rendered chicken fat think it *can't* be good for them, but actually 45 percent of chicken fat is in the monounsaturated form.

Increase Your Efficiency

You cooking will be more satisfying if you learn to be efficient. The key to efficiency is using your head instead of your time and feet. Be a thinking cook. Read all the recipes for your meal before you start cooking—preferably the night before or in the morning so you can have your strategies in mind and make sure you have what you need. Every recipe has a "night before" section that suggests what to do ahead of time to speed your cooking. A few minutes spent the night before will save a lot in time and aggravation at that difficult before-dinner time. It's a good idea to locate all the necessary ingredients, cooking pans, and utensils. Put them in a handy place, on a shelf set aside for that purpose or on the countertop. Then you can pretend you are the serene chef on a cooking show, all your needs at hand, calmly assembling your masterpiece!

Think before you cook. To finish cooking all the food on the menu at the same time, you may have to keep two or more cooking processes going at once. Consider which menu item will take the longest to prepare, like heating the water for cooking noodles, and get that started before you turn your attention another cooking task. When my assistant Clio Marsh was testing these menus, she wrote out and arranged a list of her cooking tasks. Until your cooking intuition is sharpened, you might want to do the same.

Like any artist, you need to prepare your canvas ahead of time. Your kitchen and cooking equipment need to be clean and ready, and it helps stay organized if you clean up as you go. Keep a bowl of hot soapy water handy so you can wash your hands and your utensils as they get dirty. Think about what will take the longest to cook, and get that under way first. Think about what your child can "make" while you are cooking, find an out-of-your-way place, and set him up with what he needs. Think about what other people can do to contribute to the cooking. As the main cook, you may move into the role of coordinator and supervisor while others do the preparation. As your children get older, they can make a real contribution, and you mustn't keep the more interesting cooking tasks for yourself!

PPMs (Pre-Prepared Meals)

You can increase your efficiency by cooking ahead. These recipes generally make six helpings, so you will probably have enough for lunch the next day. You might even have enough for another dinner. You can double the batch, freeze half, and have it a few weeks later when you don't feel like cooking. You will find out with experience which recipes double easily and fit comfortably into your routine—and pans—so cooking in larger quantities doesn't become too complicated.

In my university foods and nutrition classes, I learned to call these foods *pre-prepared meals*, not *leftovers*. So be it. We will call them PPMs: the leftovers of the second millennium. Whatever you call them, for PPMs to be healthful and worry-free, we will have to deal with the tiresome but vital topic of keeping food safe.

KEEPING FOOD SAFE

To keep bacteria from growing in food, it must be kept above 140 degrees (simmering or hot eating temperature) or below 40 degrees (refrigerator temperature). Between 40 and 140 degrees, bacteria can grow. To keep food safe for eating, make sure it is left at room temperature for no more than 2 hours total, including preparation, serving, and cooling-down times. After that, consider it contaminated and unsafe to eat. Throw it away, even if it looks and tastes all right, even if there are starving children somewhere.

To cool food quickly, refrigerate it in a flat pan. Leave the cover off so the air can circulate around it. After a couple of hours, put it in the storage container, cover tightly, and refrigerate or freeze it. You may keep PPMs in the refrigerator for up to three days. You may reheat them *once*. After reheating once, steel yourself to throw the food away. It gets tired, and food

bacteria have a chance to grow every time you reheat it.

The key to freezing PPMs is finding convenient meal-sized containers that can be clearly labeled with contents and dates. Freezer zip top bags work well because they have panels you can write on. Leftover cottage cheese cartons can serve as well (as long as you don't microwave them), and so can glass jars. Plastic refrigerator cartons with lids work well, either the durable kind or the low-cost, lightweight kind that you buy in packages of five or more in the plastic bag section of the grocery store. You can wash either version in the dishwasher and use them again and again until they warp or crack. Be sure they are clean and dry before you store them, though, or bacteria will grow in the wet spots.

The microwave works great for thawing and heating PPMs. You can start out with the frozen meal, and thaw it and heat it up in minutes, so you don't have to worry about contamination and wearing the food out with handling. Be sure your container is glass or microwave-safe plastic, however. Other plastics can break down and leach chemicals into the food.

Children in the Kitchen

Your children will grow up enjoying cooking, and it will hold no terrors for them when they are grown if you let them share cooking chores with you. Many of the recipes in this book have suggestions for involving children. Children love being in the kitchen with you and working with food. Older children can be a big help.

When they are young, your task is to find chores for children that are safe and interesting and that don't slow you down too much. As children get older, they can become more and more helpful. A toddler can happily play in water in the sink, with mixing cups and spoons. A toddler can more-or-less wash durable vegetables, like potatoes, carrots, and celery. A pan of rice for measuring and pouring is good for a few minutes of entertainment.

Older children can assemble simple recipes, if you help with the hot dishes and sharp knives. I have written the recipes simply, but you might want to simplify them further for a child by making a note of which pan or bowls to use. For a child that does not read, adapt written directions by drawing pictures of the ingredients. To get an idea of how to do this, see Mollie Katzen's book *Pretend Soup and Other Real Recipes* or use some recipes from Katzen's book. Older children can do most of the tasks for simple recipes and you can be the assistant.

Of course, a child can always set the table. He might enjoy doing it, and it is helpful, but don't get in a rut. To keep cooking interesting to your child, you need to share out the cooking jobs. Even when your child becomes adept in the kitchen, don't wander off. For children, the main attraction with cooking is being with *you*. If you run out of jobs to do for tonight's dinner, start on the next day's meal. Read the suggestions for the night before and work ahead.

Make sure you have equipment that will make your child's participation in meal preparation safe and fun. Children need sturdy stools to stand on. I like the little two-step folding ladders that have the waist-high, over-arching handles because they give children something to hang on to. Children need aprons. Consider cutting the arms out of a big old shirt, then button it on backward. Or check out the hardware store for the little full-length carpenter aprons. If you tie a knot in the string that goes behind the neck, it converts easily to child size.

Children at the Table

With most of the recipes, and the menus accompanying them, I have made suggestions for adapting meals for children. Being considerate in the ways I suggest is not short-order cooking. It is just setting up mealtime to help your child to be successful. Generally, the adaptation is in the *menu*. If the dish seems a little strange, like **Mostaccioli with Spinach and Feta**, it will help your child to have something familiar on the table that he knows he can manage, like corn. Remember, your child doesn't have to eat everything that is served; he can pick and choose from what you have made available. If a dish is complex, like **Marinated Chicken Stir-Fry**, I suggest making some minor modifications to serve some of the parts separately. When a child masters the parts, he will be ready to start learning to like the whole.

For the learning eater at the table, we have to be careful about shape and texture of food and about detecting food sensitivities and allergies. A young child could choke on whole, raw vegetables, like carrots or celery, or some crisp-tender vegetables, like carrots again, or broccoli. You might cook a few vegetables a little longer for your youngest eater, or give him the more tender ones, like zucchini. Before you give the beginning eater a mixed dish, try to introduce him to all the components separately. That way if he has an allergic response, you won't have to guess about what caused the reaction.

Sometimes I suggest dessert, and sometimes I don't. You don't have to have dessert; you don't have to avoid it. I have used dessert to make a meal more enjoyable and filling and to make a nutritional contribution. The desserts I suggest all have fruit; many have milk as well. When serving dessert to young children, it works best to put a single helping of dessert at each plate and let them eat it when they want to—first, last, or during. Don't give seconds on dessert. That way, dessert doesn't get to be something special you hold out for a reward at the end of the meal. When children are older and have mastered more eating skills, you can go back to the traditional method of offering dessert at the end of the meal.

Cooking and Serving Equipment

In the recipes that follow, I suggest particular pan sizes and shapes and certain pieces of equipment. I have summarized those in the the box called "A Starter List of Utensils and Equipment" on page 160 and have included some suggestions for equipping your kitchen without breaking your budget.

Serving dishes and tableware can add to your meals without being expensive. They don't have to match. Consider following the lead of a number of fine restaurants and use a hodgepodge of unmatching dishes—tableware you pick up at garage sales, discount stores, and thrift shops. If you don't have matching sets, it's not so serious when something gets broken, which helps when there are children—and adults—in the house.

RECIPE LISTING

To help you with your planning and cooking, here are the recipes from these three chapters and the page numbers.

CHAPTER 5

Tuna Noodle Casserole	78
Macaroni-Tomato-Hamburger Casserole	80
Chicken and Rice	82
Broccoli Chowder	84
Spaghetti Carbonara (Yellow Spaghetti)	86
Swiss Steak	88
Beefy Shortcut Stroganoff	90
Mostaccioli with Spinach and Feta	91
Herb-Baked Fish	92
Meat Loaf	94
Spaghetti and Meatballs	96
Spinach-Feta Frittata	97
Lemon Chicken	98
Braised Pork Chops with Sweet Potatoes	99
Wisconsin Fish Boil	100
Hamburgers	101

CHAPTER 6

Chicken Soup	104
Ricotta Dumplings for Chicken Soup	105
Beef Ragout	106
Minestrone Soup	108
Savory Black Beans and Rice	110
Marinated Chicken Stir-Fry	112
Jambalaya	114
Fried Fish	116
The Generic Casserole	119

CHAPTER 7

Dressing up Vegetables to Get Flavor, Not Be Fancy

Herbed Butter	133
Super-Quick Cheese Sauce	133
Mustard Butter	133
Olive Oil with Garlic	133
Olive-Cream Cheese Spread	134

Vegetable Recipes from the Cycle Menu

Pumpkin Custard	134
Sweet-Sour Cucumber Salad	134
Poppyseed Coleslaw	135
Poppyseed Dressing	135
Scalloped Corn	135
Panned Cabbage and Carrots	135
Glazed Carrots	136
Gingered Broccoli	136
Spinach, Red Onion, and Orange Salad with Poppyseed Dressing	136
Go-Everywhere Green Salad	137
Tomato Slices with Vinaigrette	138
Mashed Potatoes	138
Creamed Spinach	139
Greens and Bacon	139
Stewed Tomatoes	139
Herbed Peas	140
Country Summer Squash	140
Corn Pudding	140
Oven-Fried Potatoes	141
Oven-Roasted Vegetables	141
Ratatouille	141

Fruit Recipes from the Cycle Menu

Plum Cobbler	142
Apple Custard	142
Peach Crisp	143
Old-Fashioned Bread Pudding	143
Fruit with Brown Cream Sauce	144
Pineapple Upside-Down Cake	144
Microwave Chunky Applesauce	144

Tuna Noodle Casserole

INGREDIENTS

1 lb dry packaged noodles (either wide or narrow)
7-oz can water-packed tuna
10-oz package frozen peas
10¹/₂-oz can cream of mushroom soup
¹/₂ cup milk

MENU

Tuna noodle casserole
Poppyseed coleslaw (page 135)
Celery sticks, dill pickles
Crusty bread for something to chew: try toasted
or plain bagels, English muffins, or French bread
Butter
Milk
Dessert, if you like it

METHOD

Summary: Boil noodles, mix them with tuna, canned soup, milk, and peas, and then gently heat.

Fill a 4 1/2-quart pan about half to two-thirds full of water, add 1 teaspoon of salt per quart of water, and bring to a rapid boil. Add *1 pound of dry packaged noodles* and boil until al dente (see the "Cooking Pasta" box on page 79).

Meanwhile, open a *7-ounce can of water-packed tuna*, drain it, and break the tuna into flakes with a fork. Mix with a *10 1/2-ounce can of cream of mushroom soup and 1/2 cup of milk.*

Then open a *10-ounce package of frozen peas* and empty it into a colander. When the noodles are done, drain them through the peas in the colander to thaw the peas and warm them up.

Combine everything: Put the noodles and peas into the noodle pan and add the tuna-soup-milk mixture.

Turn the heat on medium low and warm the whole thing up, stirring occasionally until everything is hot.

Serve to rave reviews.

RECIPE NOTES

Fast tip: Warm the mushroom soup up ahead of time to save stirring and reheating time and keep from breaking apart and overcooking the noodles.

Serve any kind of fresh, frozen, or canned fruit for dessert. Or you can serve the bread with cream cheese and some great jam and have that be dessert.

The night before: Review the recipes for the whole menu; find all the ingredients, menu items and equipment, and put them where they will be handy.

Added touch: Add any or all of the following vegetables or herbs:
 2–4 Tbsp dried onion flakes
 1–2 Tbsp dried parsley flakes
 1 4-oz can mushroom stems and pieces, drained
 1/4 cup chopped green or black olives

Presentation: Put the tuna-noodle mixture in an ovenproof casserole dish, sprinkle on some packaged bread crumbs and some grated cheese, heat at 350 degrees uncovered for 20 minutes. If you prefer to reheat in the microwave, use a microwave-safe dish, and sprinkle with the cheese of your choice (bread crumbs will just get soggy), cover and reheat for 4 to 5 minutes on high. Uncover and sprinkle on crushed potato chips. Voilà!

Involving your children: For this meal, a preschooler can cut up the dill pickles and olives with a plastic picnic knife; he can also open the peas and pour them into the colander.

If you help with draining the hot noodles, an older child will be able to make this all by himself!

Adapting this meal for children: This meal is kid-friendly. It is all right to serve tuna noodle casserole to children who are just getting started with table food, as long as they have been previously exposed to all of the ingredients. For them, cut the noodles quite finely, mix in enough sauce to make it moist, and let them eat with their fingers. Keep in mind that a finger food is anything that sticks together long enough to get it from dish to mouth. Even preschoolers and younger school-age children make use of this technique. Often they eat with their fork or spoon—but load it with their fingers. So relax. For a young child who might have trouble chewing the celery and dill pickles, open a can of mandarin oranges. Plain bread or toast would also be easier for a toddler to chew than the bagels.

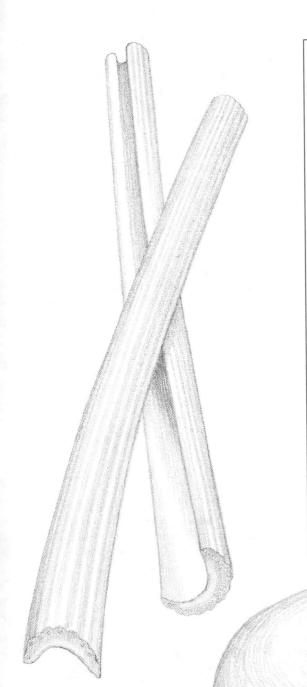

COOKING PASTA

For pasta that's well cooked and doesn't stick together, use plenty of water and keep it boiling rapidly the whole time the noodles cook. Fill a 4 1/2-quart pan half to two-thirds full of water to give room for the noodles and for the water to boil. Add 1 teaspoon of salt per quart of water to flavor the noodles. Bring to a hard, rolling boil. Add the noodles all at once, and stir to keep them from sticking together. *Watch the pot* until it boils again to keep it boiling but not boiling over. (Otherwise, it will overflow all over the stove, as mine has done many times.) Estimate the cooking time according to the package directions, but test for doneness 1 to 2 minutes before the package says to. Check by tasting. The noodles should be soft but give your teeth just a bit of resistance: that's what is meant by *al dente*. Les, a favorite baby-sitter, taught my children to test for doneness by throwing a strand or two against the wall. If it sticks, it's done. They loved it and thought of Les every time we had noodles. It may be apparent, though, why I haven't made Les's method my own.

OIL- OR WATER-PACKED TUNA

I chose water-packed tuna because that is about all I could find in my grocery stores. You may prefer oil-packed tuna, and that's fine if you can find it. Some people think it's more flavorful. Just drain the fat and throw it away. I prefer a little less flavor when I cook with tuna, so I generally run hot water through the tuna and then drain it when I'm using the oil-packed variety. Oil- and water-packed are equally nutritious.

Macaroni-Tomato-Hamburger Casserole

On the cycle menu, I have called this a *dinner of last resort*. It is the Friday night, don't-feel-like-cooking meal. We all need these meals: they are the fast and easy throw-together meals that you can practically prepare in your sleep. Keep the ingredients on hand for two or three of these last-resort meals, so you can grab and dump and have dinner. Tuna noodle casserole is a good last-resort meal because everything can be kept on the shelf. Other good last-resort meals are **Spaghetti Carbonara** and **Spinach-Feta frittata** (or any other kind of frittata). In chapter 6 I give other suggestions for quick throw-together meals.

INGREDIENTS
1 lb ground chuck
1 large onion
1/2 lb dry macaroni
28-oz can and 15-oz can diced tomatoes

MENU
Macaroni-tomato-hamburger casserole
Fruit, like apple wedges, banana chunks, canned
*   mandarin oranges, or fruit in season*
Chewy bread
Butter
Milk
Ice cream and store-bought cookies

METHOD
Summary: Boil noodles, brown ground beef and onion, and then mix it all up with toma-toes.

Fill a 4 1/2-quart pan about half to two-thirds full of water, add 1 teaspoon of salt per quart of water, and bring to a rapid boil. Add *1/2 pound of dry macaroni* and boil until al dente. Taste for doneness. Drain in a colander.

While the water for the macaroni heats, chop *1 large onion*. In a large skillet at medium heat, break up and brown *1 pound of ground beef* (a potato masher works well) and cook the chopped onion. There will be enough fat in the meat to grease the pan and cook the onion. Cook until the meat loses all its red or pink color and the onion is clear.

Combine everything: Put the macaroni back in its pan (or the frying pan, whichever is bigger), and add the cooked ground beef and onions. Add a *28-ounce can and a 15-ounce can*

of diced tomatoes (can sizes vary, so come as close as you can to this amount).

Cook the mixture over medium heat, stirring occasionally. Don't stir too energetically or you will break up the macaroni.

Serve to enthusiastic reviews.

RECIPE NOTES
Fast tip: Keep chopped onion on hand in a pint or quart jar in your refrigerator. Once chopped it lasts for a week or two and speeds up cooking time considerably. Some grocery stores carry frozen chopped onion, which tastes pretty good although not as good as fresh.To speed cooking and to save wear and tear on the macaroni, heat the tomatoes before you combine them with the beef and noodles.

The night before: Find the canned tomatoes and the cooking pan. Place the frozen ground beef in the refrigerator to thaw. Line up the other ingredients for this recipe and for the other menu items.

Presentation: For a more sophisticated pre-sentation, follow some of the suggestions I made for Tuna Noodle Casserole.

Refrigerate right after the meal. Have for lunch the next day, or freeze and have a few weeks later.

Involving your children: Children can open tomato cans and macaroni packages, and they can wash and cut up apples and bananas. If you can live with a little mangling, even a tod-dler can use a plastic picnic knife to cut up bananas and peeled apple wedges.

Adapting this meal for children: This meal is another good one for children. The casserole is moist, soft, and easy to chew. It is also slip-pery, so remember what qualifies as finger food. Again, beginning eaters may have this as long as they have been introduced separately to all of the ingredients.

Because **Macaroni-Tomato-Hamburger Casserole** has no added fat, it is a low-fat dish. Children need more fat. With this meal, you depend on butter on the bread, fat in the milk, and fat in the ice cream to give children the fat they need. Make these foods available to your children, and let them do the regulating. They will eat as much or as little fat as they need.

Variation: Use canned tomatoes with seasonings. Check out the tomato shelf in the grocery store. You will find Italian, Cajun, and Mexican tomatoes, tomatoes with onions and garlic, and others. Use a variety of macaroni and noodle shapes and sizes.

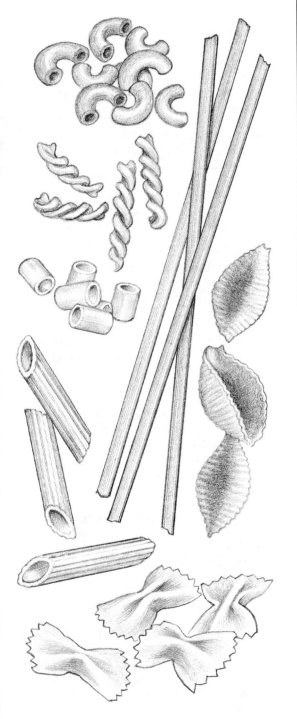

GROUND BEEF

Ground beef is out of favor these days. Well, it is and it isn't. Many people won't buy it in the grocery store because they think it isn't good for them. Then they end up at dinnertime with nothing to eat, so they scoot to the drive-through and get quarter-pounders with fries. It's crazy but understandable: if it is "bad" for you, you can eat it only when you don't think about it too much. So, *think* about it. In any case, you and your family can feel comfortable about eating ground beef. It is the key to many satisfying meals and is highly nutritious (see chapter 4, pages 56-60). Ground beef is easy for kids to eat; it cooks quickly and is easy to keep on hand. For the recipes in this book, I used ground chuck (often labeled "lean" ground beef). It is moderate in fat, but not so low that you miss out on flavor. Very little fat cooks out, so you may not even have to drain it.

Keeping ground beef on hand is easy. When you get home from the grocery store, separate it into 1-pound packages in 1-quart zipper-top bags, flatten the bags and freeze them. Flattened packages of beef thaw more quickly—but do be sure to thaw them in the refrigerator. To be tender, ground beef and other meats need to be cooked at moderate temperatures. Keeping the heat somewhere around medium also keeps fat from splattering all over your stove and wall and cuts down on cleanup. To me, "browning" ground beef means cooking until all the pink color is gone. To you, browning may mean actually cooking until it develops a brown color, which gives it more flavor but also dries it out more. If you like your ground beef really brown, you may want to cook your onions separately because they, too, will get brown and develop a pronounced caramelized flavor. On the other hand, you may like that. Who am I to say?

You don't have to be afraid of ground beef, but you do need to treat it respectfully. Ground beef is rarely contaminated with harmful bacterial, but when it is, the *E. coli 157* contamination is particularly nasty. Illness from *E. coli 157* can lead to kidney failure. Handle all ground beef as if it were contaminated. Don't let meat juices drip into raw produce, and wash your hands, utensils, and countertop with soap before and after you handle it. For more about food safety, see chapter 8, page 157.

Chicken and Rice

If you are home to put food in the oven and give it time to bake, there is no easier way to cook for a family than by making oven meals. Your food can be assembled before the just-before-mealtime jitters hit. A well-constructed oven meal does most of the last-minute work for you; you just take it out of the oven and put it on the table. You can clean up the kitchen early and know dinner is taken care of. You can also use the hot oven to prepare other foods, like warming French bread or baking a dessert.

For all those reasons, and because it *tastes* good and is filling and satisfying, chicken and rice was one of my standbys when my children were growing up. They have all, in turn, made it in their own kitchens.

INGREDIENTS

1 chicken, cut in pieces or
6 chicken breast halves, about 1 1/2 lb
1 1/2 cups uncooked enriched white rice
10-oz can cream of mushroom soup
1 1/2 cups water
1 packet dry onion soup mix
Parsley, dried or fresh

MENU

Chicken and rice
Glazed carrots or vegetables in season
French bread warmed in the oven
Butter
Milk
Apple custard (page 142) or fruit in season

METHOD

Summary: Combine uncooked rice, canned soup, dry soup mix, and water. Top with chicken, cover, and bake.
Preheat oven (see below for temperature). Mix together in a 9 x 13 glass baking dish *1 1/2 cups of uncooked enriched white rice, a 10-ounce can of cream of mushroom soup, 1 packet of dry onion soup mix,* and 1 1/2 cups of water. Sprinkle *dried or fresh parsley* over the top.

Lay *1 chicken, cut in pieces,* or *6 chicken breast halves (about 1 1/2 pounds),* over the top of the rice and soup mixture. Sprinkle on paprika and about *1/4 teaspoon of black pepper* to give a little color and flavor.

Cover the dish with aluminum foil and bake until the chicken is tender and the rice is done.

Baking time depends on the temperature: 2 hours at 300 degrees, 1 1/2 hour at 325 degrees, 1 hour at 350 degrees. To brown the chicken, remove the foil during the last 5 to 10 minutes of baking. Don't bake uncovered too long or the rice will dry out.

RECIPE NOTES

Fast tip: You can make use of the variation in cooking temperatures for your convenience in timing or to allow you to cook other foods at the same time. Cooking at 300 degrees will let you leave to run an errand. The higher temperature will let you finish baking your apple custard while you cook dinner. The French bread can be warmed at any of the temperatures, but you have to watch it more closely at the higher temperature.

The night before: Find the cooking pan and the rice. Place the frozen chicken in the refrigerator to thaw. Be sure that you put even a seemingly impervious zip top bag in another dish or pan to thaw the chicken so that if the bag leaks it won't get Salmonella all over your refrigerator and produce. Check the recipes for the other menu items and get those ingredients lined up as well.

Presentation: This is a pretty dish. Plan to put it right in the middle of the table and serve it from there. To make it easier for children to serve themselves, cut up some of the chicken breasts as you prepare this dish. They can scoop up just the right-sized piece of chicken and the rice to go with it. If you have a large, flat, oval baking dish, use it to dress up the presentation and make this recipe look festive and sophisticated. Put on a few sprigs of parsley for garnish.

Involving your children: Children can measure the uncooked rice, open the canned soup and dry soup mix, and combine them. Older children can learn about chicken sanitation and assemble the whole thing, chicken included, but an adult needs to be on hand to help ensure against cross-contamination. An adult also needs to put the dish into the oven and take it out again. That's hard for a child to do without getting burned.

A young child will be able to use a plastic picnic knife to chunk up cored apple pieces. The apple custard is a good recipe for an older child to make alone. You may have to help pour the mixture from the blender into the bowl, and you will need to put the dish in the oven and remove it when it's done.

Adapting this meal for children: Cut up the chicken finely and across the grain for young children, and mix it in with the rice. It should be quite moist, but if it is dry, add a little milk. Young children do better if some food is moist and soft. Dry, hard food seems to get stuck in their mouths.

Variation: This wonderfully convenient recipe is versatile, if you vary the liquid and spices. The trick is to keep the proportions of liquid to rice about 2 to 1. That is, it takes a cup of water to cook 1/2 cup of rice, so this recipe should have 3 cups of liquid for the 1 1/2 cups rice. For a modest variation, try golden mushroom soup instead of regular mushroom soup. Dry vegetable soup mix can also be substituted for the onion soup mix to give a change in color and flavor. Instead of soup, you can substitute chicken broth, cream or sour cream, or tomatoes. You may have other ideas. Topping each piece of chicken with a little pesto or stirring it in, adding in some Parmesan cheese—all of these possibilities will give both a chance to experiment and some variation in taste. When you have the time and want to make something a little more challenging (to eat as well as to make), you might consider trying the Jambalaya recipe in chapter 6 (pages 114-115). While the principle of cooking the rice and chicken together is the same, the variety of vegetables and seasonings makes it an altogether different dish.

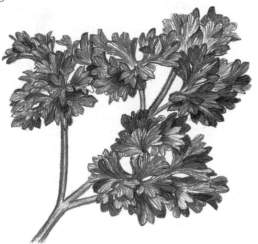

KEEPING CLEAN WHEN YOU COOK CHICKEN

Whenever I handle chicken, I have a flashback to learning sterile procedure during my dietetic-intern days. To go in the room with patients who had contagious diseases, we had to carefully gown up and put on a face mask and rubber gloves. Then, even if we didn't touch anything, we had to discard the whole works when we left. I think about it because you have to be about that careful when handling raw chicken.

Chicken won't hurt you if you handle and cook it right. However, do assume that chicken is contaminated with *Salmonella* bacteria. Unlike ground beef, which becomes contaminated only if something goes wrong in the meatpacking plant, most chicken is contaminated with *Salmonella*. It's not a big problem if you handle it right, but if you don't, it can be dangerous. Illness from *Salmonella* is unpleasant for anyone, but it's especially serious for children because the nausea, diarrhea, and fever can be dangerously dehydrating for them. Be careful not to let chicken touch or drip on food that you won't be cooking and anything you can't wash in hot, soapy water right after you finish. Rinse the chicken under cold water to start with, and consider everything that touches the raw chicken to be contaminated: your hands, the colander for rinsing the chicken, the knife and cutting board, the countertop, the sink, and the fork for turning it in the frying pan. As soon as you finish handling the raw chicken, wash all your utensils, countertop, and sink with hot, soapy water.

Do not touch *anything* before you wash your chickeny hands. *Your hands are contaminated, so keep your mind on what you are doing.* According to urban rumor, this point was made beautifully by a recent television news program. Raw chicken was coated with a substance that showed up only under ultraviolet light. A young mother was asked to get it ready for cooking. She got out her knife and cutting board and unwrapped the chicken. Then she got the shortening out of the refrigerator and the pan out of the cabinet. She washed off the chicken, and then got out the colander to drain it. Then her son came in and wanted a drink of water, so she got out a glass and filled it for him. Then she finished cutting up the chicken and started frying it. When the area was flooded with ultraviolet light, the knife, cutting board, and sink glowed purple. But, to the mother's horror, so did the drawer, cabinet, cupboard, the outside and inside of the refrigerator, the cold-water tap, the glass, and *her son's hands and mouth.* For more about food safety, see chapter 8, "Planning to Get You Cooking."

Broccoli Chowder

Here is another canned soup recipe that is easy and very good. I suggested the frozen bread with it to remind you of its availability. The dessert is more elaborate than usual because the chowder is a little sparse, as main dishes go. The peach cobbler will help you and your diners to fill up and feel satisfied. You can bake the dessert at the same time as the bread.

INGREDIENTS
4 slices bacon
1/2 onion, minced
10-oz package good-quality frozen chopped broccoli
10-oz can condensed cream of potato soup
2 cups milk
1/4 tsp salt
1/2 cup shredded Swiss cheese or cheese
  of your choice

MENU
Broccoli chowder
"Homemade" bread from frozen bread dough
Butter
Peanut butter, jam
Fruit in season
Milk
Peach cobbler (page 142) or crisp (page 143)
Ice cream

METHOD
Summary: Brown the onion and cook the frozen broccoli; combine with milk and canned soup, and then purée in batches in a blender. Heat and stir in cheese.

Cut *4 slices of bacon* into 1/4-inch pieces and cook until lightly browned. Remove the bacon and sauté *1/2 onion, minced*, in the drippings until golden.

While you sauté the onion, cook a *10-ounce package of good-quality frozen chopped broccoli* in 1/2 cup of water until just crisp-tender. Don't drain.

Combine the sautéed onion and cooked, undrained broccoli with a *10-ounce can of condensed cream of potato soup, 2 cups of milk,* and *1/4 teaspoon of salt.* While still cool, purée in the blender in batches. Return the puréed soup to the pan and heat thoroughly.

Just before serving, stir in *1/2 cup of shredded Swiss cheese* or cheese of your choice.

RECIPE NOTES
The night before: Find the canned soup and the cheese, and put the frozen broccoli in the refrigerator to thaw. For the rest of the menu, read the directions on the frozen bread dough and do what it says. Find the dessert ingredients; prepare the topping for peach crisp if that's what you plan to have for dessert.

Involving your children: Children can open the broccoli; they can also open the cream of potato soup and pour it into the pan. Then they can measure the milk into the pan. Together you can do the blending. Your young child may want to push the buttons on the blender while you do the pouring.

The bread dough is a great find for children. You can put the dough in a loaf pan and bake it as is. Or you can let your child pinch off pieces, dip them in melted butter, and put them in muffin cups to rise and bake.

An older child can make the peach dessert.

Adapting this meal for children: This meal is surprisingly easy for children to eat if you let the soup cool a bit and put it in a cup or bowl with handles so they can pick it up and drink it.

Variation: Add a cup of cooked rice after blending the soup. Substitute 2 *tablespoons of precooked real bacon bits* (which come in a can) and *1 tablespoon of butter,* or skip the bacon and use *2 tablespoons of butter.*

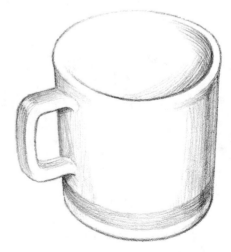

BACON

Most anyone who eats meat likes luscious bacon—and feels guilty about eating it. Bacon is one of those much-picked-on foods that have been subjected to a variety of unkind rumors over the years. Allow me to dispel those rumors. First of all, the fat: Bacon does have a lot of fat in it, and it certainly counts as your high-fat food when you have it on the menu. However, in this recipe, the bacon fat is thoroughly diluted by the soup, so the fat per serving is low. The highly flavorful bacon and bacon fat adds interest, the reason for using it.

Second, what about heart disease? The fat in bacon is the same as in (shudder, gasp) lard, a thoroughly defiled grease if there ever was one. But wait! Let us regard—*lard!* Lard is actually 15 percent polyunsaturated fat and 40 percent monounsaturated fat, so even the dietary enthusiasts must still their tongues about condemning lard. Not only that, but 30 percent of the remaining fat in lard is stearic acid, proven to neither raise nor lower blood cholesterol.

Third, what about nitrate and nitrite? There is lingering worry about bacon and other processed meats like hot dogs, luncheon meats, and sausage because they contain nitrate and sodium nitrite. (Nitrates and nitrates are chemically a little different, but nutritionally they are interchangeable.) A couple of decades ago a nitrates-and-cancer scare erupted. Frying bacon at high temperatures can convert nitrates to nitrosamine, which may contribute to cancer when you eat a lot of it. (Notice I say "may." There is epidemiological evidence of association but no clinical proof.) However, by way of being cautious without being self-sacrificing, it is better not to save bacon grease and use it for frying. If you still worry about cured meats, use it in modest amounts as we do in the recipe or eat it infrequently or both.

Sodium nitrate used in processed foods retains color and prevents spoilage. Consumers nowadays are leery of such preservatives, feeling they don't want to eat either aging food or chemicals. Not to worry. Check the "sell-by" date. Sodium nitrate is a good chemical. It retards the growth of bacteria which produce the deadly *Clostridium botulinum toxin*, a guaranteed hazard.

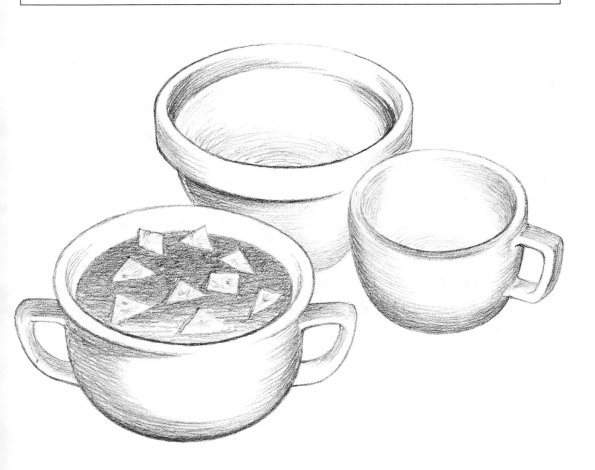

Spaghetti Carbonara (Yellow Spaghetti)

I asked each of my children, in turn, what food they remembered from their growing-up years. Each responded, "yellow spaghetti." It was my dinner of last resort, so it showed up on the menu every couple of weeks. This unlikely seeming dish has an equally unlikely name. Carbonara means "in the manner of a charcoal maker." I have served it to many people, most of them children, and have yet to be turned down. One young guest who disliked eggs was highly skeptical, but with reassurance from my children that it was good and from me that he didn't have to eat it if he didn't like it, he tasted. He liked it.

INGREDIENTS
1 lb fettucini or other spaghetti
1/2 lb bacon
6 eggs
1 cup grated Parmesan cheese (packaged or fresh)

MENU
Spaghetti carbonara
Additional grated Parmesan or Asiago cheese
Mixed vegetables
Green salad
Fruit salad
Toasted bagels
Milk

METHOD
Summary: Toss hot, drained, cooked pasta with hot, browned bacon. Add beaten eggs and cheese. The heat of the pasta/bacon mixture cooks the eggs.

Fill a 4 1/2-quart pan about half to two-thirds full of water, add 1 teaspoon of salt per quart of water, and bring to a rapid boil. Boil *1 pound of fettucini or other spaghetti* until it's al dente. Drain, shake the colander to remove the excess water, return the pasta immediately to the sauce pan, and place it back on the burner set at the lowest heat.

While the water heats, cut *1/2 pound of bacon* into 1/2-inch strips. Fry until lightly browned, separating strips as you cook. Pour off all but 2 tablespoons of bacon grease. Put the bacon back in the pan with the grease and hold over low heat.

While the bacon cooks, bring *6 eggs* to room temperature by letting them stand for 5 min-utes in your hottest tap water. (Be sure the eggs are not cracked. If they are, throw them away.) Beat the eggs with *1 cup of grated Parmesan or Asiago cheese (packaged or fresh).* (Asiago is a hard, zesty, nutty-tasting cheese.)

Timing is important here. Try to get the bacon and spaghetti cooked at the same time so they are both hot enough to cook the eggs. Because you need to put the eggs in while the spaghetti and bacon are as hot as possible, have the egg mixture ready by the time you finish cooking the bacon and spaghetti.

Assemble the dish by pouring the hot bacon and bacon fat into the cooked spaghetti. Toss to distribute evenly. Add the egg and cheese mixture, stirring and tossing the spaghetti to combine it evenly with the spaghetti-bacon mixture.

In the finished product, the egg needs to be semisolid, as in a very soft scrambled egg. It should be thick enough to cling to the spaghetti and not pool in the bottom of the pan, but not be so cooked that it turns into chunks of egg. To cook egg that is still runny, heat the pan gently to thicken it, stirring as you heat.

RECIPE NOTES
The night before: The cycle menu in chapter 8 lists **Yellow Spaghetti** for a Friday clean-out-the-refrigerator meal. The main dish is fresh, but for the other menu items, I suggest Friday as the day to do the archeological dig of the refrigerator. You may find the bits of vegetables that can be combined to make a satisfactory hot vegetable dish, or you might be able to marinate leftover vegetables in salad dressing to include in the salad. Bits of cheese can go in the salad or on the vegetables. You may have enough odds and ends of fruit to make a fruit salad, or you might have enough for **Fruit with Brown Cream Sauce** (page 144). On the other hand, if what you find in your refrigerator is not appealing, throw it away. There is nothing to be gained by traumatizing yourself and other people in the name of economy. I know a grown man who still turns green when he remembers the leftover French fries that showed up in his mother's casserole.

Presentation: Save a little crumbled bacon to sprinkle over the top of the dish.

Involving your children: Children love to crack eggs. It is especially fun to crack them by tapping them together. Surprisingly, cracking eggs together or on a flat surface makes it easier to avoid getting shell in the bowl. The Australians, who reportedly bet on anything, bet on which egg will crack first. A child could have fun predicting which egg will be the first to go. Have children crack each egg separately into a small bowl so it is easier to fish eggshell back out again and you can discard any egg that doesn't look just right. Use a clean utensil to scoop up stray bits of shell.

Adapting this meal for children: Spaghetti is only hard to eat if you are concerned about social niceties. In a child's mind, spaghetti is a finger food, so get ready. Children love to suck up strands of spaghetti, and that's fine, if you can stand it. They also love to watch you twirl spaghetti around your fork and will try to imitate you. However, they will revert to using their hands. This spaghetti sticks together, so it is somewhat easier to eat than **Spaghetti with Meatballs** (page 96). It is very tasty and can become a favorite with everyone who has been introduced to all the parts. Generally, it is best to keep the baby off egg whites and wheat until he is about 9 months old.

Variation: Instead of the bacon, you can use 3 tablespoons of butter or olive oil in this recipe. But before you reject the bacon, read the "Bacon" box on page 85. You can also use this recipe to make a version of spaghetti Alfredo that is higher in protein by virtue of substituting eggs for the cream. Save out part of the fat to sauté a variety of vegetables and then put them in with the egg/spaghetti mixture.

EGGS

Yellow spaghetti raises the issue egg safety, both from the point of view of cholesterol content and *Salmonella* contamination. About cholesterol, as I said in chapter 4, because the cholesterol in food has a minimal impact on blood cholesterol, and because eggs are so convenient and nutritious when you are cooking for a family, I recommend that you eat eggs.

I carefully researched the safety of the raw eggs in this recipe, because *Salmonella* finds its way into the yolk of about 1 in 10,000 eggs before laying. I checked with the American Egg Board and with food scientists and satisfied myself that, if you do it right, the recipe will be safe. However, you must follow the directions carefully: use only eggs with no cracks in them, put uncracked eggs in hot water for 5 minutes to bring them to room temperature before you crack them (but don't let them stand around for long at room temperature), time combining the egg mixture and spaghetti so the spaghetti is as hot as it can be, and do a final heating until the eggs are at the soft-scramble stage before you serve the dish to your family. The final heating gets the mixture up to 160 degrees or more and kills any of the few *Salmonella* germs that may be lurking around.

Whole egg soft-scrambles at about 160 degrees, the instant-kill temperature for *Salmonella*. In this recipe, the eggs are diluted with cheese, which lets them get to above 160 degrees and still be soft-scrambled. For your general information, eggs that are cooked until the white coagulates and the yolk begins to coagulate are cooked to a safe temperature.

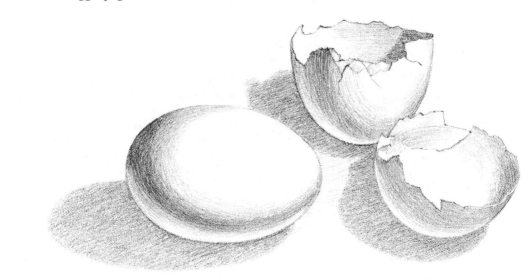

Swiss Steak

This is a good recipe for a company dinner. It looks pretty, it's easy to serve, and it can be prepared for baking ahead of time. I have also used it as a way of introducing you to clear oven cooking bags. These cooking bags are great for preparing pieces of meat and roasts. The food in the bags browns but stays moist. The recipes on the package say to set the oven temperature at 350 degrees. That works great for poultry and fish, which are tender and cook fast. However, for the tougher beef cuts, like the round steak in this recipe, I find a lower temperature allows the longer cooking time necessary to make the meat tender.

INGREDIENTS
2 lb round steak, cut in helping-sized pieces
28-oz can seasoned tomatoes
1 packet dry onion soup mix
1 small clear oven cooking bag

MENU
Swiss steak
Mashed potatoes (page 138)
Steak cooking liquid for gravy
Gingered broccoli (page 136)
Oven-browned rolls
Butter
Milk
Apple custard or another baked dessert

METHOD
Summary: Combine round steak, canned tomatoes, and dry soup mix in an oven bag and bake.

Preheat the oven to 300 degrees.

Follow the directions on a cooking bag package (except reduce the heat to 300 degrees). Usually the instructions tell you to put flour in the bag. Put the bag in a cake or jelly roll pan (10 x 15 1/2 x 1-inch pan). Place *2 pounds of round steak, cut in helping-sized pieces, a 28-ounce can of seasoned tomatoes*, and *1 packet of dry onion soup mix* in the bottom of the bag.

Close the cooking bag and cut (or don't cut) steam vents according to the package directions. Bake for 1 hour.

Remove the pan from the oven. For safety, let stand for 15 minutes before you open the bag.

RECIPE NOTES
Fast tip: This is a great way to cook and tenderize beef for other recipes. You can cut this beef into cubes, refrigerate or freeze it, and use it later in your **Beefy Shortcut Stroganoff** (page 90) or in **Minestrone Soup** (pages 108-109). You can even freeze it as is and have it weeks later as the same meal all over again.

The night before: Place the frozen steak in the refrigerator to thaw. Find the cooking bag. Line up the other ingredients. Wash the broccoli and apples, and find the rest of the ingredients for the apple custard.

Added touch: Before baking, top the steak-tomato mound with sliced mushrooms or green pepper rings.

Presentation: This looks great served straight from the cooking bag. Transfer the cooking bag to a platter, peel back or cut away the edges, and serve from the platter. Because the food is very hot, you may have to help your child get his serving, or you may be able to scooch the platter around the table. Since the steak is cut into helping-sized pieces, he can then serve himself.

Involving your children: I am a little wary of letting young children handle meat because they have a hard time remembering to wash their hands before they touch anything else. When your child can remember, he can make this whole recipe. Until then, a child can open the can of tomatoes and pour it over the beef and sprinkle the onion soup on top. He can help wash the potatoes and even mash them. He can break the broccoli into florets if you cut the stems to the length you want.

Adapting this meal for children: This meal works well for children because the meat is so tender and moist that even beginning eaters can manage it. Just cut the meat pieces across the grain to shorten the fibers. Let your child eat the broccoli with his fingers. You may find yourself doing the same!

Variations: You can add potatoes and carrots to the cooking bag and have a one-dish meal. In fact, now that you have the braised, one-dish meat idea, you can stray even further from this recipe and make that traditional favorite, pot roast. "Tough" cuts of meat, like round, sirloin, and chuck, tenderize beautifully when baked at 325 degrees for 2 to 3 hours in a covered Dutch oven, clear cooking bag (reduce the temperature to 300 degrees), or in a slow cooker for about double that time. For the braising liquid, add broth, tomato juice, beer, wine, or concentrated soup. Or add vegetables, and let them provide the liquid. You could use potatoes, carrots, onions, cabbage, or any other vegetable you fancy. Salt and pepper the vegetables as you add them. If the roast weighs 3 pounds or less, the meat and vegetables will get nicely done at about the same time. If the roast weighs considerably more than 3 pounds, you might want to give it about an hour head start before you add the vegetables. After everything is cooked, make gravy with the pan drippings using the method described in the recipe for **Hamburgers** on page 101. For an "automatic" gravy, use golden mushroom soup for the cooking liquid. For a thick gravy, use undiluted. For a thinner gravy, dilute.

COOKING BEEF TO MAKE IT TENDER

Round steak is inexpensive, nutritious, convenient, and low in fat. It is also *tough*. Like other low-fat beef (see the box "Fat in Meat" on page 170), stew meat has to be specially prepared to make it tender and enjoyable to eat. For **Swiss steak**, we braise it: we put it in a small amount of liquid and cook it for a long time at a low temperature. We could also stew it, like we do for **Beef Ragout** (pages 106-107): put it in a large amount of liquid and cook it for a long time. (Do you begin to get the principle?) It helps even more if the liquid has acid in it, like tomato juice or vinegar, because the acid breaks down the connective tissue in the meat.

For the pot roast described in the variations, the method is also braising. Crock-Pot cooking is the ultimate in braising, featuring as it does very low temperatures and very long cooking times. A pot roast in the slow cooker is a set-it-and-forget-it recipe that will let you run lots of errands while dinner takes care of itself. Since the fad for slow cooker has passed, you may not get one for a gift, but you can probably find one at a garage sale. Even new, they are inexpensive. My favorite slow cooker is the oblong one, with a separate base and roughly 5-inch-deep metal pan that fits on the base. Food cooks evenly, and the cooking pan is easy to clean and refrigerate. It doubles as a keep-warm server.

Another strategy for cooking low-fat beef is to tenderize the meat ahead of time. Presumably, you could marinate it: soak it overnight (in the refrigerator) in a liquid that has acid and seasonings. While marinades taste good, I don't find them too helpful for tenderizing. If you want to grill or broil steak, you might have to buy a cut that has more fat in it. You could also use a low-fat cut and treat it with prepared meat tenderizer. Meat tenderizers contain *papain*, an enzyme extracted from papayas that breaks down the connective tissue. Also look for packets of preseasoned tenderizer-marinade, which adds flavor as well as tenderizes. Follow the package directions to treat the meat before grilling or broiling.

Beefy Shortcut Stroganoff

This is essentially a PPM using the **Swiss Steak** from the previous recipe. In the cycle menu, the **Swiss Steak** is on for Sunday and the **Beefy Shortcut Stroganoff** is on for Tuesday. If you use the beef that quickly, you can refrigerate it. If you keep it longer, freeze it.

INGREDIENTS
2 cups leftover Swiss steak, chunked
Leftover tomatoes and sauce from Swiss steak
1/2 cup sour cream or low-fat sour cream

MENU
Beefy shortcut stroganoff
Noodles or mashed potatoes (page 138)
Green salad
Fruit in season
Bread and butter
Milk
Ice cream; store-bought cookies

METHOD
Summary: Heat leftover cubed meat and tomatoes, add sour cream, and serve over boiled noodles or mashed potatoes.

Gently heat together *2 cups of leftover Swiss steak, chunked*, and the *leftover tomatoes and sauce from Swiss steak*. Stir in *1/2 cup of sour cream or low-fat sour cream*. Add more tomatoes or tomato juice to get the consistency you want.

Serve over hot cooked noodles or mashed potatoes.

RECIPE NOTES
Added touch: Add fresh or canned mushrooms.

The night before: Locate the beef cubes; if they are frozen, put them in the refrigerator to thaw. Locate the sour cream and the other ingredients. Wash the salad greens and put them in a tight container to crisp (see page 137). Check out your fresh fruit supply. If you can't find any, check your supply of canned fruit.

Involving your children: A child can mix the ingredients for the main dish. He can also spin the greens for the salad, tear them up, and put them in the bowl.

Adapting this meal for children: This meal has a number of dishes, so your child is likely to find something on the table that he finds appealing. Don't feel he has to eat the stroganoff—noodles or mashed potatoes with butter are just fine.

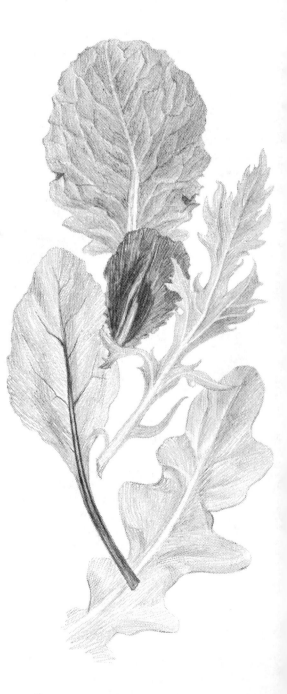

Mostaccioli with Spinach and Feta

Now we are getting fancy! This strange-sounding recipe is surprisingly appealing and popular with most people, even those who don't usually like feta cheese. Feta has a strong flavor and a distinctive, crumbly texture. It is becoming so common that you can buy it most places. Until your diners develop a taste for feta cheese, the secret seems to be in crumbling it finely—into pieces about half the size of peas. That way, the taste isn't too concentrated in any one bite. This recipe does wonderful things for spinach and lets you serve your vegetables, starch, and protein all at one time.

INGREDIENTS

10-oz package frozen chopped spinach
8 oz mostaccioli or penne pasta
3 medium raw tomatoes or 6 Roma tomatoes
6–10 green onions: bulbs and most of the tops
2 Tbsp olive oil
8-oz package mild feta cheese, finely crumbled

MENU

Mostaccioli with spinach and feta
Scalloped corn (page 135)
Toasted English muffins
Milk
Plum cobbler (page 142) or crisp (page 143) or fruit in season

METHOD

Summary: Drain thawed frozen spinach and combine with al dente pasta, raw tomatoes, and onion. Crumble in feta cheese and gently heat.

Fill a 4 1/2-quart pan about half to two-thirds full of water, add 1 teaspoon of salt per quart of water, and bring to a rapid boil. Cook *8 ounces of mostaccioli or penne pasta* until al dente.

While the pasta cooks, pour a thawed *10-ounce package of frozen chopped spinach* into a colander and squeeze out the excess liquid. Drain the cooked pasta through the spinach in the colander.

While the pasta cooks, chop *3 medium tomatoes or 6 Roma tomatoes. Chop 6 to 10 green onion (bulbs and most of the tops).*

Put the pasta and spinach back in the pan and add *2 tablespoons of olive oil*.

Combine the tomatoes and onions into the pan with the pasta and spinach and add an *8-ounce package of mild feta cheese, finely crumbled*.

Mix and warm it gently in your original cooking pan or in a glass dish in the microwave.

RECIPE NOTES

Fast tip: Have tomatoes at room temperature to speed the final heating. In general, unless they are getting too ripe, store tomatoes on the counter. Room-temperature tomatoes preserve their flavor better than refrigerated ones. A critical flavor component of tomatoes disappears when they are chilled.

The night before: Take the spinach out of the freezer and refrigerate to thaw. Be sure tomatoes are on the counter instead of in the refrigerator. Clean and wash the green onions and other vegetables. Find the corn and crackers for the scalloped corn. Make the crisp mix or find your stored jar of it in the refrigerator.

Presentation: The mostaccioli is very pretty. It looks great in a clear or white bowl.

Involving your children: Children can open the package of spinach and put it in the colander. They can toast the muffins and cut up the plums and put them in the baking pan. If you have crisp topping on hand, they can sprinkle that over the top. They can open the corn, put it in the pan, and crunch in the soda crackers.

Adapting this meal for children: As with other one-dish meals, this is a sink-or-swim meal, so be sure to give additional options. My menu is rather odd because scalloped corn doesn't really "go," but it is delicious, easy to like, and filling. The English muffin should be pretty neutral, and the dessert is filling and nutritious while it gives a serving from the fruit list.

Variation: Instead of spinach, add a variety of sautéed vegetables, like bits of carrot, broccoli, zucchini, mushrooms, green or red peppers.

Herb-Baked Fish

This basting sauce contains ginger, reportedly helpful in toning down or taking away the fishy taste of fish. Actually, if fish is fresh, it shouldn't have a strong fishy taste or odor. It should, presumably, smell like a "fresh sea breeze," and, I suppose, taste as light and delicate as that breeze smells. But for some of us even a fresh sea breeze tastes like fish, and ginger will lighten up that flavor. The menu for this meal specifies scalloped potatoes or corn pudding, both of which have fat in them. The fat in the high-carbohydrate side dish helps to balance out the relative dryness of the fish. However, even with that addition, this will be a relatively low-fat, low-calorie meal, so the **Pineapple Upside-Down Cake** helps to make this a filling and satisfying meal.

INGREDIENTS

*2 lb low-fat white fish: cod, halibut, whitefish,
    turbo, pollack, or your preference*
2 Tbsp butter or olive oil
1/2 tsp salt
1/4 tsp pepper
1/4 tsp dried thyme
1/4 tsp dried oregano
1/4 tsp ground ginger or 2 tsp fresh grated ginger
1/4 tsp onion powder
1/4 tsp garlic powder

MENU

Herb-baked fish
*Boxed scalloped potatoes prepared in oven or
microwave or*
Corn pudding (page 140)
Green salad
Whole wheat bread or toast
Butter
Milk
Fruit in season
Pineapple upside-down cake (page 144)

METHOD

Summary: Combine herbs and butter and brush the herbed butter on the fish before and during baking.

Preheat oven to 325 degrees.

Combine *2 tablespoons of softened butter or olive oil, 1/2 teaspoon of salt, 1/4 teaspoon of pepper, 1/4 teaspoon of thyme, 1/4 teaspoon of oregano, 1/4 teaspoon of ground ginger or fresh grated ginger, 1/4 teaspoon of onion powder,* and *1/4 tea-*

spoon of garlic powder to make an herb basting sauce.

Thaw *2 pounds of fish: cod, halibut, whitefish, turbo, pollack,* or *your preference,* and wash in cold water. Put the fish on a rack over a pan to catch the juices (a cooling rack over a jelly roll pan will do). Brush fish with herb sauce.

Bake for 10 to 20 minutes, brushing with herb sauce once or twice during baking.

The fish is done when it turns white and flakes easily with a fork. If you want more precise cooking times, begin with the "10-minute rule." Measure the fish at its thickest point and cook 10 minutes per inch. That is, cook a 1-inch thick piece of fish 5 minutes on each side. Double the cooking time for frozen fish that has not been defrosted. However, don't follow the 10-minute rule slavishly or the fish could get dried out. You'll learn with practice when to stop cooking.

RECIPE NOTES

Fast tip: Mix a bigger batch of the seasoning mixture and store what you don't use for the next time you make this recipe. Measure out 1 1/2 teaspoons of the mixture instead of the individual ingredients. Use 1 1/2 teaspoons of the same seasoning mixture (combined with 1/2 cup of flour) to make **Fried Fish** (pages 116-117). Since the measurement of each ingredient is the same, 1/4 teaspoon, you can make a bigger batch by using 1 or even 2 teaspoons of each ingredient.

The night before: Prepare the herb mixture. Put the frozen fish in the refrigerator to thaw. Find the scalloped potatoes or corn pudding ingredients. Find the canned pineapple.

Added touch: To serve, lay thin lemon slices on the top of the fish.

Presentation: If you would rather use a more plain carbohydrate side dish, like rice or boiled potatoes, you can make your fat source in this menu tartar sauce or a creamed vegetable dish, like creamed peas or spinach or broccoli with cheese sauce. You can also make more of the herbed butter sauce and put it on the table for family members to use on their fish and vegetables.

Involving your children: Children can tear lettuce for the salad and grate the cheese. They can also use a pastry brush to put the first layer of basting sauce on the fish. After that, the fish will be in a hot oven, so it is a job better left to a grown-up. A child will enjoy laying out the rings of pineapple and decorating with maraschino cherries for the upside-down cake. The batter for the cake is so easy that an older child could mix it up.

Adapting this meal for children: If you buy boneless fish, this is a fine meal for children. Dress the salad lightly so your child can pick it up with his fingers.

Variation: This fish tastes great cooked on the grill. Baste it as it grills, the same as you would in the oven. To make heating up the grill worthwhile, grill corn on the cob or skewer tomatoes and peppers and grill them at the same time.

You can also poach fish (simmer it in water) using the same seasonings plus a little lemon juice and lemon zest (grated lemon peel). An acid, such as lemon juice or vinegar, added to the poaching liquid keeps the flesh firmer and whiter. The 10-minute rule applies for cooking times (10 minutes per inch of thickness).

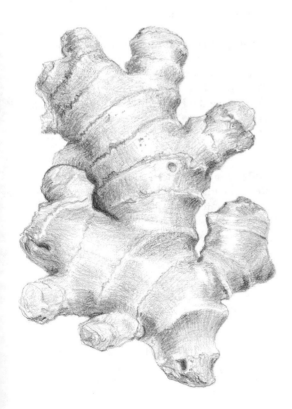

FISH

When you prepare fish, use the same clean technique that you use with chicken or other meat. Wash your hands and all utensils after you handle fish, and be careful not to touch fish and then touch anything else that you can't immediately wash in hot, soapy water. Thaw frozen fish in the refrigerator to reduce moisture loss and prevent spoilage; then rinse with cold water and dry with paper towels before you prepare it.

When you purchase fish, know what you are getting. Frozen fish is perfectly acceptable if it has an appropriate freshness date, no freezer burn, and an undamaged package (for purchasing tips, see chapter 9, "Shopping to Get You Cooking," page 170). While the word *fresh* implies that fish has not been frozen, some seemingly fresh fish in some markets is defrosted frozen fish. If you cook the fish right away, it is simply a truth in marketing issue. But if you take it home and refreeze it, both the quality and the safety will be compromised. Ask whether your "fresh" fish has been frozen and thawed, or read the fine print on the package.

Fish that is truly fresh has never been frozen. Because fish so rapidly develops off flavors and odors, fresh fish must be kept clean and cold and moved rapidly from catch to market to table. For fish that is really fresh, deal with a reputable fish market that is expert about moving fish quickly and cleanly, and cook it the day you buy it. The staff in a dedicated fish store will be able to give you advice on what to buy and how to cook it.

You can purchase fish as fillets, as steaks, or as whole fishes. Fish fillets are most common. They are sides of flesh cut from the backbone and ribs, with the skin on or off. Your supermarket frozen fish case probably includes perch, cod, and pollack fillets, lean fish with a mild flavor and white or light color flesh. Salmon, swordfish, tuna, and other large fish may be sold as fillets or as steaks, cut 1/4 to 1 1/2 inches thick. The oil and muscle development in the flesh of these moderate-fat fishes gives them a more pronounced flavor and a firm, meaty texture.

Most challenging of all—to cook and to eat—are the whole fish. If you do any fishing yourself, you know all about it. You should also know which fish taken from which waters are free from industrial contaminants and are therefore safe to eat. If you don't know, check your fishing license. The rest of us can have our whole fish by purchasing whole rainbow trout.

What about bones? All cuts of fish may or may not be boneless, depending on whether the pinbones have been removed. Your fish shop will be able to tell you. For supermarket fish you will have to look and feel. Take the bones out of your child's portion, and be careful when you eat your own. The people in a fish shop can teach you about boning fish.

Meat Loaf

Consumer research tells us that we are looking for comfort food: meat loaf, chicken soup, dumplings, mashed potatoes. Your idea of comfort food may be lots different from mine, because comfort food is good-tasting, familiar food with positive memories associated with it. Your feel-good food might be hoppin' John (rice and black-eyed peas), wonton soup, refried beans, or Twinkies.

Here is my favorite meat loaf recipe, perfected over decades. You may have one in your family as well. If you want to start a conversation with an experienced cook, ask for a meat loaf recipe!

INGREDIENTS

1 1/3 cups dried stuffing mix
1/4 cup dried onion flakes or
　　1/2 cup finely chopped onion
1 3/4 cup milk
2 lb ground chuck
1 egg
4 tsp Worcestershire sauce
1 1/2 tsp salt
1/8 tsp dried sage
1/4 tsp dry mustard
1/4 tsp black pepper

MENU

Meat loaf
Scalloped potatoes
Carrot and celery sticks
Herbed peas (pp)
Bread or toast
Butter
Milk
Bread pudding with raisins (page 143) or
Fruit in season

METHOD

Summary: Soak dried stuffing mix in milk, add ground chuck and seasonings, shape into a loaf, and bake.

In a large mixing bowl, combine *1 1/3 cups of dried stuffing mix, 1/4 cup of dried onion flakes or 1/2 cup of finely chopped onion,* and *1 3/4 cups of milk.* Soak 10 minutes.

Add all at once: *2 pounds of ground chuck, 1 beaten egg, 4 teaspoons of Worcestershire sauce, 1 1/2 teaspoon of salt, 1/8 teaspoon of dried sage, 1/4 teaspoon of dry mustard, 1/4 teaspoon of black pepper.* Mix with a spoon or with your hands.

Reserve half the recipe for meatballs or Salisbury steaks. Pack the remaining mixture into an 8 1/2-inch bread pan or mold into an oblong shape and place it on a jelly roll pan. (The bread pan gives a moister, softer meat loaf. The free-form meatloaf is firmer and has more browned crust.)

Bake at 325 degrees for 30 minutes. Use a meat thermometer and remove the meat loaf from the oven when it reaches an internal temperature of 160 degrees (if you use ground poultry, cook it to 165 degrees). If you take it out promptly when it's done, it will be juicy. If you cook it too long, all the good juices will cook out and it will be swimming in juice. Let it stand for 15 minutes to set before you serve it.

RECIPE NOTES

Fast tip: Using a #30 ice cream scoop, portion balls of the remaining meat loaf mixture onto a jelly roll pan. Refrigerate until the rest of the dinner is done. Then bake the meat balls at 325 degrees until they are done, about 20 minutes. Let cool, freeze on waxed paper on a jelly roll pan so meatballs can be separated easily, and then store in a zip top bag in the freezer. Use these ready-to-eat meatballs for **Spaghetti and Meatballs** (page 96), or take out and warm up for the occasional fast meal.

The night before: Put the frozen ground beef in the refrigerator to thaw. Find the ingredients, the bread pan, and the ice cream scoop. Wash the celery and put it in a plastic bag to crisp. Make the **Herbed Butter** (page 133) or locate your stash. Find the stale bread and cube it up for bread pudding, or set out your hoarded bread cubes to thaw.

Added touch: Squirt a ribbon of ketchup down the middle of the meat loaf before you bake it. Grate a little cheese into the mixture, or lay fancy shapes of cheese on the top.

Presentation: Serve the whole meat loaf on a platter; slice it at the table.

Involving your children: Children can wash and peel the carrots and measure the bread crumbs, onions, and milk. Some children will love getting their hands into this goopy stuff. However, to be allowed to work with raw meat, they have to be older and must have demonstrated that they know proper procedures for handling raw meat. Children will also love scooping out the meatballs and putting them on the jelly roll pan. An older child can make the bread pudding.

Adapting this meal for children: Children do well with this meal because everything is soft and easy to chew. Because children under age 2 might choke on carrot and celery sticks, give them soft, fresh fruit that has been cut into bite-sized pieces so they can eat it with their fingers.

Variation: You can also use the meat loaf mixture for making Salisbury steaks, which are simply hamburger steaks mixed with extra bread and seasonings. Form them into patties, freeze them raw on a jelly roll pan lined with waxed paper, and bag them after they are frozen. Instructions for making gravy, which you'll want to accompany your Salisbury steaks, can be found in the recipe for **Hamburgers** (page 101).

BUYING A FOOD THERMOMETER

Decisions, decisions! Even purchasing a food thermometer can be complex. Some types of thermometers can be left in foods while they cook or bake, and others can't. The ones that can be left in don't work well for thin foods like hamburgers. If you are willing to check foods at the end of cooking and *not* leave the thermometer in place while food cooks, a digital thermometer is a good, all-purpose tool. It registers the meat's temperature in 15 to 20 seconds, and because it has to be inserted only 1/2 inch deep into foods, it works well for thin foods like burgers. Thermometers that can be left in place, liquid filled or bimetal thermometers, have to be inserted 2 to 3 inches deep and take 1 to 2 minutes to get a reading. Those thermometers are best for roasts and turkeys. For meat loaf, either type would work.

SMALL ICE CREAM SCOOPS

Small ice cream scoops are great time-savers because you can quickly portion out dumplings, cookies, meatballs, or itty-bitty muffins with one hand. If yours is marked with a size, it will be on the narrow piece that sweeps out the bowl. Size 30 works well for large drop cookies, meatballs, and regular-sized muffins. Size 60 works well for dumplings and small drop cookies. The size numbers refer to scoops per quart. The 30 holds 2 tablespoons, and the 60 holds 1.

Spaghetti and Meatballs

Here is the shortest recipe in the book. It is short because you use the frozen meatballs you made when you prepared the **Meat Loaf** meal. Here you get your reward for planning and cooking ahead.

INGREDIENTS
12–16 frozen meatballs
one or two 32-oz jars prepared spaghetti sauce
dry packaged spaghetti

MENU
Spaghetti and meatballs
French bread
Butter
Tossed green salad
Apple and orange wedges or
Fruit in season
Grated Parmesan cheese: fresh or otherwise
Milk

METHOD
Summary: Heat prepared spaghetti sauce and frozen meatballs. Serve over boiled spaghetti with grated cheese.

Fill a 4 1/2-quart pan about half to two-thirds full of water, add 1 teaspoon of salt per quart of water, and bring to a rapid boil. Add *dry packaged spaghetti* (1 pound or however much your family needs), and boil until al dente. Drain and toss with a little olive oil to keep it from sticking together.

Heat up the thawed meatballs (the ones you made when you prepared the **Meat Loaf**) in the microwave. If you heat them on top of the stove, you will have to stir them, and that may break them apart.

Warm up *one or two 32-ounce jars of prepared spaghetti sauce*, whichever brand you prefer. Put the heated meatballs in the hot spaghetti sauce.

Serve sauce and meatballs over cooked spaghetti.

Added touch: Enrich the sauce with more vegetables by sautéing any or all of the vegetables in the **Marinated Chicken Stir-Fry** (pages 112-113); add them with the meatballs for the final warm-up.

RECIPE NOTES
Fast tip: Store the cheese grater in the refrigerator with the block of Parmesan cheese, and wash the grater only when you add a new block of cheese. Put the grater, loaded with cheese, on the table on a plate, and let family members grate their own.

The night before: Put the frozen meatballs in the refrigerator to thaw. Locate the spaghetti sauce. Wash and crisp the greens for the salad (see page 137). Locate fruit and French bread and put them in a handy place. Locate the Parmesan cheese and the grater.

Involving your children: Children can spin and toss the salad and peel the oranges.

Adapting this meal for children: Depending on your eaters, you may want to start by keeping the meatballs separate from the sauce. Children often don't want sauce on spaghetti, but spaghetti and a meatball makes a nice meal. Eating this meal is subject to the challenges and rewards of any spaghetti meal.

The vegetables add extra interest for those who have mastered each of them. However, do not try to sneak vegetables into your child by hiding them in the sauce. That is dirty pool—your child will be on to you in a flash, and he won't learn anything. With the tomatoes in the sauce, there are already lots of vegetables in this dish, so you do not have to resort to such a sneaky, devious, underhanded trick.

Variation: Leave out the meat, add a drained can of chickpeas (garbanzo beans), and have vegetarian sauce.

Make meat sauce by putting in browned ground beef instead of meatballs.

Cook Italian sausages, cut them up, and add them to the sauce instead of ground beef or meatballs.

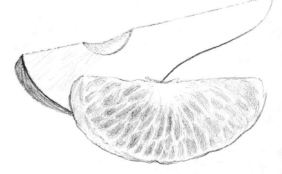

Spinach-Feta Frittata

A frittata is an unfolded omelet with vegetables or meat or both. This can be another last-resort dinner. It can also be breakfast or a Sunday brunch meal. For more about eggs, see the box on page 87.

INGREDIENTS
4–8 oz fresh spinach
1–2 tsp butter
1/3 cup water
6 eggs
4 oz feta cheese

MENU
Spinach-feta frittata
Fruit salad or
Vegetable salad
Bread or toast
Butter
Milk
Ice cream

METHOD
Summary: Beat eggs until frothy and pour them into a frying pan. Add fresh spinach and cheese; cover and cook until set.

Wash and spin dry *4 to 8 ounces of fresh spinach*, and tear it into bite-sized pieces.

Melt *1 to 2 teaspoons of butter* in a nonstick frying pan using almost-the-lowest temperature on your range.

Bring *6 eggs* to room temperature by letting them stand for 5 minutes in your hottest tap water. (Be sure the eggs are not cracked. If they are, throw them away.) Crack the eggs into a deep glass bowl. Add 1/3 cup of cool water (1 tablespoon per egg). Beat with an electric mixer until the eggs are frothy. Pour mixture immediately into the frying pan.

Gently press the fresh spinach into the eggs, putting in as much as can be coated with egg, and finely crumble *4 ounces of feta cheese* over the eggs.

Cover and cook for 10 to 20 minutes or until the eggs are set to your liking.

Slip the frittata onto a plate, slice, and serve.

RECIPE NOTES
Fast tip: Frittata *is* a fast tip. It is a busy person's version of an omelet. With frittata, you don't have to hover and check and fold and check again. Write down the setting and burner you used and how long you cooked the frittata. Next time you make it, you can set the timer and forget it.

The night before: This can be a clean-out-the-refrigerator meal. Investigate your resources for vegetables for the frittata or for fruit or vegetables for a salad.

Presentation: Serve the frittata on a pizza pan and slice with a roller-style pizza cutter.

Involving your children: Let children crack the eggs, wash and spin the spinach, and with *clean* hands, press the spinach into the frittata.

Adapting this meal for children: Be sure to have plenty of toast, milk, and a popular fruit. Even if they don't like fritatta, children will survive.

Variation: Almost any vegetable would work well in a frittata, and almost any cheese. Brown pre-prepared hash browns, add chopped onions and cook them until they are clear, substitute grated cheddar cheese, and you will have a whole different dish. Or warm up leftover vegetables from the refrigerator, add them to the beaten egg, and top with any kind of grated cheese you choose. My favorite is leftover **Ratatouille** (page 141) and Swiss cheese. Use your imagination!

For a big crowd, you can double this recipe and bake it in a 9 x 13-inch pan at 325 degrees for 20 minutes.

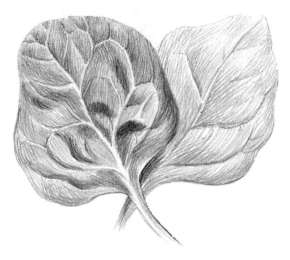

Lemon Chicken

This is a fast, easy, and wonderfully tasty chicken recipe that features prebrowning in store-bought mixed seasoning and olive oil or butter, then braising to get the chicken done inside. Other mixed seasonings work equally well and give an entirely different taste. Try Creole or Greek seasoning and throw in a few olives. Peruse the spice shelves at the grocery store to get other ideas. Lemon chicken makes a handy PPM. Put it on a bun for a hot or cold sandwich, or cut it across the grain into thin slices and toss the slices with a green salad for a quick lunch. Simply super.

INGREDIENTS
2 Tbsp butter or olive oil
2 tsp lemon pepper
6 chicken breast halves (3–4 oz each)

MENU
Lemon chicken
Oven-fried potatoes (page 141)
Creamed spinach (page 139) or
Vegetables in season
Peach cobbler (page 142) or crisp (page 143)
Fruit in season
Bread or toast
Butter
Milk

METHOD
Summary: Brown chicken in seasoned oil. Add water to the pan, reduce heat, and cover. The steam finishes the cooking.

Heat *2 tablespoons of butter* at medium temperature in a nonstick frying pan. Add about *2 teaspoons of lemon pepper*.

Wash and drain *6 chicken breast halves (3 to 4 ounces each)*. Immediately add the chicken and brown on both sides. When the browning is finished, add 2 tablespoons of water and cover.

Reduce the heat to low and let the steam finish cooking the chicken—probably another 15 minutes. It's done when the chicken is white in the middle. Don't overcook it or it will get tough and dry.

RECIPE NOTES
The night before: In separate pans, place the frozen chicken and spinach in the refrigerator to thaw. Locate the potatoes, maybe wash them. Line up the ingredients and the pan for the oven-fried potatoes. Find the peaches and locate the dry ingredients for the cobbler (mix them up and put a plate over the top of the bowl), or locate your cache of crisp topping.

Presentation: Garnish with thin lemon slices.

Involving your children: Children can scrub the potatoes, mix up the potato topping, unwrap the frozen spinach, put it in the colander, squeeze out the water, and put it in the cooking dish.

Adapting this meal for children: This is an easy meal to put on serving dishes, and your children will enjoy serving themselves. Cut some of the chicken breasts up into child-sized helpings as you put them on the platter. Let your children eat the potatoes with their fingers. Put the spinach in little bowls so they can eat it easily with a spoon.

Variation: Make mock fried chicken by flouring chicken pieces with a mixture of 1/2 cup of flour, 1 teaspoon of salt, 1/4 teaspoon of pepper, 1/2 teaspoon of poultry seasoning, and 1/2 teaspoon of paprika. Brown the pieces at medium heat in butter, reduce the heat to low, and cover them to finish cooking for 5 or 10 minutes.

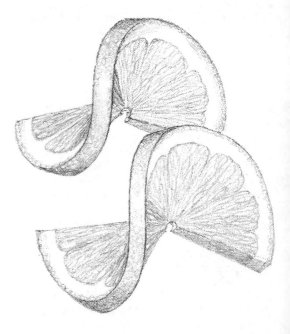

Braised Pork Chops with Sweet Potatoes

Consider putting pork chops on your menus. Fresh pork is delicious, reasonably priced, high in protein, and particularly high in thiamine. Because grocery stores have difficulty convincing consumers to buy pork, prices are often extremely reasonable. Today's pork is low in fat and is trichina-free. It is tender and cooks quickly, and you don't have to overcook it and dry it out to make it safe. Like other meats, cooking to an internal temperature of 160 degrees, or until the pink color is just gone, is enough and will still leave it juicy, tender, and appealing.

Adding sweet potatoes to this dish makes it tasty and expeditious. Not only are the potatoes an excellent source of vitamin A and carotene, but they are also filling and complementary to the taste of pork.

INGREDIENTS

4 sweet potatoes
1–2 Tbsp butter
1–2 tsp dried sage
6 3/4-oz boneless or bone-in loin pork chops
Salt and pepper to taste
1/2 cup chicken broth or apple juice

MENU

Braised pork chops with sweet potatoes
Microwave chunky applesauce (page 144)
Bread or toast
Butter
Milk
Ice cream

METHOD

Summary: Brown pork chops in butter and sage. Parboil sweet potatoes. Combine everything, cover, and braise until done.

Peel the *4 sweet potatoes* (which may also be called *yams*), wash them, and cut them into 1-inch slices. Parboil (partially boil) the sweet potatoes by cooking them for 10 minutes in boiling water salted with 1 teaspoon of salt per quart. When the potatoes are beginning to soften, remove them from the heat and drain.

While the potatoes cook, melt *1 to 2 tablespoons of butter* at low to medium heat in a large frying pan that has a tight-fitting lid. Sprinkle *1 to 2 teaspoons of dried sage* into the melted butter or rub on the pork chops. With the lid off, brown the pork chops on both sides and remove them from the pan.

Pour off excess grease from the frying pan and add *1/2 cup of chicken broth or apple juice*. Lay the parboiled sweet potatoes into the frying pan, lay the browned pork chops over the sweet potatoes, add *salt and pepper to taste*, cover, reduce the heat to low, and cook for an additional 10 to 20 minutes or until both the pork chops and the sweet potatoes are cooked through.

RECIPE NOTES

Fast tip: Once you master cooking pork chops, they can be your fast tip. Pork chops are ready to cook, and they cook quickly.

The night before: Place the frozen pork chops in the refrigerator to thaw. Find the potatoes, peel them, and cover them with water to keep them from darkening. For the microwaved apples, find and wash the apples and locate the dish for cooking them.

Involving your children: Children can peel the potatoes. A preschooler can cut up the apple wedges for the applesauce. An older child can make the applesauce, except for getting it in and out of the microwave.

Adapting this meal for children: This meal works great for children because the meat is so tender and the vegetables are appealing.

Variation: You can make braised pork chops to combine with other menus by using the same technique given in the **Lemon Chicken** recipe. Brown the chops in seasoned butter or oil (you can experiment with a variety of seasonings—or use none at all), and finish cooking by braising: Add a small amount of liquid and cook with the lid on the pan. As with the chicken, you can also make mock fried pork chops by flouring them before you brown them. Some people prefer the flavor and texture they get from frying the pork chops until they get completely done, without braising at the end. That method is also fast and acceptable, although it is harder to finish cooking the chops without drying them out.

Wisconsin Fish Boil

This is a variation on poached fish. I have given it to you this way because fish boil is a traditional meal in Door County, a lovely vacation spot that makes up the "thumb" of Wisconsin. For the full treatment, fish boil needs to be prepared in a huge cooker over an open fire. The vegetables go in first and the fish later. Since cherries are a big product of Door County, the meal is only complete with a cherry dessert.

INGREDIENTS
1 1/2 lb cod or haddock
6 medium boiling potatoes
6 small whole onions
1 1/2 lb carrots

MENU
Poached fish
Potatoes
Carrots
Onions
Melted butter
Bread and butter
Cherry cobbler (page 142)
Ice cream

METHOD
Summary: **Boil potatoes, onions, and carrots in salted water. Add fish and simmer.**

Fill an 8-quart pan about two-thirds full of water, add 1 teaspoon of salt per quart of water, and bring to a rapid boil. Fish boil works best if you use a soup pot with a steamer basket, but a vegetable steaming rack set down into the boiling water works pretty well too.

Prepare the following: *1 1/2 pound of cod or haddock*, cut into helping-sized pieces, *6 medium boiling potatoes, 6 small whole onions, 1 1/2 pounds of carrots*, peeled and cut into chunks, or baby carrots left whole.

Begin cooking the vegetables first by putting them in the salted, boiling water. Because you need to leave room for the fish, the water level needs to be 2 to 3 inches above the top of the vegetables.

When the vegetables have been boiling for 15 minutes, put in the rack and lay the fish into it, lower the temperature to a fast simmer, cook for 10 more minutes, remove everything from the water, and serve.

RECIPE NOTES
Fast tip: To remove the fish, lift out the rack. Drain the vegetables in a colander, and you are ready to serve!

Added touch: Melt butter and put it in a pitcher to serve. This is not really "added." It is essential!

The night before: Thaw the frozen fish in the refrigerator, find the cooking pot, and determine what you will use as a steamer basket for the fish. Locate the vegetables. For the cherry cobbler, find your can of cherries or put the frozen cherries in the refrigerator to thaw. Locate the dry ingredients and mix them up.

Presentation: As artfully as you can, arrange the fish and vegetables on a platter and add a few slices of lemon and a few sprigs of parsley to dress it up. This meal is hard to arrange to make it look pretty, but if you don't forget the melted butter, it won't matter.

Involving your children: Children can help clean the vegetables and make the cherry cobbler.

Adapting this meal for children: As long as the fish is boneless, this is a great meal for children. The menu has a number of items, and they are all moist, soft, and easy to chew.

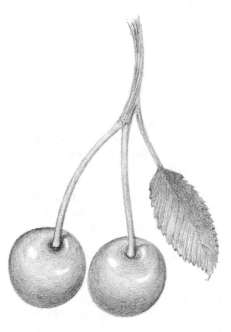

Hamburgers

Once you master your method, your table can be the place to get the best burgers in town. The key to juicy, flavorful hamburgers is cooking them until they are done—but no more.

INGREDIENTS
1 Tbsp butter
2 Tbsp Worcestershire sauce
1 1/2 lb ground chuck

MENU
Hamburger on a bun
Dill pickle slices
Lettuce
Tomato slices
Chopped onion
Mayonnaise
Ketchup and mustard
Potato chips
Carrot and celery sticks, pickle spears
Fruit in season
Milk

METHOD
Summary: Shape hamburger patties and fry them until they are done to your liking.

In a nonstick frying pan, heat *1 tablespoon of butter* and *2 tablespoons of Worcestershire sauce* at medium temperature.

Form *1 1/2 pounds of ground beef* into six 4-ounce patties (which will cook down to 3 ounces).

Fry the hamburgers until they are brown, turn them *only once*, and cook them until brown on the other side. To be as juicy as possible but still be safe, meat needs to be cooked until it is done but not overdone. Test for doneness with a meat thermometer—final cooking temperature should be 160 degrees.

RECIPE NOTES
The night before: Put the frozen ground beef in the refrigerator to thaw. If they've been refrigerated, put the tomatoes on the counter so they come to room temperature. Locate the condiments and potato chips. Find the ketchup, mustard, mayonnaise, potato chips, and pickles; clean and crisp the celery and carrots. Chop the onions and refrigerate them in a tightly closed jar.

Fast tip: To keep hamburger patties on hand in the freezer, make them when you get home from the grocery store, lay them out on a jelly roll pan lined with wax paper, freeze them, and then break them apart and store them in a zip top bag.

Added touch: Sprinkle a little dill weed on these burgers as you begin to cook them. Search for some *great buns*. Buns make all the difference between just a hamburger and *a great hamburger*.

Presentation: Put out toppings and let family members doctor their burgers to taste.

Involving your children: Once your child is reliable about cleanliness when working with raw meat, like washing hands before and after and not putting meat-juicy hands in his mouth, let him help shape hamburger patties. Making an initial or a shape can be a fun treat occasionally, but don't get caught up in making food cute to capture your child's interest . If you do, you are probably trying to get your child to eat, and even though your attempts are creative and playful, they will backfire.

Adapting this meal for children: These hamburgers are big, so you might want to cut them in half to serve them to children. If you can find little buns, make the hamburger patties smaller. Kids enjoy food that is "their size."

Variation: In their cookbook *Desperation Dinners*, Beverly Mills and Alicia Ross lament the difficulty of keeping hamburger buns on hand. So when good buns aren't available, they recommend making hamburger steaks with mashed potatoes and gravy. To make the gravy, shake up a mixture of 1 1/2 cups of water and 3 tablespoons of flour in a pint jar. Move the hamburger patties to a plate, and pour the flour and water mixture into the pan drippings. Stir constantly with a wire whip, scraping the bits of meat crust and juice off the pan as you stir. Boil for about 1 to 2 minutes to thicken. You will have—gravy! Add 1/4 teaspoon of pepper and salt to taste—1/4 teaspoon should do it. If the gravy lacks flavor or color, add a little beef broth concentrate. Serve with **Mashed Potatoes** (pages 138-139).

Keep Up the Good Work

- Tune in to your cooking and learn to enjoy it.
- Try preparing some dishes that are a bit more complex (they may also be more rewarding). The recipes in this chapter will build on what you've learned so far.
- Keep ingredients on hand for a few "grab-and-dump" meals for nights when you have very little time to prepare dinner. Experiment with a few prepackaged convenience foods to discover what works best for you and your family.
- Get creative in the kitchen! Learn to put together your own casseroles with the generic casserole formula.
- Consider taking a cooking class or getting a new cookbook to help you to continue learning new cooking skills.

CHAPTER
6
HOW TO KEEP COOKING

It's time to take a look at your progress. Are you having some successes by now with your cooking, and—even more wonderful—are you starting to get some real pleasure from cooking and from food you make yourself? Rather than finding cooking a mysterious and alarming business, are you developing rhythms and intuitions with food? Are you making some dishes automatically, without even having to get out the recipe? When someone asks you for a recipe, are you puzzled about what you really *did* do? That means you are turning into a cook. Congratulations!

I do hope the process of food preparation holds some satisfaction for you, at least some of the time. If not, why not? Are your standards too high? Does your attitude need adjustment? Would you benefit from setting aside time occasionally to enjoy cooking? Like eating, cooking can be a creative act that gives you a change of pace and restores your energy. Why not let it be that for you? Take a clue from your meditating friends, and let your cooking be mindful. Tune in on it, enjoy it, and let it be restorative.

Can you make a few things well? Give yourself a pat on the back. Things didn't turn out the way you had hoped? Keep it to yourself. Your apologies just make other people uncomfortable. You're not forcing anybody to eat, so they can take care of themselves. Make notes in your cookbook for how to make it better the next time, and forget about it. After more cooking failures than I care to think about, I finally concluded that if something turned out well the first time, I was lucky. If it turned out well the second or third time, it was because I knew what I was doing—I had adapted the recipe to

my stove and my pans and my methods and it had become *mine*. No matter how good a recipe is, the nature of working with food is variation. As you develop your cooking skill and intuition, you will be able to take those variations in stride.

More Recipes and Cooking Possibilities

The recipes in this chapter are a bit more complex than the ones in chapter 5 and give you opportunities to learn about cooking dry beans, making soup (with its all-important broth), choosing and cooking rice, and frying. Although they have a few more steps, the recipes are still simple and accessible. Because we are cooking ahead to make PPMs (pre-prepared meals, otherwise known as leftovers), and because they keep well and taste even better the second day than the first, some of the recipes also make bigger batches. The **Beef Ragout, Chicken Soup**, and **Savory Black Beans and Rice** will make about 12 helpings, roughly twice the number as the recipes we have worked with before.

Along with more steps, we will talk about fewer steps. In this chapter, you will find "last resort" ideas like grab-and-dump and prepackaged "convenience" meals. We'll talk about cookbooks and cooking classes that help you continue to improve your cooking skills. Finally, in the discussion about the **Generic Casserole** we'll eke out some general principles of food composition and recipe construction that you can use when you want to improvise your very own signature one-dish meal.

103

Chicken Soup

This recipe makes a double batch so you can eat it for lunch or freeze it for another dinner. The surveyors tell us that chicken soup, like meat loaf, is one of the comfort foods that we long for. Chicken soup is also prized for curative powers—the source of which is a mystery to medical science. Whatever its appeal, there is no doubt that knowing how to make a pot of chicken soup comes in handy. Winter or summer, soup makes a convenient and satisfying meal.

INGREDIENTS
2 large (46-oz) cans chicken broth
2 chicken breasts, about 12 oz each
1 1/2 cups carrots, shredded
1 large onion, chopped
1/2 lb celery, chopped
8-oz wide egg noodles

MENU
Chicken soup
Chewy bread
Butter
Fruit in season
Milk
Ice cream and cookies

METHOD
Summary: To make this soup, first poach chicken breasts in broth and set them aside. Boil carrots, other vegetables, and noodles in the broth. Cut up the chicken and add back to the broth. Thicken the soup if desired.

Poach 3 chicken breasts, about 12 ounces each: Bring chicken and *1 large (46-ounce) and 1 small (15-ounce) can low-salt chicken broth* to a boil in a large Dutch oven or soup pot, then reduce heat to a *simmer*, cover and cook the chicken for 20 minutes, 30 minutes if it is frozen.

Using a long-handled slotted spoon, remove the chicken from the broth. Bring the broth back to a rolling boil and add *1 1/2 cups of shredded carrots* and any other vegetables that can cook in about 5 to 10 minutes, like *1 large chopped onion* and *1/2 pounds of chopped celery*. While you put in the vegetables, add a *16-ounce package of wide egg noodles*.

Reduce the heat to a steady boil and cook until the noodles are al dente.

Just as the noodles finish cooking, you can thicken the broth if you want to. In a covered jar, shake together 4 tablespoons of flour and 1/2 cup of water until the lumps disappear. Add the flour mixture slowly to the boiling broth, stirring the broth all the while with a wire whip. Bring the soup to a boil, stirring occasionally as it thickens.

Meanwhile, cut up the cooked chicken into bite-sized pieces, using a sharp knife and a cutting board.

When the noodles and vegetables are done, reduce the heat and add the cut-up chicken. Put in some fresh or dried parsley to give it a little color.

Reheat if you want to before you serve it.

RECIPE NOTES
Fast tip: To make this recipe even easier, buy canned, deboned chicken. The quick-blending flours, like Wondra or Shake & Blend, may help you avoid lumps when you thicken the broth.

The night before: In the refrigerator, thaw the frozen chicken in a pan to catch the drips. Unearth the soup pot. In my house, it is in the basement. I use it infrequently, so I store it in an out-of-the-way place. Wash and chop the onion and celery.

Presentation: Keep your eyes open at garage sales for an interesting soup tureen to serve this and other soups in.

Involving your children: Children can help wash celery and peel onions. Chopping onions is tricky, so keep that job for yourself. A child can mix up the flour and water, an older child can make the dumplings (for the variation). A child can separate the cooled chicken from the bones.

Adapting this meal for children: Adding in the by-now-cooled chicken will bring the soup temperature down to where children can eat it comfortably. You may want to remove your child's portion before you reheat it. For a young child, you can use a slotted spoon to dip out the vegetables; let him eat them with his fingers and then drink the broth from a cup. Or you can give your child less liquid or add crackers to thicken it so it's easier to eat with spoon or fingers.

Ricotta Dumplings for Chicken Soup

Leave out the noodles and make dumplings, instead. Since the dumplings cook somewhat into the soup, the dumplings do the thickening for you.

After cooking for 30 years, I discovered that the secret of keeping dumplings from falling apart in the broth is to let the mixed-up dough sit for a few minutes before spooning it into the boiling broth. Don't peek while the dumplings cook, or they will get hard. Hard is the way I like them, so when I was a little girl I regularly sneaked into the kitchen to lift the lid off the pot. However, that is not prescribed dumpling-making technique.

INGREDIENTS

2 cups all-purpose flour, stirred before you measure
1 Tbsp baking powder
1 tsp salt
1/2 tsp dried thyme
1 Tbsp dried parsley flakes
1/2 cup ricotta cheese
1/4 cup milk
1 egg

METHOD

Summary: Combine the dry ingredients in one bowl and the wet ingredients (the cheese, egg, and milk) in another. Mix the two together to form a dough. Drop dumpling-sized spoonfuls into boiling broth and simmer.

In a medium-sized bowl mix together *2 cups of all-purpose flour, stirred before you measure, 1 tablespoon of baking powder, 1 teaspoon of salt, 1/2 teaspoon of dried thyme, and 1 tablespoon of dried parsley flakes*.

In a small bowl, beat together until the egg is well mixed *1/2 cup of ricotta cheese, 1 egg, and 1/4 cup of milk*.

Add the wet ingredients to the dry ingredients. Stir just until the dough holds together; if you stir the batter too much, the dumplings will be tough.

Let the dough rest for 15 minutes.

Using a tablespoon or a #60 ice cream scoop (60 scoops to a quart, or 1 tablespoon each), form dumplings and drop them into the gently boiling broth. Dip the utensil in the boiling broth each time to set the dumplings into the broth more easily. Cover and cook 15 minutes.

Variation: Make dumplings using the recipe and directions on the Bisquick box.

POACHING AND SIMMERING

Chicken cooks fast in water. The instructions say to *poach* it in simmering water separately from the noodles because noodles need to be boiled and boiling can make chicken tough and stringy. Poaching the chicken in the broth gives both chicken and broth a little more flavor. Liquid simmers when the bubbles rise slowly to the surface and just barely seem to break.

BROTH

The stock is the essential ingredient of making good soup, so don't skimp on it. This recipe calls for canned broth, which is tasty. The "real cook's" way of making a soup base is to cook bones and vegetables for a long time, simmer the cooking liquid down to concentrate it, then strain it. I won't teach you that because I do not know how. After years of trying, I had a major breakthrough when I gave up. I discovered the broth-concentrate paste. Some places have it in bulk; I can only find it in jars. It is very flavorful but often salty, so you have to be careful about how much broth base and added salt you use. Your grocery store might have frozen soup base or broth, and if it does, you might have a choice of salt-free which, for most of us, is unnecessary. You might like bouillon cubes or crystals. To me, they taste artificial, but that might just be my taste buds. Explore until you find a soup base that you like. It will open up a whole world of soup-making possibilities for you.

Regular canned chicken broth has 1,000 milligrams of sodium per cup, which is high. Even the low-salt variety has 700 milligrams of sodium per cup. That's a reasonable amount unless you are on a salt-free diet. If you follow the package directions to substitute broth concentrate or bouillon cubes, you will get about 500 to 600 milligrams of sodium per cup of reconstituted broth.

SIFTING FLOUR

Because flour packs down in the bag or canister, many baking recipes call for sifted flour. To be measured properly, flour has to be sifted or fluffed up again. I find that stirring fluffs it enough and is a whole lot faster and easier than sifting.

Beef Ragout

This recipe makes a double batch, is good warmed over, and freezes well. I thought you might enjoy it because what could be more sophisticated than a French dish? The word *ragout* comes from a French word meaning "to revive the taste." I can only assume the recipe originated as a way to use up leftovers. I was going to leave out the wine to make it easier to keep the ingredients on hand, but as nearly as I can tell, the difference between a *ragout* and a *stew* is *wine*—and possibly *mushrooms*. Oh, yes, the stew has potatoes. And mushroom soup instead of broth. And not all those seasonings. Oh well, I guess they *are* quite different.

Anyhow, you can put in the wine or not. It adds an interesting flavor and the alcohol cooks off so you don't have to worry about inebriating your children. However, it also tastes good without it, and your family won't know if they are eating a less-than-authentic ragout.

This recipe calls for cooking at low heat on top of the stove, but it will cook equally well in a slow cooker.

INGREDIENTS

1–2 Tbsp butter, stick margarine, or cooking oil
2 tsp dried thyme
1/4 tsp black pepper
2 lb stew beef, cut into 1-inch cubes
4 cloves garlic, minced
4 cups beef broth or
*4 cups water with 4 tsp to 2 Tbsp beef broth
    concentrate*
15–20 peeled baby carrots
2 medium onions, cut in wedges
1/2 cup dry red wine (optional)
8 oz fresh mushrooms, sliced or
16-oz can mushroom stems and pieces, drained

MENU

Beef ragout
Buttered noodles
Chewy bread
Butter
Canned peaches or fruit in season
Cucumber slices
Milk
Pumpkin custard (page 134)

METHOD

Summary: Season cubed stew beef and brown in butter. Add garlic, beef broth, carrots, and onion (and wine if you want to). Simmer or bake until meat is tender. Add mushrooms and serve.

In a large, nonstick frying pan or Dutch oven, heat *1–2 tablespoon of butter, stick margarine, or cooking oil* at medium temperature until sizzling.

Mix together in a container with a shaker top (an empty spice container works well) *2 teaspoon of dried thyme* and *1/4 teaspoon of black pepper*. Sprinkle spices evenly over *2 pounds of stew beef cut into 1-inch cubes*.

Brown beef in butter at medium temperature until it is light brown. At the very end of browning, add *4 cloves of minced garlic*. Cook garlic briefly until it is golden but not brown. Add 4 cups of beef broth or *4 cups of water with 4 teaspoons to 2 tablespoons of beef broth concentrate* (read the package directions; use less concentrate than recommended, and taste to see if you need to add more).

Heat to boiling, scraping the sides of the pan to get all the good stuff off the pot and into the broth (if you want to be fancy, call this "deglazing"). Add *15 to 20 peeled baby carrots, 2 medium onions, cut in wedges, and 1/2 cup of dry red wine (optional)*.

Bring everything to a boil. Reduce heat to low, cover, and cook for approximately 1 1/2 hours until the beef cubes are tender (check now and then to see whether you need to add more water). You can also bake it in a 350-degree oven for 1 hour (this is rather a hot oven to let you bake the pumpkin custard at the same time). Keep an eye on the ragout to be sure you don't overcook it. Or, cook in a slow cooker at medium temperature for about 3 to 4 hours, or at low temperature for about 5 to 6 hours.

Just before serving, add *8 ounces of fresh sliced mushrooms* or a *16-ounce can of mushroom stems and pieces, drained*.

If you like, thicken the broth with a mixture of 4 tablespoons of flour and 1/2 cup of water.

RECIPE NOTES

Fast tip: Instead of cutting up onions, you may use canned or frozen tiny onions. It makes a nice touch and saves crying over onions. Add them midway through cooking so the flavor can blend with the other ingredients without overcooking the onions. To save cleanup, buy several pounds of beef cubes, cut them up, and freeze them in 1-pound zip top bags. Thaw them, and put them directly into the frying pan. You wash the knife, counter-top, and cutting board only once.

To make this dish faster to cook, ask the butcher for cubed sirloin, which will cook ten-der in about 30 to 45 minutes. It will cost about half again as much. You could also ask for his recommendation for a faster-cooking, still-not-terribly-expensive cut of meat to use for beef cubes for braising or stewing.

The night before: Put the frozen beef cubes in the refrigerator to thaw. Locate the beef con-centrate, the other ingredients, the wine. Taste the wine to be sure it is okay. (Just kidding.) Get out the slow cooker.

Presentation: This is a juicy dish, and the juice is wonderful. Why not set the table with flat bowls and eat it with spoons instead of forks? Added touch: Garnish with parsley. Adults can drink the rest of the wine. Children may have grape juice for a treat.

Involving your children: Your children can count out the baby carrots, wash the potatoes, and pound the garlic, once they learn to do it gently. Mushed garlic still tastes like garlic, but it's a little hard to scrape up.

Adapting this meal for children: Everything in this meal is soft and easy to chew. Children like eating plain cucumber slices and consider them finger food.

Variation: Using this cooking method, the car-rots get quite soft. If you prefer crisper carrots, add them about halfway though cooking. Beef stew is the American version of this recipe. To make beef stew, brown the beef, substitute one can of golden mushroom soup for the broth, add about two dozen baby carrots, a pound of potatoes (peeled or scrubbed and quartered), and two onions, quartered. Add water to make as liquid as you like. Make a batch of refriger-ated baking powder biscuits. Um-umm!

BROWNING MEAT

You brown meat, fish, and poultry to develop the flavor. Prescribed meat cooking technique is to brown at high temperatures to sear the meat and seal in the juices. However, the high temperatures makes the fat splatter more, and I think it is dangerous and messy to do it that way, especially with children in the house. So I use a medium temperature. Generally when you brown, the food is not fully cooked—the cooking has to be finished another way. Whether you cook at medium or high tempera-ture, you will notice that at first, water and juices cook out. The water and juices bubble up, making a soft, gurgling, water-in-a-brook sound. As the water cooks off, the sound changes to a more high-pitched, fat-splattering sound. That's when browning occurs. At that point, watch the food carefully, because it browns quickly. Brown to your taste. I find if I get beef cubes too browned it dries them out too much, so I settle for only lightly browned. Butter browns foods more easily than other fats and adds a lovely flavor. However, it also burns more easily, so you have to watch it more carefully during browning.

GARLIC

Garlic tastes better if it is lightly cooked before you put it in a recipe. An easy way of getting the skin off garlic and beginning the mincing at the same time is to put the garlic clove on a cutting board and pound it lightly with a meat mallet or the bottom of a jar or squash it with the flat side of a knife. That breaks away the skin so you can remove it easily with your fin-gers. Then you can use a garlic press or a knife to finish the mincing job. With a sharp knife, cut off the clove ends and discard. Cut cross-wise into thin slices, and chop the slices up as finely as you want. OR forget the whole thing and buy garlic in jars or garlic powder. The container will tell you how much to substitute for cloves of garlic.

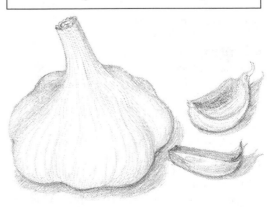

Minestrone Soup

This recipe makes enough for two meals. I generally double it when I make it, but here I cut it down so you could try it out to see if you like it before you produce it in such quantities. Minestrone soup freezes and warms up well, so having some in reserve is both a treat and a help.

Cooking dry beans is quite easily done with a little planning and preparation. The main strategy in this recipe is to cook the beans and beef at the same time and let them flavor each other. Using canned beans, however, is perfectly legitimate, so don't feel obligated to start with dry beans if you don't want to.

INGREDIENTS

1/2 lb dried kidney beans
1 lb beef stew meat
1–2 Tbsp butter
15-oz can tomatoes with Italian seasonings
1 medium onion, chopped
2 cloves garlic, minced
2 oz carrots, shredded
1 potato, diced
2 oz cabbage, shredded
2–3 Tbsp olive oil
1 tsp salt
1/4 tsp pepper
2 tsp dried Italian seasoning
1 cup cooked spaghetti, broken into 1-inch segments
  (5–6 oz dry)

MENU

Minestrone soup
Oyster crackers
Variety of snack crackers
Chewy bread
Butter
Milk
Apple wedges, orange slices

METHOD

Summary: Soak beans and simmer slowly with browned beef 3 to 4 hours. As the liquid cooks away, replace it with canned tomatoes. Add sautéed vegetables, seasonings, and cooked spaghetti.

Wash and soak overnight *1/2 pound of dried kidney beans.*

Brown *1 pound of beef stew meat in 1 to 2 table-spoons of butter.*

Drain the beans and put them into a large Dutch oven or soup pot with the browned beef. Cover the beans and beef with water (about 3 inches to spare), and add 1 teaspoon of salt per quart. Put a little water in the frying pan you used for the beef and cook it to get up the brown drippings from the meat. Add this to the soup, too.

Cook the beans and beef slowly for 3 to 4 hours until the beans and meat are tender. As the water cooks down, replace the liquid with a 15-ounce can of tomatoes with Italian seasonings.

Sauté *1 medium onion, chopped; 2 cloves of garlic, minced; 2 ounces of shredded carrots; 1 diced potato; and 2 ounces of shredded cabbage in 2 to 3 tablespoons of olive oil.* Add vegetables to the soup at the very end of cooking.

Also at the end of cooking, add about *1 teaspoon of salt* (adjust this depending on your taste), *1/4 teaspoon of pepper, 2 teaspoons of dried Italian seasoning, 1 cup of cooked spaghetti, broken into 1-inch segments (5 to 6 ounces dry),* and the rest of the canned tomatoes.

RECIPE NOTES

Fast tip: To make a fast minestrone, use left-over beef from Swiss steak (1 cup, finely cubed) and 1 15-ounce can of beans instead of dry beans.

To substitute canned beans for dry beans, double the weight. That is, instead of a pound of dry beans, which you then cook, use 2 15-ounce cans. Drain them before adding to the pot. You can substitute one kind of canned beans for another, depending on what you like. Get creative by using beans in any combination: red kidney beans, garbanzo beans (chickpeas), white beans, or pinto beans.

The night before: Put frozen beef cubes in the refrigerator to thaw, sort and soak the beans, locate the other ingredients, and find the stew pot. Chop the onions and put them in a tightly covered jar in the refrigerator.

Added touch: Grate fresh Parmesan or Asiago cheese over the soup.

Presentation: Serve this in a tureen or stew pot so you can dish it up at the table. Your children can tell you how much to put in the bowl for them. Be sure to listen—when you are doing the serving, they lose control and won't eat as well unless you pay attention to their directions.

Involving your children: Children can sort the beans. Since you definitely don't want to bite into a rock or a clump of dirt, make a routine of picking the beans over twice. You can take turns being the first one to do the picking. Children can also open the carrots and put them in the pot, cut up the potato, clean the garlic, and break up the spaghetti before you cook it.

Adapting this meal for children: This is generally an easy meal for children to eat, as long as you don't serve it too hot. All the tips for chicken noodle soup apply to minestrone, as well (see page 104).

Variation: To make this recipe meatless, skip the stew beef, use a vegetarian soup base, and add an extra can of beans and 1/4 cup olive oil.

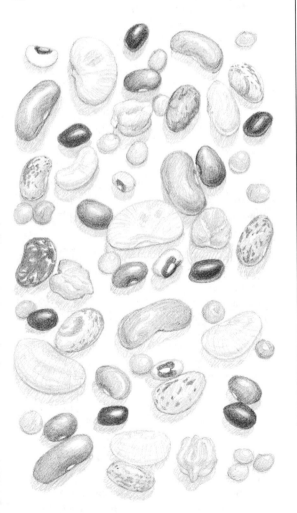

COOKING DRY BEANS
Dry beans need to be sorted, washed, soaked, and then cooked, generally for a couple of hours.

To sort: Spread them out by the handful on a plate and look them over carefully to weed out the rocks, sticks, and blighted beans. Dump the plateful into the cooking pot full of water, and sort through another handful until you are done.

To wash: Let sit in the water for a couple of minutes to loosen any dirt. Stir or swish briskly, then pour through a colander, rinse again by running water through the colander, and then put the beans back in the pot. Cover with water to a couple of inches above the top of the beans.

To soak: You can use the hurry-up or overnight method.

Hurry-up: Bring washed beans to a boil. Boil 1 minute, turn off power, cover and let soak for 1 hour. Drain and replace the water.

Overnight: Let the beans sit in water overnight. The next morning, drain and replace the water.

Presumably, changing the water after you soak beans makes them less gassy. That is, you have less intestinal gas after you eat the beans. Even for your children, intestinal gas is a social, not a physical or medical dilemma. Presumably #2: If you eat beans a lot, gas is less of a problem. I am not sure if this is because your intestine adjusts—or your nose does.

SAUTÉING VEGETABLES
Sautéing vegetables cooks them and gives them extra flavor. The strategy here is to sauté them until done—to the crisp-tender state—and then add them to the soup without cooking them any more. That gives the soup a fresh flavor and more texture than if you simply cooked the vegetables in the soup in the first place. It also adds a step, so you might not think it is worth it. In that case, put the raw vegetables directly into the soup and let them simmer for 20 minutes.

Savory Black Beans and Rice

I like this recipe because it reminds me of my friend June, who taught me that children eat what I think of as challenging food. June came back from several years in Brazil with a craving for black beans and rice and a conviction that this to-me-exotic dish was, to Brazilian children, simply a familiar and well-liked food. Comfort food, you might say. It has since occurred to me that *gourmet* cooking is, in most cases, our attempt to duplicate some other country's everyday cuisine.

When first presented with black food, my children varied in their responses. Curt, always the adventurous one, tried it willingly, immediately loved it and ate it in great quantities. Luke, the skeptical one, took a look and said he didn't like it. One of June's boys said, "Try it, it's really good." Luke tried it and he, too, loved it and ate it in great quantities. Kjerstin said, "No, thank you." On black-bean nights, Kjerstin ate rice.

"The darker the beans, the greater the flavor," said June, an excellent cook. If June said it, it must be so. However, these beans and the liquid they cook in are really black, so they might be a little challenging for your eaters at first. To make this recipe more accessible, you can start out using red beans instead. Red beans may be easier to manage than black ones, especially when used in the variations I have suggested. I do acknowledge that black bean tacos are a little strange.

INGREDIENTS

1 lb dry black beans or
  2 15-oz cans black beans, drained
1/4 lb bacon cut into 1/2-inch pieces
1 large onion, chopped
2 cloves garlic, minced
3/4 tsp dried leaf oregano
1/2 tsp dried rosemary, squashed
1/4 tsp dried thyme
1/4 tsp black pepper
2 dried chilis (whole red peppers)
1 tsp salt

MENU

Savory black beans
Rice
Corn pudding (pages 140-141)
Bread and butter

Orange rounds with parsley sprigs
Add a side dish of cooked sausages (your choice)
  if you have a dedicated meat eater at the table
Milk
Ice cream

METHOD

Summary: Combine cooked bacon and sautéed onion and garlic with presoaked or canned black beans. Season, simmer a couple of hours, and serve.

Wash, soak, and drain *1 pound of dry black beans* (see the "Cooking Dry Beans" box on page 109 for soaking methods) or use *two 15-ounce cans of black beans, drained*.

Cook *1/4 pound of bacon cut into 1/2-inch pieces* until golden brown. Use a slotted spoon to move the bacon into the beans. Use the bacon fat to cook *1 large onion, chopped*, and *2 cloves of garlic, minced*, until clear.

Measure into the beans *3/4 teaspoon dried leaf oregano; 1/2 teaspoon dried rosemary, crushed; 1/4 teaspoon of dried thyme; 1/4 teaspoon black pepper; 2 dried chilis (whole red peppers)*; and *1 teaspoon salt*.

Put enough water into the pot to cover the beans with an inch or two to spare.

Reduce the heat and simmer about 2 hours until the beans are tender. If you started out with canned beans, simmer about 1/2 hour to blend the flavors.

The night before: Wash and soak the beans. Locate the bacon, onion, and garlic. Locate and line up or mix up the spices. Line up the ingredients for the corn pudding.

Presentation: Spruce up the presentation with chopped green onions and a dollop of sour cream. What, you may say, is a dollop? Well, it is a glob. Always attentive to your image, I can tell you that you will seem like a far more sophisticated cook if you use a *dollop* rather than a *glob*.

A dish of orange rounds (peel the oranges and cut crosswise) with snips of parsley is the traditional Brazilian accompaniment to this dish. The sweet, slightly tart flavor complements the beans, and the color and shape dress up the plate.

Involving your children: Children can pick over the beans. Children can also crush the rosemary and measure the spices and herbs into a little dish so they are all ready to put into the beans. They can peel the oranges and tear the parsley into sprigs. An older child can mix up the corn pudding.

Adapting this meal for children: With the menu I have suggested, there are plenty of choices so your children will be able to pick and choose and have a meal even if they don't feel ready to tackle the beans. The food in this meal is all soft and easy to chew, so even your least-experienced eater will be able to manage it, provided she has been previously introduced to all the parts separately. For a younger child, you might want to mash the beans with a fork to make them easier to mouth and swallow. A child who has mastered eating table food with his fingers can pick up the beans and rice and make a lovely meal of it—and a lovely mess as well. Wait to clean up until after the rice dries and it will sweep or vacuum up easily and take no time at all. This is a little spicy, but most children are not put off by that nor does it hurt them. In fact, they like it. Southwestern and Mexican children develop a preference for spicy foods at quite a young age.

Variation: If you don't want to use bacon, substitute 3 tablespoons of butter or cooking oil.

This makes a big recipe, so you will have enough for a second meal. On the cycle menu I suggest black bean soup, which you make by simply adding more water or broth. Other possibilities are refried black beans (mash them and add a little more fat), black bean tacos, and black bean burritos. You get the idea.

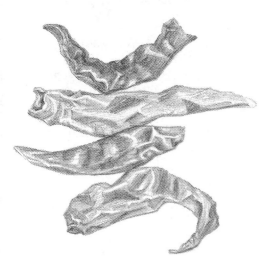

RICE

You have lots of choices with rice, all of them good. The quickest way to cook rice is to use minute or instant rice, which is available in either the white or brown variety. Short-grain or long-grain brown rice, as well as relative newcomers wehani and basmati, are available in the bulk foods case. These are flavorful choices, and since only the hull is removed in the milling process, the B vitamin- and fiber-containing bran and rice germ remain. For regular white rice, converted white rice is a good choice because it is more reliably nutritious that other white rice. In the conversion process, rice is parboiled before milling, which forces the B vitamins in the outer coating into the grain itself, thus increasing the nutritional value of the rice. For *polished enriched rice*, white rice is fortified by spraying with a solution of B vitamins. To conserve nutrients on the surface, don't rinse the rice, and cook it in as little water as possible.

The cooking method, as well as the finished product, depends on the rice you start with. Quick-cooking rice takes about 10 minutes, and directions are specific to the product: read the box. With most other rice, cook rice in double the amount of water (that is, one part rice to two parts water). However, read the directions on the bin at the bulk foods case for the whole-grain rices. Bring the salted water to a boil (1 teaspoon of salt per quart of water), add the rice and stir, cover and turn the heat to low. Converted rice and polished white rice take 20 to 25 minutes, and whole-grain (brown) rice takes about 40 to 45 minutes. If you like whole-grain rice and don't have time to cook it, consider cooking a large batch and freezing it in meal-sized quantities.

Quick-cooking, converted and whole-grain rices tend to be dry, flaky, and easily separated when cooked. Polished rice may be dry or sticky, depending on its origin. *Indian* rice is long grained and easily separated, whereas *Japanese* rice is short grained and sticky when it is cooked.

FLAVORING BEANS

Black beans taste good on their own, but making them savory requires added fat, salt, herbs, and chilis. The fat from 1/4 pound of bacon may seem like a lot, but it is not—it figures out to about two teaspoons of fat per cup of beans. This amount of fat conforms to the magic number of 30 percent or less calories from fat. Do not be tempted to delete the fat; it is important for flavoring the beans and gives them their stick-to-the-ribs quality. If beans are fat-free, they are only carbohydrate and protein, which don't stay with you that long. Herbs provide depth and complexity to flavor, and chilis add a gentle bite. They bite hard, however, if you happen to get one in your mouth! Use them for cooking, then fish them out before you serve.

Marinated Chicken Stir-Fry

To keep stir-fry from turning out like Chinese stew, use a medium-high temperature and cook vegetables quickly and lightly to the crisp side of crisp-tender. You don't need a wok; a large fry pan with a tight-fitting lid will do.

INGREDIENTS

1 1/2 lb chicken breast strips
1/3 cup rice vinegar
3 Tbsp chopped garlic
3 Tbsp soy sauce
2 Tbsp dark-brown sesame oil
1/4 tsp black pepper
1 Tbsp peanut or canola oil
3 cups raw vegetables, including
  carrot sticks
  broccoli florets
  cauliflower pieces
  green or red pepper strips
  whole fresh or frozen snow peas
  zucchini rounds
  mushroom slices
  green onion, crosscuts
  bean sprouts

MENU

Chicken stir-fry
Rice
Fruit in season
Bread or toast
Butter
Milk
Bread pudding (pages 143-144)

METHOD

Summary: Make a marinade and combine it with chicken breast strips. Refrigerate for 24 hours. Stir-fry chicken and vegetables, boil remaining marinade, and add to the cooked dish.

Make a marinade by mixing together *1/3 cup rice vinegar, 3 tablespoons of chopped garlic, 3 tablespoons of soy sauce, 2 tablespoons of dark-brown sesame oil,* and *1/4 teaspoon of black pepper.*

Combine *1 1/2 pounds of chicken breast strips* with marinade in a zip top bag. Refrigerate for 24 hours, turning occasionally.

In a large nonstick skillet or wok, heat *1 tablespoon of peanut or canola oil* on medium high. Empty the chicken into the skillet, brown

it, add a little marinade, and steam for 2 to 3 minutes to finish cooking.

Pour the rest of the marinade from the bag into a saucepan, heat to boiling, and boil gently for 3 minutes (this is to kill any *Salmonella*). Put in a separate dish and serve on the side.

After the chicken is done, remove it from the pan, add 1 to 2 tablespoons of boiled marinade, and begin cooking any or all of the vegetables in the ingredients list. The ones that need to cook longest are at the top of the list. Put those in first. Aim for a total of about 3 cups of vegetables.

Add the cooked chicken to the cooked vegetables, heat, and serve.

RECIPE NOTES

Fast tip: The rice vinegar is a fast tip. It has a sweet flavor and provides the sweetness for this sweet-and-sour marinade. Drain the marinade from the chicken strips by snipping the corner off the zip top bag and letting the marinade drip into a small sauce pan.

Along with the other marvelous helps you can find in the meat section of your grocery store, you can probably find chicken cut up into bite-sized pieces and ready to go into stir-fry. It might be fresh or frozen. Either is a worthwhile investment because it saves you time, energy, and mess.

Two nights before: Refrigerate frozen chicken (in a pan) to thaw.

The night before: Get the chicken started marinating. Locate the vegetables you will use. Clean the vegetables, and perhaps even cut some of them up.

Presentation: Serve the rice and stir-fry in separate dishes so your diners can pick and choose. Until your children become accustomed to this dish, you might even serve the chicken and vegetables separately.

Involving your children: A child can wash vegetables and help break the pieces apart. She can also mix up the marinade.

Adapting this meal for children: Everything at this meal is soft and easy enough to chew for children over age 2. For the toddler, you may want to keep out the harder, chewier bits. The first few times you have this, your children will probably just eat the rice, and that's fine. Then, they may have a small helping and eat just the foods that look familiar. Still fine. Serving food that they may not immediately like gives them an opportunity to learn to quietly push what they don't eat to one side and leave it. Then, they may want to paw through the serving bowl and find what they like. Not fine. That can spoil the dish for others at the table. Children need to learn to respect others' wishes and needs at mealtime as well as their own.

Variation: This marinade also tastes good with pork, which you can buy finely sliced and ready to cook. To give your butcher the opportunity to make your life easier, call the day before you shop and ask to have stir-fry meat ready for you. Develop a relationship with your butcher people. You will find they use much ingenuity to prepare foods ahead of time and get them ready for you to cook.

SESAME OIL
The oil in this recipe is often called "toasted" sesame oil, although it may not say that on the bottle. It is dark brown, comes in a small bottle, and has a pronounced flavor. Experiment. If you think this marinade is too strongly flavored, cut the sesame oil to 1 tablespoon and use peanut oil for the other tablespoon. You can also buy clear sesame oil for general purpose. It is nearly flavorless and behaves about the same as other seed oils.

Jambalaya

Jambalaya is a famous Creole-Cajun dish. The word "jambalaya" is probably derived from "jambon," both Spanish and French for the ham typically used as an ingredient. The "a-la-ya" is probably an African exclamation.

INGREDIENTS

4 slices bacon
1 1/2 lb boneless chicken breasts or combination
    of boneless breasts, legs, and thighs
1 tsp salt
1/4 tsp black pepper
4 tsp Creole seasoning
4 cloves garlic, minced
1 green or red pepper, chopped
1 cup chopped celery
1 large onion, chopped
1/4 cup chopped fresh parsley or
    1 Tbsp dried parsley
1 tsp dried thyme
1 bay leaf
15-oz can chicken broth
15-oz can diced tomatoes
1 1/2 cups uncooked enriched white rice

MENU

Jambalaya with rice
Glazed carrots (page 136)
Sweet-sour cucumber salad (page 134)
Cornbread and butter
Apple custard or fruit in season

METHOD

Summary: Fry and remove the bacon and use the fat to sauté chicken and vegetables. Combine with the seasoning, hot liquids, and rice; bake covered in the oven.

Cut the *4 slices bacon* into 1/4-inch pieces and cook in a large Dutch oven until lightly browned. Set the bacon aside to drain and leave the drippings in the pan for browning the chicken and sautéeing the vegetables.

Wash the chicken pieces, dry with paper towels, cut into roughly 1-ounce chunks, and sprinkle with *1 tsp salt* and *1/4 tsp black pepper*. Cook the chicken in the bacon fat. Add *4 tsp Creole seasoning* to the drippings (being careful not to breath any vapors from the hot spice). Brown the chicken pieces in the seasoned bacon fat. Remove the chicken to drain.

In the remaining fat in the Dutch oven, sauté all together until the onion is clear: *4 cloves*
garlic, minced; 1 green or red pepper, chopped; 1 cup chopped celery; 1 large onion, chopped. Toward the end of cooking, add *1/4 cup chopped fresh parsley or 1 Tbsp dried parsley* and *1 tsp dried thyme.*

While you sauté the chicken and vegetables, heat one *15-oz can chicken broth* and a *15-oz can diced tomatoes* to nearly boiling. Add the browned chicken, bacon, sautéed vegetables, and bay leaf.

Cover and bake at 325 degrees for 30 minutes; check once during baking to add more hot broth or water if the jambalaya begins to dry out. Remove the bay leaf, adjust the salt and pepper, and serve. Put hot sauce or crushed red peppers on the table for any family members who don't think it's hot enough unless they cry.

RECIPE NOTES

The night before: Find the cooking pan and the rice. Locate the spices and put them where you can find them easily. Clean the vegetables, and perhaps even chop them. Put the frozen chicken in the refrigerator to thaw. Find the bacon. Check the recipes for the other menu items and get those ingredients lined up as well.

Presentation: This is a beautiful, hearty, colorful dish. Bring it to the table in a hearty-looking pan, like your Dutch oven.

Involving your children: Children can wash and dice the vegetables, measure the rice, and open the cans of broth and tomatoes.

Adapting this meal for children: While this dish is mildly seasoned, it is seasoned. Given the seasoning and the mixture of a number of foods, this may be a challenging dish for your children. However, Cajun children eat it enthusiastically. Your children may, too, or they may need time to get accustomed to the mixtures and the seasonings. Eating bread or drinking milk with spicy dishes helps cool the burning sensation out of the mouth. Fruit with the meal gives a cooling side dish.

Make the meal more accessible by cooking the rice plain, then combining all the other ingredients as a sauce and serving separately. Children can generally manage the rice even if the jambalaya itself is too challenging.

Variation: Make ham and chicken jambalaya. Cut the amount of chicken down to a pound, and add 1 cup diced ham just before you put it in the oven. You can also use shrimp in jambalaya, either alone, as a substitute for chicken, or with the chicken and/or the ham.

I put glazed carrots on the menu because they are easy to like and give a sweet contrast to the spicy flavor of the main dish. The traditional but more challenging vegetable with this meal is greens. For experienced eaters, try substituting **Greens and Bacon** (page 139) for the carrots, then add back the sweet flavor by using **Sweet-Sour Cucumber Salad** (pages 134-135) or simply have some sweet pickles.

Fried Fish

Fried fish is last on the list of recipes because it is the most difficult. While restaurants make it seem so simple, it is tricky to fry food well and safely. I debated about whether to include this recipe and finally decided to leave it in for its teaching value. Fried food, like other food that is relatively high in fat, is perfectly acceptable some of the time. Anything can be good for you—or not so good. It all depends on the dose and frequency. You can overdose on *water*, if you drink too much of it.

My developmental editor, Paulette Sharkey, says she would never fry fish. When it's time for fried fish, says Paulette, it is time to eat out or stop at the seafood market for some of theirs. Well, I can understand that. It makes a mess and it stinks up the house. In Wisconsin, restaurants and churches have wonderful fish fries on Friday nights, a heritage of our German-Catholic forebears. However, like a lot of foods, I like fried fish better if I make it at home, so I think it is worth the mess and the smell.

If you fry even once in a while, you need to know what you are doing. Frying involves using relatively large amounts of fat, heated to a relatively high temperature. That can be dangerous. Use a fresh liquid oil that has a relatively high smoke point, such as peanut, soybean, cottonseed, or safflower oil. These oils have smoke points that are 60 to 100 degrees higher than cooking temperatures. Food needs to be fried at 350 degrees.

The smoke point is very close to the point at which oil bursts into flames. If you use fresh oil and keep the cooking temperature around 350 degrees, you shouldn't have trouble with fire. However, to put out an oil fire, slap the lid on the pan, use a fire extinguisher, or sprinkle salt or baking soda on the fire. *Don't* use water—it will make the fire spread. You can prevent grease fires by not reusing fats. Even one use of fat at a high temperature can decrease by 100 degrees the point at which it will burst into flame.

To have the coating adhere well to the fish, make sure the eggs are cold and the fish is dry. The fat should be about 1/2-inch deep in the pan so that the fish will float in the hot oil rather than being immersed in it.

INGREDIENTS

2 lb boneless fish fillets: cod, halibut, whitefish,
  turbo, pollack, or your choice

1/2 tsp pepper
1/2 tsp dried thyme
1/2 tsp dried oregano
1/2 tsp ground ginger
1/2 tsp onion powder
1/2 tsp garlic powder
1/2 cup flour
2 eggs
2 Tbsp cold water
1/2 lb saltines

MENU

Fried fish
Tartar sauce
Baked potatoes with sour cream
Green salad
Fruit in season
Bread or toast
Butter
Milk
Cherry cobbler (page 142)

METHOD

Summary: Season the fish fillets with the herb and spice mixture, and then dip fish pieces three times: first into seasoned flour, then into egg, and finally into cracker crumbs. Fry in hot oil.

Thaw *2 pounds of boneless fish: cod, halibut, whitefish, turbo, pollack, or your choice.* Wash in cold water, cut into helping-sized pieces, drain, and pat dry.

Make an herb and spice mix by combining *1/2 teaspoon pepper, 1/2 teaspoon dried thyme, 1/2 teaspoon dried oregano, 1/2 teaspoon ground ginger, 1/2 teaspoon onion powder, and 1/2 teaspoon garlic powder.* Sprinkle half of the mixture over the fish.

Get out three shallow bowls for dipping the fish. In the first, combine the remaining herb and spice mixture with *1/2 cup of flour.* In the second bowl, thoroughly blend *2 eggs* with *2 tablespoons of cold water.* In the third bowl, spread cracker crumbs that you have purchased or made. (In the blender, blend *1/2 pound of saltines* on high until they become fine crumbs. It's best to use regular salted saltines with salted tops.)

Begin heating the oil so it is hot by the time the fish is coated. Frying temperature for fish is 350 degrees. To gauge the temperature, use an electric frying pan set to 350 degrees, use a frying or candy thermometer, or test the temperature with part of the egg-cracker coating. The oil will be hot enough when the coating floats, sizzles, and slowly browns. If it brown immediately, it is too hot.

To coat the fish, dip each piece in the flour, then in the egg, then in the cracker crumbs. As each piece is coated, immediately place it in the hot oil. Use a pancake turner or serving tongs to keep your fingers safe. Fry until bubbles start to appear on the upper surface of the fish, then gently turn one time only. The fish will be done when it is white and flakes easily, about 10 minutes per inch of thickness. If fish is thinner than one inch, fry it only briefly on the second side, just to cook the egg coating. Drain the fried fish on paper towels.

RECIPE NOTES

The night before: Find the potatoes and wash them. Wash the greens, spin them, and return them to the refrigerator, in the spinner, to crisp.

You can purchase already-prepared tartar sauce. I prefer the flavor and texture of one I make quickly myself, with 1/2 cup Miracle Whip, 2 to 3 tablespoons of sweet pickle relish, 2 to 3 tablespoons of dried onion flakes, and 2 to 3 tablespoons of dried parsley flakes. Mix it together (I use a jar) and add extra milk to make it soupy (hydrating the dried onion and parsley thickens it). Let it stand in the refrigerator for a half hour and add more milk if it needs it. You can keep this tartar sauce for a month or two. It can be mixed with tuna to make great tuna salad sandwiches.

Presentation: Serve the fish on a pretty platter and garnish with lemon wedges.

Involving your children: Children can break and beat the eggs, wash and pierce the baked potatoes, spin the salad greens, and tear them into bite-sized pieces.

Adapting this meal for children: Children generally do well with this meal because they like fried food. Choose boneless fish. Dress the salad lightly so they can eat it with their fingers. Show your child how to mash some butter or sour cream into the potato.

Variation: This fish warms up great in a toaster oven or in the microwave. Have it again for lunch the next day or make it into a sandwich with lettuce and tartar sauce.

Try making sautéed fish for a tasty variation on fried fish that takes less fat, less heat, and

makes less of a mess. Dip washed, drained, and blotted fillets in a mixture of 1 1/2 teaspoons of spice mixture (from the fried fish recipe above or from the **Herb-Baked Fish** on pages 92-93), 1/2 teaspoon of salt, and 1/2 cup of flour. Sauté in 1 to 2 tablespoons of butter in a nonstick frying pan at low-medium to medium temperature until the fish is nicely browned on both sides and flakes easily. Serve immediately.

PEANUT OIL

I hesitated about recommending peanut oil because some children are allergic to peanuts. However, the Food Allergy Network says that peanut oil doesn't carry the peanut allergen unless it is cold-pressed. (To contact the Food Allergy Network, check their Web site at www.foodallergy.org or call 800/929-4040.) Peanut oil is really the best for frying. Heat doesn't break it down easily, and it browns well. Butter burns too easily, margarine breaks down, and hydrogenated vegetable oils are out of favor because they are high in trans fatty acids, which aren't good for you. Lard is good and it browns well, but not everyone likes its smell.

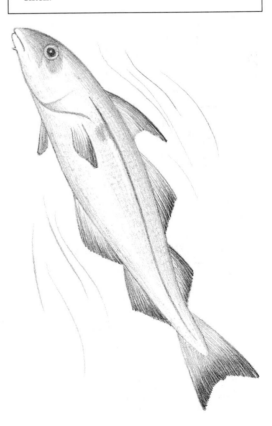

Grab-and-Dump Meals

The early menus in chapter 5 are so simple that it may be hard to imagine scaling them down, but it can be done. Every cook needs a few meals to keep on hand that require little or no thought or preparation to throw together quickly. Here are my ideas; you undoubtedly will have your own. These are real meals; you can serve them and feel you have done your job of getting a meal on the table.

Consider these possibilities, all of which are nutritious:

- Hot dogs, canned baked beans, and potato chips—with ice cream for dessert.

- Macaroni and cheese (packaged Kraft dinner) and canned green beans. You can put tuna in the Kraft dinner to increase the protein.

- Bologna sandwiches with lettuce and mayonnaise, canned grapefruit slices, store-bought cookies for dessert.

- Tuna salad sandwiches or hot tuna sandwiches on a bun (foil-wrap tuna salad and cheese on a bun, bake 15 minutes at 325 degrees), canned peaches.

- Canned "hearty" soups with oyster crackers (read the label to find ones that have at least 5 to 7 grams of protein per serving), ice cream for dessert.

- Canned beef stew with Bisquick dumplings or canned biscuits, canned fruit.

- Canned spaghetti dinners, like SpaghettiOs (aggressively orange and slippery, these are more popular with children than with adults), pineapple cottage cheese salad, instant pudding for dessert.

- Corned beef hash, poached eggs, canned apricots.

- Rice meal from the recipe on the box of herb-seasoned rice or minute rice (they tell you the protein to add), canned fruit or vegetable.

- Boxed bean dishes, like red beans and rice. Add sausage if you like; put together a dish of grapefruit sections and orange rounds.

- Pancakes with syrup or applesauce-yogurt topping and sausages on the side.

- Pancakes with chicken or hamburger gravy.

- Toaster waffles and scrambled eggs, orange juice.

Prepackaged "Convenience" Meals

Prepackaged meals jump-start your cooking by giving you ideas and gathering up the ingredients for you, and they may require reduced cooking times. For instance, if you have a package of Tuna Helper on your shelf, you can lean on the cupboard door and get an idea for dinner. All the ingredients (except the tuna, of course) are pulled together in one place so all you have to do is find the pan, the colander, the tuna, and the water. If you were to use the recipe in chapter 5, you would also have to find the noodles and the cream of mushroom soup. Tuna Helper costs only about 10 percent more than the tuna noodle casserole you make yourself, and it has about 10 percent more salt, still a reasonable amount. You still might want to add more noodles as well as more vegetables. Is it worth it to buy the mix? You decide. Only you know how you feel when you are leaning against the cupboard door seeking dinner. If you have gone into survival mode, rounding up noodles and mushroom soup may be more than you can bear.

Of course, the preassembled idea can be taken to a ridiculous extreme, such as in the prepackaged bowl, spoon, cereal and milk I saw in the dairy case the other day. I suppose that could be helpful when you are out camping or on the road and looking for a quick breakfast at a picnic bench, particularly since the milk is processed at ultrahigh temperatures so you don't have to refrigerate it until after it's opened. However, the advertising implies that you can just hand these to your kids in the morning and expect them to eat while you do something else. That's like feeding a dog. It takes the nurturing out of feeding.

The same is true of the special kids' meals that the food industry promotes. The idea with kids' meals is that you feed your child a separate, special dinner. With these products, the food industry is pandering to consumer research that says family meals are going the way of the covered wagon. Ironically, with all the advertising, parents get the idea that it is okay to feed kids this way, whereupon advertisers promote the concept all the more. Not a good idea. Handing kids food takes the loving out of feeding, and I don't recommend it.

However, you have my blessing to buy any prepackaged meals *for the whole family* that take your fancy. The important issue is having family meals, and doing what you have to in order to make those family meals happen. Using prepackaged meals will cost you extra, but, surprisingly, not always that much extra. Buying mixes is *certainly* less expensive than eating out. The "helper" mixes, as I said earlier, cost about 10 percent more than preparing your own comparable dish. The freeze-dried soup starters cost about 20 percent more than making a comparable soup from scratch, and they save time and trouble—they take just a few minutes to mix up and 90 minutes to simmer until done. Frozen vegetable and vegetable-and-pasta mixes cost about 20 percent more than such dishes you assemble yourself; They give you menu ideas and save some time and trouble. Of course, there are also the frozen dinners where everything is included: you just bake or microwave.

The Generic Casserole

Nutritionally, a casserole is like an ordinary sandwich, which gives you two slices of bread, 2 to 3 ounces of protein (poultry, fish, peanut butter, cheese, etc.), about 2 teaspoons of fat (butter, mayonnaise, or margarine), and maybe some vegetables (lettuce, tomato, pickles, etc.). From a serving of casserole you hope for the same: 2 servings from the bread group, 2 to 3 ounces of meat, 2 teaspoons of fat, and some vegetables. Prepackaged casseroles, soups, and mixes are good meal substitutes if they give you the nutritional equivalent of a sandwich.

Like all of our children who learned to run the day after they learned to walk, you are now ready to turn cooking skills into *improvising*! You can turn that bit of sandwich-equivalent information into a Generic Casserole formula that you can use to throw together your own casseroles from whatever you happen to have on hand. You can also use it to evaluate other recipes, to determine whether they are likely to work.

Generic Casserole is *not* the alarming dish that shows up on the table after someone cleans out the refrigerator. It is a potentially new and delightful creation. It may become the dish your children fondly remember when someone says to them, "What food do you think of when you remember eating meals at home?"

THE GENERIC CASSEROLE FORMULA
Each helping of casserole gives the following:

2 ounces of meat, poultry, fish, dry beans,
   eggs, or nuts
1 cup of bread, cereal, rice, or pasta
   (2 servings on the Food Guide Pyramid)
A liquid of some sort: concentrated soup,
   canned tomatoes, white sauce
About 1/4 teaspoon of salt
About 2 servings of fat

To make Generic Casserole, first you have to figure out how much raw food to cook to make a helping. Well, actually, first you have to figure out what a *helping* is. Remember that a helping is a unit of measurement, like a gallon of gas. It is not a prescription but a neutral term without any value judgments attached. It's fine to eat three helpings, if that's what you need to get filled up. Some cars are gas guzzlers, some get 50 miles to the gallon.

The starch for Generic Casserole: Figure that a portion of the bread, cereal, rice, and pasta group, after it has been cooked, is—tah-dah!—1 cup!

Coming now to the crux of the matter, *how much is that before it is cooked?*

Starchy Ingredients: What Cooks to Make a Cup?
1/3 cup of uncooked rice
4 ounces of uncooked macaroni
4 ounces of uncooked noodles
3 to 4 ounces of uncooked spaghetti
8 ounces of potato
1/4 cup of dry beans

Now, the alert reader, to steal Dave Barry's words, will note that *potatoes and beans are not cereals!* Well, who cares? They are starchy, and that is what we are after for our Generic Casserole: a source of complex carbohydrate to mix in with the protein. In scalloped potatoes and ham, you use potatoes for the starch. In baked beans and ham, you use beans for the starch. You'll get a higher protein casserole if you use meat and then cooked dried beans for starch, but it won't hurt you.

The Protein for Generic Casserole: Coming to another crux of the matter, if you will allow me the liberty of two cruxes, what about the protein? To answer that question, it is easier to talk about ounces than servings. For Generic

Casserole you need about 12 ounces of cooked meat equivalent, or about 1 pound raw. Ounce-sized portions of high-protein foods are given in the following list. Each contains about 7 grams of protein. Notice that the ever-versatile beans show up yet again, this time as a source of protein.

Protein Ingredients: What Counts as an Ounce?
1 ounce of cooked meat, poultry, or fish
1 egg
1 ounce of hard cheese (like cheddar)
1/2 cup of cooked dried beans, peas, or lentils (1/4 cup dry)
2 to 3 tablespoons of nuts or seeds
1/4 cup of cottage cheese
2 tablespoons of peanut butter
1/3 cup of tofu

The fat for Generic Casserole: By now you may have figured out that you are getting lessons in *food composition*, and that is all to the good. Knowing about food composition can set you free. Knowing about fat can *really* set you free. To talk about substituting one fat for another, it is easiest to think in terms of equivalents for a teaspoon of butter or margarine.

A teaspoon of butter or margarine gives about 5 grams of fat, a modest amount. So does 3 tablespoons of half-and-half, a tablespoon of sour cream, and 1/3 cup of cream of mushroom soup. You can estimate fat by reading the nutrition label. It will tell you how much *total fat* there is in a serving and give it to you in grams. Amounts of fatty foods that give 5 grams of fat per serving are summarized below. No, I am not turning on you and becoming a fat-gram policewoman, but knowing the numbers and what they mean will give you more freedom in your food selection. The truth is in the details. How do you think I got to the point where I can give my blessings to almost anything? Just look at how much half and half or sour cream you can substitute for a teaspoon of butter!

Fatty Foods: What Substitutes for What?
1 teaspoon of butter or margarine
1 teaspoon of cooking oil or solid shortening
1 teaspoon of mayonnaise
1 tablespoon of Miracle Whip
1 tablespoon of cream cheese
2 tablespoons of Neufchâtel (looks and tastes like cream cheese)
3 tablespoons of half and half

1 tablespoon of whipping cream
1 tablespoon of sour cream
3 tablespoons of low-fat sour cream
1/2 cup whole milk
3 tablespoons of medium white sauce or gravy
1 tablespoon of hollandaise sauce

Isn't this fun? My nutritionist friends will tell me it's a little odd to put whole milk on this list. Clearly whole milk has more protein in it than other fatty foods, but I want you to know that 1/2 cup of whole milk has the same amount of fat as a teaspoon of butter and gives you another way of adding fat to your mashed potatoes and cream soups.

In view of all the hysteria about fat and the conviction that *less is better*, you may be tempted to forgo fat altogether or to substitute the fat-free versions of say, margarine, sour cream, or mayonnaise. *Don't do it!* You will ruin the taste and texture of the recipe and discourage yourself from being a cook. Fat makes food taste good and contributes to browning and texture. If you don't get fat at home, you will have to sneak off frequently to get a grease fix at the local fast-food place. Most of us need those fixes from time to time, but if yours get too frequent, something is the matter with your strategies for making meals at home.

The following table lists the possibilities for your very own Generic Casserole. Combining these foods in the amounts suggested will give you about six helpings.

You will notice that some of the liquid ingredients, like cheese sauce or mushroom soup, add fat. Others, like tomato sauce or broth, do not. Generally, that isn't a problem because most of the protein ingredients have fat in them. However, if you are making a casserole using only beans as the protein ingredient, you could end up with a fat-free main dish, which is not good. Fat-free food doesn't taste good, and it gets digested quickly and leaves you hungry very soon. To get enough fat in an all-bean dish, add one serving of fat for each 1/2 cup of cooked beans. For the Generic Casserole formula, you would add 12 teaspoons of butter or cooking oil. Since 3 teaspoons = 1 tablespoon and 4 tablespoons = 1/4 cup, you would add 1/4 cup fat to the recipe. This startling amount figures out to only 1 teaspoon of fat per 1/2 cup of beans.

GENERIC CASSEROLE		
Select one item from each column. Combine in a 2-quart casserole dish, bake at 350° for 30 to 45 minutes. Makes six helpings.		
Protein ingredients	**Liquid ingredients**	**Starchy ingredients**
1 lb raw weight 12 oz cooked weight, or 1 1/2 to 2 cups cubed or chunked	1 1/2 to 2 cups	6 cups

Tuna fish
Canned meat or chicken
Cooked meat or poultry:
  Chicken
  Ground beef
  Sausage or sausages
  Beef
  Pork
  Turkey
  Ham
Hard cooked eggs
Dried beans or peas
  (3 cups cooked
  or 1 1/2 cups dry)
Cheese
	Broth or bouillon
	Milk
	Cheese sauce
	Canned tomatoes
	Cream soups:
	  Mushroom
	  Potato
	  Broccoli
	  Celery
	  Chicken
	  Cheese
	Tomato soup
	Tomato sauce
	Shredded cheese plus milk
	Evaporated milk
		Bread, cubed
		Cooked rice
		Cooked macaroni
		Cooked spaghetti
		Cooked noodles
		Cooked barley
		Cooked bulgur
		Cooked potatoes

Cooking Classes

Cooking classes can inspire you, give you support for your commitment to cooking, dignify your art, teach you shortcuts, and help you find like-minded people. What could be better? Look for cooking classes at vocational schools, cookware stores, and cookware departments in department stores. Sometimes grocery stores give cooking classes as part of a promotion for certain foods. Cooking classes for kids are fun and helpful, too, if you remember that the point is not to teach your child how to cook dinner *for* you, but rather how to cook dinner *with* you.

University extension, technical schools, and community colleges offer cooking classes—look them up in your city or county telephone directory. "We promote the Food Guide Pyramid," say my friends in these programs. "How can you recommend our programs and still disagree with what we teach?" I recommend them because I know they have far more to offer than teaching the rules—they teach cooking, planning, budgeting, and shopping. Some programs even go into homes to teach food skills.

Cookbooks

Where does this leave you? Do you want to learn more about cooking, or have you had enough? With what you have learned in these two chapters, and with what you *will* learn in chapter 7, you will have an adequate and flexible tool kit to manage family dinners. I encourage you to keep working with these tools until you feel comfortable with them and can make a few meals without much stress and strain. Work up to planning and cooking at least a week of menus at a time. It will help you even more if you can manage 3 to 4 weeks at a time. The cycle menu idea may please you, or you may want to start over with your recipes, food advertisements, and menu requests in hand each time you plan.

If you want to learn more, the choices are vast, but we can narrow them down a bit. For books that deal with cooking at about the same level as these chapters, you might consider *Desperation Dinners* by Beverly Mills and Alicia Ross, or *Now You're Cooking* by Elaine Korn. Written by authors of a food column of the same name, *Desperation Dinners* emphasizes "home-cooked meals for frantic families in 20 minutes flat." In *Now You're Cooking,*

Elaine Korn identifies failure to cook as a bad habit, offers "everything a beginner needs to know to start cooking today," and begins by teaching how to make egg salad. How-to-cook books for older children make great primers for adults as well as being a good introduction to cooking for youngsters. Micah Pulleyn and Sarah Bracken's *Kids in the Kitchen* and Marion Cunningham's *Cooking with Children* are both good choices in this category.

A step up from the beginner books—quite a big step—are the standard, all-purpose cookbooks, like *Better Homes and Gardens, Betty Crocker*, and *The Fannie Farmer Cookbook*. It helps to have at least one all-purpose cookbook on hand for looking up obscure questions like "How do you make muffins so they don't have tunnels?" or "How do you poach an egg?"

Still another step up, into books that emphasize fine cuisine rather than straightforward good cooking, consider *The New York Times Cookbook*. As editor Craig Claiborn comments in his preface, "Cooking is one of the simplest and most gratifying of the arts, but to cook well, one must love and respect food." Also consider *Vegetarian Cooking for Everyone* by Deborah Madison, who observes that in her cooking classes, "many students regard cooking as a quirky process that's hard to grasp. Unnerved, they fail to notice that . . . cooking is guided by common sense and even logic." In the cuisine category, my regional favorite is Suzanne Breckenridge and Marjorie Snyder's *Wisconsin Herb Cookbook*, which includes "recipes to challenge and recipes to start you on your way to confident (herb) cooking." The

authors tell how to grow herbs as well as how to cook with them. They comment enticingly, "Herbs have a sneaky way of becoming an obsession when given half a chance."

I feel the same way about cooking. If you have been bitten by the food and cooking bug, you might want to challenge yourself in another direction, with a couple of books that are for the scientifically curious. Shirley Corriher, author of *CookWise*, bills herself, justifiably, as a "culinary food sleuth." A research biochemist, food scientist, and accomplished chef, Corriher gives recipes that "not only please the palate but demonstrate the roles of ingredients and techniques." Corriher accessibly teaches the science of food and cooking.

If you like your science straight, with no recipes, also check out Harold McGee's classic, *On Food and Cooking: The Science and Lore of the Kitchen*. McGee's book blends culinary lore, scientific explanation, and historical and literary anecdotes to examine the history and makeup of food, as well as what happens when it's cooked. McGee's huge, fact-packed book makes a great reference for anyone who has wondered about food. It would be a wonderful resource for a teacher who wants to inject fascination into the food lessons presented in chapter 10, "Raising a Healthy Eater in Your Community."

Even though we have been talking about other authors, our own lessons on food and cooking aren't done yet. In the next chapter, "Enjoy Vegetables and Fruits," you'll find still more easy and nutritious ways of making your meals satisfying and delicious.

Expand Your Repertoire!

- Don't try to trick children into eating fruits and vegetables, but rather help them learn to enjoy them by offering a wide variety of good-tasting choices.
- Feel free to use fresh, frozen, or canned vegetables and fruits. Canned or frozen varieties are often as nutritious as fresh, and sometimes are more so. They are also more convenient and have a long shelf life.
- The recipes in this chapter will help you and your family develop a healthy appreciation for a wide variety of fruits and vegetables.

CHAPTER
7
ENJOY VEGETABLES AND FRUITS

In the now-I've-heard-everything-category, I received an e-mail the other day that was pushing fruit and vegetable gummi bears. According to the enthusiastic dispatch, "Each little gummi bear actually consists of a serving and a half of selected vine-ripened vegetables and is flavored with real fruit extract. Children who refuse to eat their vegetables may benefit from these exceptional gummi bears."

Well, I wouldn't argue that these gummi bears aren't exceptional, if by "exceptional" you mean "odd," "peculiar" or "strange." However, much more important than getting vegetables into your child today is helping your child enjoy vegetables for all his tomorrows. Can't you just see him growing up and going out to the work site or to the classroom, and at lunchtime pulling out his gummi bears?

It isn't good to trick children into eating. Come to think of it, it isn't possible. Children are not stupid. If you trot out vegetable-laced gummi bears, they will know something is up and will react in a way that you won't enjoy. Children don't need to have their food look like toys. They are capable of learning and growing, even in the area of eating vegetables. If you cook vegetables, offer them, and enjoy them, your children will learn to eat and enjoy them as well.

No, I didn't keep the address of where you can get those gummi bears, so don't ask me. If you want to go that direction, you are on your own. However, if you want to enrich your food environment with vegetables and fruits, read on. We are going to *enjoy* vegetables and

fruits. The recipes in this chapter will *enhance* rather than *disguise* them.

Use Fresh, Canned, Frozen, and Dried Vegetables and Fruits

Use a variety of vegetables and fruits. Your children are more likely to learn to appreciate them if you offer many different choices over time. Also, feel free to use canned, frozen, and dried vegetables and fruits as well as fresh. Processed varieties are at least as nutritious as fresh if not more so.

FRESH VEGETABLES AND FRUITS
Some fresh vegetables and fruits are standbys of many menus: Potatoes, onions, carrots, celery, greens for salads, bananas, apples, oranges. Other fresh vegetables and fruits are available in a more limited way, but they come canned, frozen, or even dried, so you have a choice: Consider corn, peaches, or mushrooms. Most times, it is a matter of choice. Some people emphasize fresh produce over other kinds because they prefer the taste, texture, and look.

When vegetables are in season, why not buy and use fresh? There is nothing like an August meal of fresh sliced tomatoes, corn on the cob, and cucumbers in sour cream or a sweet-sour dilled cucumber salad. When fruits and vegetables first come to market, they taste so good, you don't even miss the main dish. Ah, the luxury of a bowl of fresh strawberries in June! Makes your mouth water, doesn't it?

Fresh vegetables and fruits carry memories in a way that no other food does. I got hives the spring I was 4 years old from eating too many strawberries. A coven of aunts, feeling sorry for me because my mother was away for a few days, plied me with strawberries. Every June, I get nostalgic about the time we were in the Yakima Valley in Washington State when the bing cherries were ripe. We ate bing cherries by the carton. Luckily, no one got hives. I'm sure you have your own examples. To make more memories, consult the discussion about seasonal fresh vegetables and fruits in chapter 9 (pages 171-172).

Fresh vegetables and fruits are not necessarily the most nutritious. It depends on how they have been handled between the farm and your plate. Produce loses nutrients every day it travels from the farm to the supermarket to your table. Losses become even more dramatic if the produce is mishandled in any way, say, if it is transported in a hot truck or stored unrefrigerated. Even if "fresh" food is refrigerated, if it sits for a few days before you eat it, nutrients can decrease significantly.

However, I'm not saying that you should stop eating fresh vegetables and fruits. Even if the quality has degenerated a bit, you can make up for nutritional losses by eating a variety. Eat fresh, frozen, and canned and even dried vegetables and fruits. What one lacks, the other will offer.

CANNED VEGETABLES AND FRUITS

Now you know better, but if you thought fresh produce was best, you had lots of company. Eight out of 10 consumers believe that fresh is superior to processed and that frozen foods are more nutritious than canned foods. Some believe that canned vegetables contain less fiber than fresh. The fact is that canned vegetables and fruits provide the same fiber and more of certain nutrients than their fresh or frozen counterparts. Most nutrients survive the canning process well and are stable during the 1-year shelf life of canned foods. Some vitamin C, folate, and other water-soluble nutrients dissolve in the cooking liquid and can be recovered by using the liquid to make soups, sauces, and gravies.

Canned produce can be nutritionally superior to fresh because produce for canning is picked at the peak of ripeness, when nutrient content is at its highest, and rushed through processing immediately after harvest. Packers strive for the best-tasting, best-looking food that will arrive in your kitchen as appetizing as possible. With vegetables and fruits, being tasty and appetizing goes right along with preserving vitamins and minerals.

Canned vegetables and fruits have a distinctive taste and texture, and they are wonderfully easy to keep on hand and convenient to use. I know a food scientist who loves canned peas and prefers them to the frozen or fresh variety. I love canned corn, both the whole kernel and cream-style variety, and I appreciate the convenience of opening a can and warming it up. I could not live without canned tomatoes and appreciate the variety of canned-tomato products. Canning methods are being refined, and the resulting products are crisper and have less water in them than those canned using traditional methods. As I write this, you can buy Del Monte Freshcut corn and green beans, and they are wonderful. You can buy diced and crushed tomatoes and tomatoes with Mexican, Italian, and Cajun flavorings.

If you hesitate to use canned vegetables and fruits, it may be because you have heard they are not good for you. Bosh. All the nutrients of vegetables and fruits are in the can. Canned vegetables have salt added to them strictly for taste, as consumers prefer the taste of salt. The amount is modest and reasonable: about 200 to 300 milligrams per 1/2 cup. In chapter 5, I suggested that about 250 milligrams of sodium per 1/2 cup of food is standard and tastes right to most people. The problem with canned vegetables and fruits has been political, not nutritional.

The difficulty arose when one bureaucracy tried to talk to another. The U.S. Food and Drug Administration (FDA) set out to do its labeling job. The task was to define the word "healthy" to conform to the Dietary Guidelines of the U.S. Department of Agriculture and U.S. Department of Health and Human Services. The FDA decided that the word *healthy* could appear on a food label only if certain conditions were met: (1) the food had to be low in sugar, fat, and saturated fat; (2) it had to meet limits for sodium and cholesterol; and (3) it had to contain at least 10 percent of certain vitamins and minerals. Such standards ruled out scallions, iceberg lettuce, mushrooms, and a host of other foods.

More recently, the FDA recognized that vegetables and fruits in general have a place in a healthy diet and allowed all produce as well as canned fruit to be called healthy. However, because they contained the dreaded sodium, regularly canned vegetables still can't be called healthy. Despite their considerable nutritional value, and despite the greater nutritional importance of eating vegetables than avoiding sodium, canned vegetables are still condemned by the nutrition enthusiasts as being too high in sodium. The Dietary Guidelines imply that target sodium levels should be 2,400 milligrams per day, a level that is more appropriate for nutritional *medicine* than for normal healthy people and is too low to allow general use of canned vegetables. And *that*, in turn, is a nutritional mistake of the sort that comes about when we base our standards on food avoidance rather than food seeking. The standard for what constitutes healthy food is so unrealistic that even these wonderfully nutritious foods can't qualify!

These convoluted standards are bad, particularly for low-income people, who are most likely to use canned vegetables and fruits. Like the rest of the population, low-income people have learned their nutrition lessons. They have learned that what they can afford to feed their families, keep on hand, and *prefer* is inferior. In an article about hunger and food insecurity, a Cornell University researcher quoted a low-income mother who lamented, "I buy canned vegetables to substitute for a vegetable. You can get them cheaper, but I don't like them. I rinse them, but I still don't like the thought of it." Making people feel this way isn't good nutritional policy, it's nutritional bullying.

Many low-income people walk to the grocery store, and because they're on foot, they may have to walk to a higher-priced neighborhood grocery store where food is more expensive and fresh produce is especially expensive. They don't have the money for a freezer to store frozen vegetables and fruits. So they buy canned and feel sorry because they think they aren't doing the best for their families. Making people feel bad about eating perfectly good food doesn't help. It harms.

If it's not already apparent to you, I'll tell you that I am angry. It bothers me enormously when nutritional politics undermine people's relationship with food and make it hard for them to enjoy their eating. You wouldn't think anybody could get so worked up about canned vegetables, would you? I am a little surprised

myself. But getting down off my soapbox and back to the issue at hand, I recommend that you use canned vegetables and fruits if you like them. Use them, secure in the knowledge that you are doing something good for your family.

You can buy canned fruits that are packed in light syrup or in fruit juice, but it isn't necessary, and they generally cost extra. The fruit juice in canned fruit is generally concentrated grape juice; it has doubtful nutritional value and is actually high in sugar. It isn't necessary to avoid regular sugar syrup. The syrup makes the fruit taste good and preserves its shape and texture. Sugar helps fruits and vegetables retain their texture longer by slowing down the breakdown of what are known as pectic substances, the glue that holds cell walls together. Sugar syrup on fruit pulls water out of the fruit and maintains the "glue" and therefore the structure of the cell walls. In canned fruit, water comes out of the fruit rather than sugar going in. As a consequence, a canned peach has about as much sugar as a fresh peach. The syrup is extra. A tablespoon of syrup on canned fruits gives about 50 calories. If that 50 calories worries you, you don't have to eat the syrup.

Packers use sugar and salt the way good cooks have always used sugar and salt—to make food taste good, to improve the texture, and to make it appealing. Most of us, children especially, are not on such nutritional tightropes that we can't afford a little extra salt and sugar, especially if it comes hooked onto nutritious, delicious vegetables and fruits. So settle down, and I will too.

FROZEN VEGETABLES AND FRUIT

Like their canned counterparts, frozen vegetables and fruits are processed at the peak of ripeness, freshness, and nutritional value. As long as they are held throughout the storage period at zero degrees (Fahrenheit) or below, the food will stay nutritious and of high quality.

In most cases, vegetables are frozen without added salt. Lima beans, peas, mixed vegetables, and corn have a light salt brine to keep them from sticking together during freezing.

Frozen vegetables taste more like their fresh counterparts and are a breeze to cook and serve—there is no cleaning or sorting. Just put them in a covered pot, boil or microwave, doctor them up however you want to, and *voilà!* Dinner is served.

There are lots of products in the frozen vegetable case that producers call "value-added." That is, they have something done to them that will make you willing to part with more money to buy them. Potatoes are a helpful value-added frozen vegetable that let you make fried potatoes or hash browns in your own oven. Some stores carry frozen chopped onions, which taste pretty good and save time and tears. With other value-added vegetables, the helpfulness is less clear. Vegetables with sauces save you the time of *making* the sauce, but often you get more sauce and less vegetable than if you made your own sauce and bought the vegetable plain. Mixed vegetables with added pasta give you the idea and assemble the ingredients for you, but often the combination is a simple one and you pay extra for it. Meal starters, both with and without pasta, have you "just" add the protein, which is the most expensive ingredient. Only you can decide if the value-added feature is valuable to you. Periodically, when you have a little extra time, it is worth exploring the frozen vegetable case to find any new products that can help you—for a price you are willing to pay

Keep in mind that if you know the rudiments of planning and cooking, many of the products will be unnecessary. Manufacturers are increasingly catering to people who don't know the first thing about cooking. Many people plan dinner by pulling something out of the freezer. There is nothing wrong with that, but when you know how to cook and plan, you have more choices. Often, it is so easy to duplicate a manufacturer's ingredients and recipes at home that you may not feel you need to buy the product.

DRIED VEGETABLES AND FRUITS

Ah, now you put me to the test! What are some dried vegetables? Well, potatoes, of course. Mashed potatoes are dried, and so are scalloped potato mixes. Most dried vegetables are freeze-dried—you can tell because they are paper-dry and lightweight. Freeze-dried vegetables are often included in soup mixes; dried onions, garlic, chives, and parsley can be found on the spice shelves. Camping and backpacking outfitters offer a whole array of freeze-dried foods. They are expensive but lightweight versions of dinner for you to take with you into the wild. And of course, widely available these days are the gourmet dried tomatoes, which are generally lightly salted and dried in the sun. Roma tomatoes, or Italian plum tomatoes, are usually used for drying because their solids content is two to three times that of regular tomatoes.

Freeze-drying is vacuum drying at temperatures far lower than those used for standard freezing. Ice crystals in the food go directly into a vapor, which keeps the cell membranes from rupturing. Reconstituted freeze-dried products have the taste, texture, and nutritional value of frozen foods. As long as products are stored dry, are reasonably cool, and are protected from crushing, they hold up well.

Some of the more familiar dried fruits are raisins (dried grapes), prunes (dried plums), dates, figs, and apricots. Unless you live in a tropical area, you may not eat fresh figs, but almost everybody knows about figs in the form of Fig Newtons. Some vitamin C may be lost in drying, but other nutrients are relatively unaffected.

You can find dried apples and bananas in the bulk foods case or in the baking aisle. The cranberry people have struck it rich with their new dried snack Craisins. These good-tasting fruits are wonderful for both eating and cooking and extend the short fresh-cranberries season. Other dried fruits, as well, make great snacks and wonderful ingredients for baking.

Prune puree is showing up on the market and being touted by nutrition enthusiasts as a low-fat baking ingredient. Pureed prunes are used as a substitute for fat in recipes because they hold moisture and mimic the tenderness and moistness that the product usually gets from fat. It won't surprise you that I think those products are unnecessary. You *can* tell the difference; baked products that substitute prune puree for shortening are *not* as good. In my view, if you are going to bake, it makes more sense to make something truly delicious and enjoy it to the maximum. You can't trick your eaters into thinking they are getting something they are not. If you want to use prunes in baking, ask me for the wonderful prune cake recipe I got from my mother!

When my children were small, I did far more baking than I do now. I found that for most recipes I could cut the sugar and the fat by about a third or a fourth without sacrificing quality. Twenty-five years ago, when my children were small, I found that most recipes went way over what was reasonable in sugar and fat. Now I find most recipes go way under.

Enlisting Your Children's Help

In chapter 5, many of the suggestions for how children can help with meal preparation have to do with fresh fruits and vegetables. I have also included a few specific suggestions with the recipes in this chapter. A child can wash apples, peel bananas, and spin salad fixings. If you give him a plastic picnic knife to work with (and if you can tolerate the results), even a young child can cut up apples for applesauce or chunk watermelon for a salad. Children can help a lot with making salads: they can spin and tear the greens, peel oranges, and break apart onion rings. Here are some other ways children can help:

- They can empty canned fruit into a serving bowl.
- They can paint vegetables with butter.
- They can separate broccoli florets.
- They can mix up simple vegetable and fruit recipes.
- They can shave butter with carrot peeler (e.g., see the **Plum Cobbler** recipe on page142).

Do remember, however, that even fresh vegetables can have harmful microorganisms on them. Particularly if those germs get on other foods and are allowed to grow and multiply, bacteria can reach high enough levels to make someone ill. Read more about food safety in chapter 8, page 157.

Preparation of Fresh Vegetables

Wash vegetables well before you cook them. Unless they are clearly labeled "prewashed," assume that there is something on them that you would rather not eat.

Here is a bit of do-as-I-say-not-as-I-do advice: When cooking vegetables, especially the low-starch varieties, pay attention to be sure they don't cook too long. I tend to be a put-it-on-then-do-something-else cook. In my own defense, I was raising children during my most intense cooking years, and children have a way of *seeing to it* that you do something else. Statistics show that with toddlers around, a parent is interrupted about every 6 minutes. Back to the point. Pay attention, and take the vegetables off as soon as they are done. Other dishes can wait and can get overcooked without hurting them too much. Vegetables suffer though, especially the green ones. Yellow, orange, and red fruits and vegetables can tolerate longer cooking times than green vegetables can.

When green vegetables are cooked, the cells break down so that the chlorophyll in the cells comes in contact with natural acids in the vegetables. The chlorophyll breaks down and the color turns from bright green to olive green and, eventually, to brown. Generally, this color change takes place after about 7 minutes of heating, but the time varies because some vegetables have tougher cells than others; some have more or less acid. To get your vegetables done in the critical 7 minutes, cut them into small pieces. With cabbage family vegetables like broccoli, cauliflower, brussels sprouts, and, of course, cabbage, to preserve the mild, sweet taste, keep the cooking time even shorter: closer to 5 than 7 minutes if you can. The extra 2 minutes *doubles* the amount of hydrogen sulfide gas (which smells like rotten eggs) that the vegetable produces. To keep cooking time down, cut the vegetables into small pieces before cooking them.

Cooking methods that dilute out the acids also help to keep vegetables green. Steaming lets the volatile acids evaporate or drip to the bottom of the cooking pan. Cooking uncovered in a large amount of rapidly boiling salted water lets the acids evaporate as well as dilutes them as they cook out. (The salt helps preserve the pectic substances, or "glue," between the cells and protects the vegetables' texture.) An iron skillet or tin-lined pan makes green vegetables turn brown. Copper pans turn green vegetables a vivid green from the formation of a copper chlorophyll, but it may not be safe to eat that much copper.

Because they were blanched before freezing, frozen vegetables are easier to keep green than fresh. Blanching removes some of the acids in the vegetables that change the color to olive drab. Microwaving creates fewer volatile compounds than other methods. A microwaved whole artichoke or an unpeeled onion, turnip, or beet is delicious.

High-Starch and Low-Starch Vegetables

In nutritional components and in the way they are cooked, vegetables break down roughly into two categories: high starch and low starch. With high-starch vegetables, with the exception of corn, we eat the root. With low-starch vegetables, we eat the upper part of the plant, the fruit or the leaf.

High-Starch Vegetables	Low-Starch Vegetables
Beets	Asparagus
Carrots	"Cruciferous"
Corn	Broccoli
Parsnips	Brussels sprouts
Potatoes	Cabbage
Rutabagas	Cauliflower
Squash	Collards
Sweet potatoes	Kale
Turnips	Swiss chard
	Green beans
	"Greens"
	Beet
	Mustard
	Spinach
	Turnip
	Mushrooms
	Peas
	Zucchini

Both high- and low-starch vegetables can be cooked by boiling, microwaving, or baking. Both need to be cooked with moisture. For both, cooking tenderizes cell walls. There the similarities end. High-starch vegetables need to be cooked in more water to hydrate and cook the starch. For boiling, you add water. For baking or microwaving, the water in the vegetable itself is retained within the vegetable to cook the starch.

Low-starch vegetables are relatively high in water, have tender cell walls, and generally cook faster than high-starch vegetables. (The exception is cabbage-family vegetables, which have tough cells that need to cook longer.) It is easy to break the cell wall with too much heat or too much handling and to make them mushy. Low-starch vegetables can be cooked in a small amount of water by steaming, boiling, and microwaving. They can also be baked, but the baking dish has to have a lid on it to retain the moisture.

PREPARING HIGH-STARCH VEGETABLES
Boiling high-starch vegetables: Peel or scrub the vegetables and remove blemishes. Cut them into similarly sized pieces—the smaller the piece the quicker the cooking. Rinse the vegetables with cold water. To keep them from

blackening, cover potatoes with cold water until you are ready to cook them. Choose a pan with a lid, large enough to leave head room for boiling water. To preserve nutrients, the best method is to start the water boiling first (add 1 teaspoon of salt per quart) and then add the vegetables. Boiling water immediately inactivates the vegetables' enzymes that would otherwise break down the nutrients. Reduce the heat to keep the water boiling rapidly but not boiling over. Don't use hot tap water because it is higher in lead than cold water.

Boil until the vegetables are as done as you like them. Drain them, put them back in the pan, and put the pan back on the turned-off burner to let the rest of the water evaporate. Boiling vegetables generally takes about 10 to 15 minutes.

Baking high-starch vegetables: Heat the oven to 425 degrees. Prepare the vegetables as you would for boiling. Put them on a baking sheet to catch drips (squash will drip). Line the sheet with aluminum foil for easy cleanup. Bake until done. A medium baked potato will take about an hour. So will half a medium squash, a beet, turnip, or rutabaga. Since parsnips and carrots are more slender and are subject to drying out, watch them carefully during baking or put them in a covered dish to bake.

Microwaving high-starch vegetables: High-starch vegetables do well in the microwave. Prepare vegetables as you would for the other methods. If you are leaving the vegetables whole, puncture several times with a fork to let out steam and to keep them from exploding. Check your microwave book for directions about cooking times, power settings, and standing times. As with everything else you prepare in the microwave, the more food you cook, the longer it takes.

Corn on the cob can be microwaved without even shucking it. Four ears of corn can be cooked in 8 to 10 minutes, plus five minutes of standing time. As with anything you microwave, to cook the food evenly it is a good idea to stop halfway through rearrange it. To prepare corn for microwaving, peek inside to be sure no worms are riding along, pull off a little silk if you must, leave the cob end on to give something to grab onto when you serve and eat it, and microwave away. You don't have to add water because the husk retains the moisture. Once the corn is cooked, the silk comes off easily when you peel back the husk.

PREPARING LOW-STARCH VEGETABLES
To retain nutrients, flavor, and texture, be fast and conservative about water when cooking low-starch vegetables (with the exception of strong-tasting ones like brussels sprouts). Use as little water as you can, and get the vegetables done as quickly as you can.

Clean the vegetables well. With all their little blossoms and wrinkles, low-starch vegetables are harder to clean than high-starch ones. Sort the vegetables by removing tough stems and blighted areas. Soak them in a pan of cold water to loosen up the dirt and sand. Swish them around, and then place them in a second pan of water. Rinse them off, being careful to run water through all the areas where sand might be hiding. You might find a colander helpful for this purpose. There is nothing worse than getting a gritty mouthful of sand when you are trying to enjoy your spinach or asparagus.

Steaming or boiling low-starch vegetables:
Vegetables are done when they are crisp-tender; green vegetables are done when they are bright green but not gray-green or olive green. Generally, when people think of steaming, they think of using a vegetable steaming rack or a special insert in a pan to get the vegetables up and out of the water. The more finely divided the vegetables, the more quickly they will get done. To keep times below the 5- or 7-minute limit, make the pieces small and uniform.

Vegetables vary a lot in how long they take to cook. Fresh spinach takes just a couple of minutes. On the other hand, turnip greens take as much as 20 minutes to cook. Some vegetables that we *call* greens, like kale and chard, aren't greens at all but members of the cabbage family. Those "greens" take as long or longer to cook than turnip greens. Confusing, isn't it? As you become more familiar with cooking these vegetables, it won't seem so confusing.

Some nutrients, like carotene and minerals, hold up well with cooking. Others, like vitamin C and B vitamins, migrate into the cooking water or are broken down somewhat. Consequently, the less water you use, the less you throw away, the fewer nutrients you lose. That principle makes my next bit of advice seem pretty strange.

To introduce children to the strong flavors of cruciferous vegetables (like cabbage, cauli-flower, broccoli, and brussels sprouts), tone them down by cooking them with extra rapidly boiling salted water and leaving the lid off the pan during cooking. Cut them small enough to get the cooking done within 5 minutes. Cruciferous vegetables contain sulfur, but the word *crucifer* comes from the Latin word meaning "cross," because these vegetables bear a cross-shaped flower. Some research indicates that these vegetables may be helpful in protecting against certain forms of cancer.

Despite their presumed health-giving qualities, learning to like these cabbage-family vegetables is challenging because of their strong taste and smell. Cooking them in lots of water with the lid off the pan helps to cook off the sulfur and dilute the flavor. Putting vinegar in the cooking water helps to preserve the color and improves the taste. But even with expert cooking, some children are particularly sensitive to the flavors in cruciferous vegetables and don't like them at all. Studies of taste show that this aversion is *real* and it is *unpleasant*. With any food, but with cruciferous vegetables in particular, don't try to get your child to eat if he doesn't want to.

Microwaving low-starch vegetables: Often, the water from washing is enough to cook low-starch vegetables in the microwave. At most, put in 1/4 cup of water per pound of vegetables. Use a glass dish with a cover for cooking. Depending on how much you are cooking, 3 to 4 minutes cooking time plus 2 to 3 minutes standing time may be enough. Stir the vegetables halfway through cooking.

Baking low-starch vegetables: You hardly ever bake low-starch vegetables. If you do, the principle is to keep the vegetable moist. Cabbage wedges taste great in a pot roast, and they cook slowly enough so they can be put in with the other vegetables. On the other hand, to include zucchini or mushrooms in a stew, it would be better to wait and add them toward the end of cooking.

Cooking Frozen Vegetables

Cooking frozen vegetables is a snap. Keep them frozen until you put them in the pan. Use minimal water, minimal time, and *attend*. Stop cooking the vegetables the instant they are done. As I said earlier, it is easier to keep the color bright in frozen vegetables because they were blanched before they were frozen. Blanching gets rid of some of the color-destroying acids.

STOVE-TOP COOKING

Place the amount of frozen vegetables you want (blocks of vegetables are usually 10 ounces, bags are usually 14 to 16 ounces) in a covered pan. Add the amount of water called for on the package or *less*. Experiment to see how little water you can use. Extra water just gets thrown away, and along with it, a few nutrients.

Begin by adding 1/4 teaspoon of salt per 10 ounces of vegetables. Cook on medium high for 3 to 4 minutes or for as long as it says to on the package. Check during cooking and stop when vegetables are crisp-tender, even a little underdone. They will continue cooking in the hot pan or serving bowl. Add butter or other seasoning. I like to put in the butter by "coloring" the hot vegetables with the exposed end of a cold stick of butter. That distributes the butter well without dousing the vegetables too heavily. Check the taste, and add pepper and more salt if you think it needs it. Another 1/2 teaspoon or less should do it.

MICROWAVE COOKING

Place the desired amount of frozen vegetables in a covered glass casserole dish. Do not add water, even if the package says so (with the exception of lima beans). Begin by adding 1/4 teaspoon of salt per 10 ounces of vegetables and dot with butter. Stir once during cooking to assure even heating without overcooking some portions. Add butter before or after cooking. Add 1/4 teaspoon of pepper and more salt to your taste.

You can even prepare frozen vegetables (10 ounces) in the original package. Pierce top of package and set it on glass saucer. If vegetables are frozen in pouches, pierce the top of the pouch also. If packages are foil wrapped, remove the foil.

Cooking Canned Vegetables

Don't boil canned vegetables. They are already cooked and just need to be warmed up. Canned vegetables are very tender. To keep

them from breaking apart and getting mushy, stir and heat as little as you can.

To prepare vegetables in cans, drain the liquid into a saucepan and bring it to a boil. Add the vegetables, turn down to the heat to medium high, and heat through for about 2 minutes without boiling. When preparing dishes that involve combining them with other ingredients, add the canned vegetables last.

Some of the nutrients from the canned vegetables are in the liquid. Most canned vegetables have more liquid than you would generally consume. There are, however, some varieties of canned vegetables, packaged in 13-ounce cans, that contain considerably less liquid. They are good tasting, and well worth looking for, but they aren't available everywhere.

To keep from having to throw away water-soluble nutrients (vitamin C and folic acid) with the liquid, you can boil the liquid down a bit before you put in the vegetables. If there is less liquid, you'll be more likely to eat it rather than throw it away. Of course, the boiling breaks down the nutrients some, but otherwise you would throw them away . Boiling down also concentrates the flavor, which is a plus.

To cook canned vegetables in the microwave, do the same thing as with stove-top cooking. Boil the liquid first in a glass dish, add in the vegetables, and heat. Don't stir; let stand for a minute or two to equalize the temperatures. You won't need any more salt, but you might enjoy the taste of a little pepper.

Dressing Up Vegetables

Below, I give you many recipes for fruits and vegetables. You don't have to use them. You do not have to be fancy. If you cook vegetables properly and put in a little salt and butter, they will be tasty and appealing. If you open a can of fruit and put it in a nice bowl, it will become an attractive part of the meal. In fact, if you make a main dish that requires time and energy, it would be better if you *didn't* go to a lot of trouble with the other parts of the menu. Putting too much on yourself with food preparation will just defeat you, later if not sooner. Many experienced cooks plan vegetables and fruits for a meal by leaning on the pantry door or peering into the freezer.

However, you do need to add some salt and

fat to vegetables for them to taste their best. To me, a moderate amount of salt is about 1/8 teaspoon of salt and 1 to 2 teaspoons of butter or fat equivalent (see page 120) per 1/2-cup serving of vegetable. In my recipes, I recommend starting with 1/4 teaspoon of salt before cooking, and then adding salt carefully after cooking, tasting after each addition. The amounts of salt and fat in each of my recipes are reasonable and prudent; they enhance flavor without drowning it. Use these amounts as rules of thumb for evaluating recipes in other cookbooks as well.

A child will enjoy "coloring" the hot vegetables with the opened end of a stick of butter. The lightly buttered result will give about 1 teaspoon per serving—and a *lot* of flavor. You might like bottled cheese spreads, like Cheez Whiz, on your vegetables. Or you can make your own **Super-Quick Cheese Sauce** (page 133) to put over broccoli, cauliflower, or any other vegetable you like.

If you are a novice eater of vegetables and fruits, the enticements of toppings and sauces may help you. You can also turn to our recipe section for more ideas to help you and your children be successful with vegetables and fruits. Glazed carrots are still carrots. The sweet flavor makes them more appealing to people just beginning to establish a relationship with carrots. Fruits can be baked into desserts. The **Plum Cobbler** (page 142) has all the nutrients of fresh plums, with some added enticements.

HERBED BUTTER

Mix the following ingredients together:
1/4 cup softened butter
4 Tbsp fresh herbs of your choice: dill, chives, mint, basil, and parsley

Store the mixture in a covered jar in the refrigerator and use as needed for flavoring vegetables.

To keep fresh herbs on hand, wash them and then freeze them in water in an ice cube tray. When you are ready to use them, thaw as many cubes as you need and blot the herbs with a paper towel.

SUPER-QUICK CHEESE SAUCE

This is essentially a white sauce, but instead of putting milk and butter in separately, I use half-and-half. The fat content comes out the same as for a medium white sauce, and it is easier and faster. This sauce works great for broccoli, cauliflower, and potatoes. It can also be multiplied and mixed with macaroni for a fast homemade macaroni and cheese.

Combine the following ingredients in a small saucepan or microwave-safe bowl:
1/2 cup half-and-half
2 tsp flour (regular or quick-mixing flour like Wondra or Shake and Blend)

Heat gently until the mixture boils; reduce the heat still more and boil gently for one minute to cook the flour and thicken the cream.

Add the following to the thickened cream:
1/4 cup shredded sharp cheddar cheese
1/4 tsp salt
1/4 tsp dry mustard

Here are some other simple ideas for toppings you can mix up and keep on hand indefinitely in the refrigerator. Like the cheese sauce, you can use these toppings on any vegetable.

MUSTARD BUTTER

This is good with peas, brussels sprouts, cauliflower, broccoli, and green and wax beans.

Mix the following together well:
1/2 stick soft butter
1 tsp herb or Dijon mustard
1/2 tsp lemon juice

Add the following to the mixture and mix well:
1 tsp dill weed, fresh
1 tsp chives, minced
dash pepper
dash salt

Store the mixture in a covered jar in the refrigerator.

OLIVE OIL WITH GARLIC

Try this on peas, green and wax beans, brussels sprouts, cauliflower, and broccoli.

Combine the following ingredients in a blender:
8 cloves minced garlic
1/4 cup olive oil

Heat gently in a frying pan or in the microwave until the garlic bits are light brown.

Store the mixture in a covered jar in the refrigerator.

Variation: Toss vegetables with the mixture, then add 1/2 cup prepackaged Italian seasoned bread crumbs, and toss again.

OLIVE–CREAM CHEESE SPREAD

This works well as a dip for pretzels or raw vegetables. It also melts nicely on hot vegetables. It is surprisingly tasty with brussels sprouts. The strong flavor of the topping competes nicely with the strong flavor of the vegetable.

Finely chop 1 tablespoon of stuffed green olives. Mix with 1/4 cup of cream cheese or Neufchâtel, including a couple teaspoons of olive juice.

Store in a covered jar in the refrigerator.

Vegetable Recipes from the Cycle Menu

The two criteria for choosing these vegetable recipes are that they taste *good* and they are *fast and easy*. I hope you find at least one recipe among this group that will become a family standby. My main contenders are **Creamed Spinach** and **Gingered Broccoli. Glazed carrots** and **Scalloped Corn** are so sure-fire and easy that it is embarrassing to even call them recipes. Once you get the idea, you'll find your own favorites. But let's start with a surprise: a vegetable recipe that isn't eaten as a vegetable at all, but rather as a dessert. Pumpkin!

PUMPKIN CUSTARD

Beat the following together in a large bowl:
1 15-oz can pumpkin
1 15-oz can milk (use the pumpkin can to measure the milk)
3 eggs
Mix the following together in a separate bowl:
1 cup sugar
1 tsp cinnamon
1 tsp nutmeg
1 tsp ginger
1/4 tsp cloves
Pinch (about 1/8 tsp) salt

Combine the two mixtures and pour them into a 2 1/2-quart glass casserole dish. Bake uncovered at 400 degrees for 1 hour. Serve plain or with whipped cream.

RECIPE NOTES

Fast tip: Leaving the crust off the pumpkin pie is the fast tip. If you are a whiz at making pastry (or you've found a good store-bought pastry) and your pumpkin pie isn't the same without it, go for it.

Variation: Pumpkin is a wonderful vegetable that's high in vitamin A. It doesn't have to be relegated to dessert. Double this recipe and put it on the table for breakfast. Pumpkin custard has eggs, vegetables, and milk, so it is really quite nutritious. Serve it again for dessert the next night: it will fill any corners that are left after the tuna-noodle casserole.

SWEET-SOUR CUCUMBER SALAD

This is a variation on a traditional Scandinavian dish. You can keep the sweet-sour sauce for up to a week, adding more sliced cucumbers as you eat them.

Scrub or peel (see fast tip) and slice as thinly as you can (paper thin, if you can manage):
2 large European-style cucumbers (often called burpless)
or 4–5 slim cucumbers, 7 or 8 inches long

Bigger, thicker cucumbers have coarser seeds and don't taste as good. If you can find dill-pickle-sized cucumbers, they are the best. The skins are often tender and the seeds are small.

Place the slices in a medium-sized bowl. Make a sweet-sour sauce, by mixing together the following ingredients until the sugar is dissolved:
1/2 cup white wine vinegar
1/4 cup sugar
1/2 tsp salt
Dash pepper
4 tsp chopped fresh new dill
or 1 tsp dried dill weed

Pour the sauce over the cucumbers and refrigerate for 3 hours to allow the flavors to blend. Drain the cucumbers, garnish with dill sprigs, and serve. After you eat these cucumbers, you may add more to the sauce and have

Cucumber Salad for another meal.

RECIPE NOTES

Fast tip: You don't have to peel cucumbers if the skins are tender and good tasting. The only way to tell whether they're good or not is to taste them. If you object at all to the skin flavor, peel them.

Stemmed, cleaned, spun-dry fresh dill can be kept fresh and tasty in a zip top bag in the refrigerator for a week or more. To keep it longer, try chopping it up and freezing it into ice cubes.

Variation: Serve your cucumbers plain and more thickly sliced, or cut them into wedges. Your children might enjoy them more that way.

POPPYSEED COLESLAW

If you can, make this about 30 minutes to an hour before mealtime to give the flavors a chance to blend. Check the package on the preshredded vegetables to see if you need to wash them again. Many are not prewashed.

Chop the vegetables until they are as fine as you like them:
6 oz prechopped cabbage
4 oz prechopped carrots

Mix in a large bowl and, if you like, add 1/2 cup raisins. Mix in **Poppyseed Dressing** (recipe follows) to taste.

POPPYSEED DRESSING

Not only does this dressing taste great on the coleslaw, but it is wonderful on the **Spinach, Red Onion, and Orange Salad** (pages 136-137). It is also good with fruit salad. You'll have your own ideas.

In a blender, combine the following dry ingredients with the vinegar:
1/3 cup flavored vinegar (red wine, raspberry, etc.)
4 tsp sugar (for a sweeter dressing, use up to 3 Tbsp sugar)
1 1/2 tsp dry mustard
1 tsp salt

Add the following fresh or dried vegetables and herbs to the blender and blend until they are finely minced:
2 Tbsp chopped green onions
1 Tbsp onion
1/4 cup fresh chives (To use dried chives, read the bottle to find out how to substitute dried for fresh.)
1 1/2 tsp poppyseeds
Finally, drizzle the oil into the blender, mixing constantly at low speed:
3/4 cup cooking oil

Fast tip: Double or triple this recipe and keep it in a glass jar in the refrigerator. It will be all ready to use for a sweet vegetable salad or fruit salad.

SCALLOPED CORN

Mix the following ingredients together:
1 15-oz can cream-style corn
1/2 cup slightly crushed soda crackers (approximately 10)
1/4 cup milk or half-and-half
Pinch of pepper, salt to taste
(You can also put in dried parsley and onions, if you like.)

Heat the mixture gently on low, stirring as little as possible to avoid breaking up the crackers.

Variation #1: For a baked version of scalloped corn, add *1 beaten egg* to the corn mixture. (Beating the egg ahead of time makes it mix in more easily so the crackers won't get broken as much.) Pour the mixture into an ovenproof baking dish. Bake at 350 degrees for 45 minutes. Keep this recipe in mind when you have the oven already going for another dish. With the milk and egg, it is almost a meal on its own.

Variation #2: For corn and broccoli bake, add *1 10-oz package frozen chopped broccoli, thawed and drained,* to the baked scalloped corn.

PANNED CABBAGE AND CARROTS

For this recipe, you can use the same shredded vegetables that you did for the coleslaw.

In a large frying pan with a lid, heat *2 to 3 teaspoons of butter* over medium heat.

When the butter is hot, add the following ingredients all at once and sauté for 3 to 4 minutes.

8 oz prechopped cabbage, red or white
4 oz prechopped carrots
1/4 tsp salt
A few drops of flavored vinegar: balsamic,
  wine vinegar, or rice vinegar

Cover the frying pan and finish cooking for another 1 to 2 minutes until the vegetables are tender but still a little crisp. Add *1/4 teaspoon of pepper*. Taste for salt and add more as needed. Another 1/4 teaspoon should do it.

GLAZED CARROTS

Even without added sugar, cooking carrots makes them taste sweeter than when they are raw. The brown sugar makes them even sweeter. Because almost everybody likes sweets, this recipe is a great way to introduce kids—and grown-ups—to carrots.

Combine all the following ingredients and heat:
2 cups hot cooked carrots: fresh, frozen, or canned
2 Tbsp brown sugar
1 Tbsp butter
salt to taste (about 1/2 tsp)

Notes: I like fresh carrots best for this recipe. You may peel carrots and make carrot rounds or sticks, or use the little prepeeled carrots and cook them whole—or cut them up.

GINGERED BROCCOLI

Sauté *1 pound of broccoli florets in 1 tablespoon of toasted sesame oil* at a high to medium temperature until the broccoli is warmed and slightly cooked.

Remove the broccoli from the pan. In the sauce pan, combine the following ingredients and heat to boiling:
2 Tbsp water
1/4 tsp broth concentrate or bouillon crystals
1 tsp soy sauce
1/8 tsp powdered ginger
1/8 tsp powdered garlic

Put the broccoli back in the pan with the broth and seasoning mixture, and cover it with a lid. Cook until the broccoli is crisp-tender but still bright green. It should take about 3 to 4 minutes, but check it as it cooks.

SPINACH, RED ONION, AND ORANGE SALAD WITH POPPYSEED DRESSING

Here's another use for your poppyseed dressing. You can find the very small red onions in early summer. They taste good and add a beautiful, festive appearance.

Trim, wash, and spin dry *10 to 12 ounces of fresh spinach*, and tear it into bite-sized pieces. (Salad needs less dressing if the greens are dry.) Slice *1 small red onion or 2 to 3 very small red onions* thinly, and break the slices apart into rings. Peel *2 oranges*, halve them end-to-end, and slice. Crumble *1 cup of blue cheese*.

Combine all ingredients, dress lightly (don't use all the dressing, it will be way too much). Dressing makes the lettuce wilt, so don't add it until the last minute. Use a small amount of dressing—less than you think you will need. Toss well until all the leaves have some dressing on them. Taste and add salt or more dressing as needed.

RECIPE NOTES
Fast tip: Prepare the dressing and put the amount needed in the bottom of the salad bowl. Cross long-handled serving fork and spoon on top of the dressing, then pile the prepared greens on top of the crossed utensils. The fork and spoon keep the greens from touching the dressing. Cover the salad bowl with plastic wrap and refrigerate until serving time. Toss just before serving.

It is particularly worth purchasing prewashed spinach. Spinach has so many little wrinkles that can hold on to sand and dirt, and it takes so many changes of water to get it all out that it can be quite discouraging to cook with fresh spinach.

Adapting this dish for children: Dress this salad lightly or not at all so children can eat it with their fingers.

About the blue cheese: It's always a mistake to assume children won't be able to handle something and start adapting the dish before children have been given an opportunity to learn to like the food. However, the blue cheese in this salad might be a little challenging for many children. Unlike the purple onions, which will also be challenging, they can't eat around it. It permeates everything. To start with, why not put the crumbled blue cheese in a separate little bowl and pass it.

Logistically, it might work even better if you sprinkle it on the *top* of your salad dish rather than letting it sink to the bottom of the serving bowl.

However, even as I write this, I wonder. I could see a child relishing the strong flavors and colors of this salad—blue cheese and all. I leave you to try it out—and observe.

Variations: Vary this salad by using different fruits, greens, and cheeses. For instance, try a spinach-grape-feta cheese salad with poppy-seed dressing. Or substitute green lettuce for the spinach.

Make this into a main-dish salad by adding cold, thinly sliced cooked chicken. The **Lemon Chicken** (page 98) works great with this recipe.

GO-EVERYWHERE GREEN SALAD

Now that you have the sweet salad, you also need a savory salad. You will develop your family favorites and standbys for green salads. Many families have the same salad over and over again and don't seem to get tired of it. You can vary it by changing the salad greens or by dressing it up with herbs or a variety of cheeses.

I like to make my own dressing because I don't like bottled dressings. This dressing is simple and keeps as long as you want it. The milder taste of the wine vinegar lets you use less oil than the usual two parts oil to one part vinegar, and the grated cheese adds a surprising amount of flavor. For many children, a very light dressing or none at all works well because it makes it easier to pick the food up with their fingers. However, you and your child may like bottled salad dressing and plenty of it, and that's fine. As an alternative to the salad dressing in this recipe, you can use bottled dressing or packets of premixed salad dressing seasonings that you mix yourself with vinegar and oil.

Rub a wooden salad bowl with a *clove of garlic,* and sprinkle with *salt.*

Add cleaned and spun-dry salad greens, enough for your family. Choices can include romaine, garden lettuce, iceberg lettuce, spinach, or combinations. Sprinkle *freshly grated Parmesan or Asiago cheese* over the top, and sprinkle with pepper if you like it.

Just before you serve, put on dressing to taste mixed by these proportions: *1/3 cup red wine vinegar* and a *generous 1/2 cup cooking oil.* Toss to coat all the vegetables with dressing, but don't drown them.

Variation: To the basic salad recipe, you can add croutons, grated carrots, thinly sliced green onions, thinly sliced red onions (very

---

PREPACKAGED SALAD GREENS OR DO-IT-YOURSELF?

It is up to you whether you buy bagged, prepackaged salad fixings or the type you have to core, sort, and wash. Prepackaged salad is a value-added product that costs more per portion than the do-it-yourself variety. The salad greens that offer the dressing and other condiments are the most costly. With the plain salad greens, the difference is smaller and may be smaller than you think when you consider what you have to throw away when you buy in bulk. Your time is also worth something. Whether or not you have to *wash* these prepackaged products depends on what it says on the package. The words to look for are "washed," "prewashed," or "ready-to-eat." Harmful bacteria have been removed from the varieties that are "washed" and "ready to eat." Large manufacturers use a state-of-the-art cleansing process that kills bacteria better than you could at home.

Don't be put off prewashed greens by scary television and newspaper reports about high bacterial counts. Uninformed reporters sounded the alarm on prepackaged fruits and vegetables when their laboratories found high bacterial levels in many packages of precut vegetables. "You're probably better off eating raw ground beef than you are eating this produce," warned one newscaster. What reporters didn't know,—what they didn't bother to find out—is that the bacteria they were finding were completely harmless. Anything that is grown in the ground has germs on it. Only a few of those germs will make you sick, and those germs were *not* present in the prepackaged produce.

However, that is not to say that you can relax about washing your greens. If you don't see specific words that say products are washed, wash the greens yourself before you eat them. Bulk lettuce should always be washed, even if it looks ready to eat and even if the display box says "washed." Any product that is sold out in the open, where people can touch it or sneeze on it, is subject to contamination. By the way, it's a good idea to wash greens you get from the farmers' market, even those that are spun dry.

pretty), parsley, chives, black or green olives, cucumbers, tomatoes, leftover cooked vegetables marinated in salad dressing.

Some combinations benefit from more salt, as does this wonderful combination: Thinly sliced cauliflower, crumbled blue cheese, thinly sliced black olives, and thinly sliced small purple onions.

You can also make a main-dish salad by adding chopped hard-cooked eggs, thin slices of cold leftover meat or poultry, and chunks or shreds of cheese.

TOMATO SLICES WITH VINAIGRETTE

When tomatoes are farm fresh and vine-ripened, they don't need any help to make them taste wonderful. Just slice them and serve with salt and pepper or with sugar. However, toward the end of the season, if you or your neighbor have a tomato plant that just won't stop, you might appreciate pepping up those tomato slices with this vinaigrette.

You can keep this vinaigrette in the refrigerator, and just before you serve it, take out a portion and add fresh herbs. The fresh herbs become strong and unpleasant if they are left in the oil for any length of time.

In a blender, combine and mix the following ingredients well:
1/4 cup wine vinegar or lemon juice
3/4 tsp salt
1/4 tsp freshly ground black pepper
1/2 tsp prepared mustard
1/2 tsp dry mustard

Gradually drizzle *3/4 cup of cooking oil* into the vinegar/seasoning mixture, blending as you add it.

Just before you use the dressing, take out 1/4 cup of dressing and add *1 tablespoon of chopped fresh herbs.* Experiment with herbs to find out what you like and write it down. I have used dill, basil, parsley, and chives. Occasionally I use thyme, but only in a very small amount because it has a strong flavor.

MASHED POTATOES

It is certainly okay to use boxed mashed potatoes. I have gone through many a box of Potato Buds in my life, probably because as a hungry child, when I would whine to my mother, "When is dinner going to be ready?"

she would invariably say, "As soon as the potatoes are done." For my children, instant potatoes prevented the trauma, but I undoubtedly traumatized them in other ways.

Even though the boxed varieties are convenient, nothing compares with the taste and texture of mashed potatoes you make from scratch. Mashed potatoes are enjoying a comeback at the finest restaurants. Try making them with Yukon Gold potatoes—they are yellow and have a buttery flavor.

Peel and quarter or cut into 1-inch slices *2 lb Russet potatoes* or other white or all-purpose potatoes. Heat salted water (1 teaspoon of salt per quart) until boiling, and put in the potato slices or chunks. Reduce the heat to a moderate boil and cook for about 20 minutes or until they are fork-tender. Drain off the water by cracking the lid and pouring it through the crack, or use a colander. Put potatoes back into the pan and put the pan on the turned-off-but-still-hot burner to let the extra water evaporate.

Meanwhile, measure out and arrange to have hot when the potatoes are done, *1/2 cup half-and-half.* In the cooking pan, mash the potatoes with a hand masher or put them through a device called a ricer. (An electric mixer is also all right, but it will tend to make the potatoes more gluey.) When the potatoes are mashed to your liking, mix in the cream a little at a time until the potatoes are the consistency you like. You may prefer your potatoes more coarsely mashed, with little lumps in them. There are no rules. Taste, add *1/4 teaspoon of pepper* and as much *salt* as you need— 1/4 to 1/2 teaspoon should do it.

RECIPE NOTES
Fast tip: Peel the potatoes the night before and let them stand in cold water (so they don't get black). Cook and mash the potatoes ahead of mealtime and set the bowl or pan in another pan of simmering water to keep them warm so you don't have the last-minute rush of getting them ready.

Variations: Mashed potatoes can be prepared many ways to keep them interesting. Cook the potatoes with the skins on and mash the skins right in. (Be sure to thoroughly wash them and remove the blemishes and green patches.) Make garlic mashed potatoes by stirring in 4 to 5 cloves of chopped and sautéed garlic. Use milk instead of cream and stir in 2 to 3 tablespoons of Neufchâtel cheese. Use buttermilk

instead of cream—it is surprisingly good!
Don't heat the buttermilk or it will clump up
and separate. When you begin cooking dinner,
set a cup of buttermilk on the counter to let it
come to room temperature.

Alternate method for mashed potatoes: If
your mashed potatoes get too gluey, consider
Shirley Corriher's method from her book
Cookwise. Corriher recommends cooking the
potatoes ahead of time, cooling them, then
reheating them in hot water when you are
ready to mash and serve them. Using this
method, you can heat up cold, leftover potatoes and make mashed potatoes.

Corriher points out that boiling potatoes
makes their starch granules swell. Cooling
after cooking lets the starch granules in the
potatoes recrystallize so they aren't soluble in
water and don't break down as readily when
you mash them. When you make potato salad,
this bit of food chemistry is very helpful.
Cooking and cooling potatoes before you slice
them for salad helps slices keep their shape.

POTATOES
High-starch potatoes like Russett Burbanks (also
known as Idaho Russetts or just Idahos) are
excellent for mashing and baking because they
have a dry, mealy texture. Yukon Golds are a
little lower in starch but still have enough to be
good baking potatoes as well as good boiling
and mashing potatoes. A relatively new variety
of potato on the American market, Yukon Golds
have a golden yellow flesh and buttery taste.
Red potatoes and some round white potatoes
are firm and waxy. They make good scalloped
potatoes and potato salad. Round reds are all-
purpose potatoes—you can either bake or boil
them. Of course, the sky wouldn't fall if you
boiled a Russett potato, but it would cook apart
more than a red potato. If you bake a red potato, the texture will be somewhat soggy rather
than dry and mealy.

CREAMED SPINACH

This is my nomination for a recipe you will
make again and again. I discovered it in a fine
eating establishment in Birmingham, Alabama.
I don't remember what I had for the entrée,
but I do remember the spinach!

Thaw and drain two *10-ounce packages of
chopped frozen spinach* in a colander. Empty into
a microwave-safe glass dish. Heat in the

microwave until the spinach is hot (not to cook
it though, as it is already cooked enough).

After heating the spinach, add *1/4 cup half-
and-half or whipping cream,* and *1/4 cup grated
Parmesan or Asiago cheese.*

RECIPE NOTES
The night before: Put the frozen spinach in
the refrigerator to thaw. Leave it wrapped
until you're ready to use it. In case the packages leak, thaw them in the dish you will use
for cooking.

Variation: Leftover creamed spinach tastes
great with poached eggs for breakfast or for an
easy lunch or dinner.

GREENS AND BACON

This is a quick version of traditional salt pork
and greens. Once again, even though we use
bacon and bacon fat, there is only about 1 teaspoon of fat per serving in this dish. The salt in
the bacon may do the last-minute salting for
you. Taste and decide if you need more.

Following package directions, cook a *16-
ounce package of frozen collards, chard, or turnip,
beet, or mustard greens with 1/2 teaspoon of salt.*
Some greens require as much as 35 minutes to
cook. When the greens are done, drain them
thoroughly in a colander and return them to
the pan.

Meanwhile, cook *4 slices of bacon* at a low to
moderate temperature until they're as crisp as
you want and crumble them. *Don't drain!* Add
the bacon and bacon fat to the greens, toss,
and serve. Add *freshly grated Parmesan cheese* if
you like.

RECIPE NOTES
Fast tip: Keep bacon in the freezer. When you
want a small amount for a recipe like this, saw
two or three 1/4-inch slices off the end of the
frozen block. Break apart as you cook.

Variation: Cook 1/4 cup chopped onion in
the bacon fat after you remove the bacon and
add it to the dish. Try the bacon and onion
trick with waxed beans as well. It adds flavor
to an otherwise bland dish.

STEWED TOMATOES

This is a homey, easy vegetable recipe that
tastes surprisingly good. My daughter,

Kjerstin, remembers it fondly.

Tomatoes have protective properties, thanks to a high content of *lycopene*, an antioxidant that may help guard against digestive tract and prostrate cancer. But don't let that tidbit turn tomatoes into medicine for you. Tomatoes are a mainstay of our diet because almost everyone eats spaghetti and pizza.

Heat a *15-ounce can of stewed tomatoes* (the can will say "stewed") until hot in the microwave or on the stove. Add *1 cup of tough or dried-out bread cubes*. Let stand a minute or two for the bread to soak up the tomato juice.

Serve in sauce dishes or custard cups.

HERBED PEAS

Cook the peas using your preferred method, and add salt and sugar during cooking (the sugar gives the peas a just-picked taste):

10-oz package frozen peas
1/2 tsp sugar
1/2 tsp salt

After cooking, drain the peas and stir in the following:

1 Tbsp butter
1 Tbsp fresh herbs of your choice: dill, chives, mint, basil, and parsley all go well with peas

RECIPE NOTES
Variations: Combine the cooked peas with pearl onions (you can buy them frozen), cooked carrots, or mushrooms. The added vegetables can be sautéed fresh or canned (if canned, drain them first).

More variations: Sauté *2 cloves of minced garlic in 1 tablespoon of olive oil*. Pour the following into the hot cooked peas or peas and onions:

1/4 cup freshly grated Parmesan cheese
1 cup flavored croutons

COUNTRY SUMMER SQUASH

This recipe is from Shirley Corriher's *Cookwise*. I have depended on Corriher's expertise for making sure my vegetable and fruit recommendations are technically correct.

This recipe is a bit tricky because you have to cook the bacon and onion in time for the squash to be done so you can put it all together while it's hot. As with stir-fry, it works best if you get the vegetables prepared and the bacon in the pan before you actually start cooking. Everything will probably come out together if you start cooking the bacon at the same time as you start heating the water for the squash, then put the squash in to boil about the same time as you get the onions in the bacon fat to cook.

Wash and prepare *6 medium or 8 small (about 2 1/2 pounds) yellow crookneck squash, cut into 1/2-inch slices*. Bring water (with *1 teaspoon of salt* and *1 teaspoon of sugar* per quart) to boil in a large saucepan. Add the sliced squash and cook until the squash is very tender when pierced with a fork, about 10 minutes. When the squash is cooked, drain it in a colander and mash thoroughly with a potato masher. Set aside. This weeps, so you might want to put it back in the colander to drain again.

In a large frying pan, cook *4 slices of bacon* over low heat until they're as crisp as you want. Remove bacon from the pan, crumble it, and set it aside. Leave the bacon drippings in the frying pan and cook *2 large coarsely chopped onions* until they are clear and beginning to brown.

Add the cooked and mashed squash to the onions and cook for several minutes, stirring constantly. Season to taste with *1/4 teaspoon pepper* and *1/4 to 1 teaspoon of salt*. (Add additional salt 1/4 teaspoon at a time, tasting between additions.)

Finally, add the crumbled bacon.

CORN PUDDING

This is a more sophisticated version of scalloped corn. You may have seen this recipe with cornbread mix instead of the dry ingredients. I tried that cornbread-mix recipe and thought it was a little sweet, so I figured out this one. If you want to save a few steps, use a package of Jiffy cornbread mix instead of the dry ingredients I have listed.

Start the oven at 350 degrees.

Mix together the wet ingredients in a large mixing bowl:

15-oz can cream-style corn
15-oz can whole kernel corn, liquid and all
1 Tbsp melted butter
1 cup low-fat or regular sour cream
2 beaten eggs

Mix together the dry ingredients in a small mixing bowl:

3/4 cup cornmeal
3/4 cup flour

1 tsp sugar
1/4 tsp salt
2 1/2 tsp baking powder

Stir the dry ingredients into the wet ingredients until mixed. Beat with a spoon for one minute. Pour into a 2-quart casserole dish. Bake at 350 degrees for 45 minutes until it is golden on top, or at 325 degrees for an hour. Adjust the temperature depending on what else you are baking.

OVEN-FRIED POTATOES

These are wonderful newly made or reheated. They satisfy the need for French-fried potatoes without having to heat up a large vat of oil.
Start the oven at 375 degrees.
Thoroughly wash *2 1/2 pounds of Russet potatoes*. Remove blemishes and green patches. Cut the potatoes into chunks and dry them with paper towels. Toss with *3 to 4 tablespoons of cooking oil* in a large bowl, coating well.

Mix together seasonings for potatoes:
5 Tbsp grated Parmesan cheese
1/2 tsp salt
1/2 tsp garlic powder
1/2 tsp onion powder
1/2 tsp paprika
1/4 tsp black pepper

Pour the seasonings into the oiled potatoes and toss well. Pour them out on a jelly roll pan. Bake for 40 to 45 minutes, until potatoes are tender when you push a fork into them. Stir once with a pancake turner during baking.

OVEN-ROASTED VEGETABLES

Preheat oven to 425 degrees.

Mix together the following ingredients:
3 Tbsp olive oil
1 Tbsp lemon juice
1/2 tsp dried rosemary, crushed
1/4 tsp pepper
2 cloves garlic, chopped
1/2 tsp salt

Clean and prepare the following:
2 large onions, coarsely chopped
2 yellow summer squash, cut in slices
1/2 cauliflower, broken or cut into small florets
2 potatoes, cut into large chunks

Arrange vegetables in a shallow 9 x 13 baking pan. Drizzle the oil mixture over them. Bake for 20 minutes or until vegetables are as tender as you like them. Stir during baking with a pancake turner. Serve hot with grated Parmesan cheese, if desired.

Variations: Instead of the rosemary, use fresh basil. Just before serving, toss with 3/4 cup of slivered fresh basil leaves. Basil is an easy herb to grow fresh and keep on hand. To easily sliver them, roll several leaves into a long cylinder and slice them across the grain.

RATATOUILLE

Delicious hot or cold, by itself or on top of a frittata, ratatouille is nothing more nor less than mixed vegetables. This version cooks in 30 to 45 minutes in a pan on the stove top. To set it and forget it, you can also make a slow-cooker version. It is a wonderful late summer dish, when the locally grown tomatoes, summer squash, peppers, and eggplant are ready. Salting the eggplant and letting it sit gets it to "weep" out some of the bitter flavor.
Cube *1 medium eggplant*; salt it in layers in a colander and let it stand for 30 to 60 minutes. Then squeeze the cubes to get rid of the bitter, salty juice and rinse.

Combine the following in a saucepan:
cubed, rinsed, and drained eggplant
15-oz can Italian tomatoes
2 small zucchini, sliced
2 small yellow summer squash, sliced
1 medium onion, coarsely chopped
1 large red or yellow bell pepper, cut in
  thin strips
2 cloves garlic, finely chopped
1 tsp dry basil, finely crushed,
  or 1/4 cup fresh, shredded
3 tsp Italian seasoning, crushed
2 Tbsp dried parsley or 4 Tbsp fresh
1 tsp salt
1/2 tsp pepper
1 Tbsp olive oil

Bring to a boil, reduce heat, and cook on low for 30 to 45 minutes. Check periodically, and when zucchini and yellow squash are about half done (the colors will be bright and the vegetables not quite crisp-tender), put in *8 ounces of sliced fresh mushrooms* for the last 10 minutes of cooking.

Taste for seasoning and add more salt and pepper if you think it needs it. For a more zesty flavor, you might try adding a few drops of *balsamic vinegar*.

Slow-cooker variation: Cook at medium to low temperature. At medium, this should be done in 2 to 3 hours, but every slow cooker is different.

This recipe calls for only 1 tablespoon of olive oil, which isn't very much. I think that's all it needs. You may think otherwise. Anything up to 1/4 cup of olive oil qualifies for our definition of moderate fat use.

PEPPERS
Sweet bell-shaped peppers can be green, red, yellow, orange, brown, or purple, depending on the variety and stage of ripeness. The **Ratatouille** calls for red or yellow peppers primarily because of the color, although the sweeter flavor blends well with the other milder-flavored vegetables. Most peppers are sold at the mature green stage—fully developed but not ripe. As they ripen on the vine, green bell peppers turn red and become sweeter. Because they lack the capsaicin contained by their hotter cousins, bell peppers have no "bite." All peppers are excellent sources of vitamin C, with at least twice as much of the vitamin as citrus fruits.

Fruit Recipes from the Cycle Menu

Now it's time for the cycle-menu fruits. Fruit is, of course, perfectly presentable plain. Fresh fruit makes a wonderful dessert or meal accompaniment, as does canned or frozen fruit. It is surprising that although most people like fruit, food consumption surveys say we don't eat much of it. Not only that, but much of the fruit we consume is in the form of juice.

So it is clear we could use a little enticement. These fruit desserts add little in terms of time, and they add a great deal in terms of taste. We all like our sweets, so why not hook sweets onto something nutritious, like fruit?

PLUM COBBLER

Wash and cut *25 Italian plums* in quarters or slice *10 purple plums* to yield about a quart of fruit altogether. Spread fruit evenly on a 10 x 6-

or 8 x 8-inch baking pan. Sprinkle *2 tablespoons of sugar* and *1/4 teaspoon of cinnamon* over the fruit. Dot with little shavings of *butter* (the carrot peeler works well for shaving butter).

Mix together the dry ingredients:
1 cup flour (you may use half white and half whole wheat)
1 cup sugar
1 1/2 tsp baking powder
1/2 tsp salt
2 Tbsp Saco buttermilk powder
1/4 tsp baking soda

Add and stir the following ingredients until evenly blended:
1 egg, beaten
1/2 cup cold water
1/4 cup cooking oil

Pour the mixture evenly over the plums. Be sure to get the topping into the corners. Bake at 375 degrees for 45 minutes. The cobbler is done when the top is evenly brown and the plums pierce easily with a toothpick. Check the cobbler toward the end of baking, as it burns easily. Depending on what you have in the oven, you can get away with baking this at 400 degrees, 350 degrees, or even 325 degrees. Adjust the baking time accordingly.

Variation: Substitute an equal volume of other fruits for the plums.

Rhubarb: Sprinkle with 1/4 to 1/2 cup sugar.
Peaches: 4–5 fresh peaches, peeled and sliced, or 16-oz bag frozen peaches, or 28-oz can sliced peaches, drained (you may not need the 2 Tbsp sugar).

APPLE CUSTARD

In our family, this is known as "Gross Dessert" because I got the recipe from Annette Gross who put it in a crust and called it

---

BUTTERMILK
Buttermilk tenderizes baked goods and gives them a pleasant flavor. If you choose not to use buttermilk, substitute milk for the water and leave out the soda. Saco buttermilk powder is a great dried product; it's easy to keep on hand and is made from the whey of the butter-making process. You may also use 1/2 cup fluid buttermilk and omit the water.

"Dutch apple pie." Many of my recipes are named for the person who gave them to me. Cooking connects people and carries sweet memories.

Combine the following ingredients in a blender until the apples are finely chopped:

2 cups milk
4 eggs
2/3 cup sugar
1/4 tsp salt
3/4 tsp cinnamon
4 tsp flour
2 medium apples, washed and cored

Pour mixture into a casserole dish. Bake at 425 degrees for 10 minutes, then at 350 degrees for an additional 40 minutes. The custard is done when a clean knife inserted near the center comes out clean.

COOKING APPLES

The produce manager can tell you which are the cooking apples, and maybe even which ones keep their shape with cooking and which get mushy. Some common brands are McIntosh, Rome Beauty, Golden Delicious, and Cortland.

Whether you have mushy or firm cooked apples also depends on when you add the sugar. Adding sugar first makes for chunky applesauce. Cooking in water and adding sugar last makes for mushy applesauce. Choosing brown versus white sugar does the same. Brown sugar, which contains calcium, helps to preserve the "glue" between cells and keeps the chunks firmer. Tomato processors put calcium in tomatoes to preserve their texture, and you can use the calcium nutritionally.

PEACH CRISP

Put *3 cups sliced fresh, frozen, or canned peaches (drained)* in the bottom of a 10 x 6- or 8 x 8-inch baking pan.

Mix the dry ingredients together in a large mixing bowl:

1/2 cup brown sugar, packed
1/2 cup flour
1/2 cup oatmeal
1 1/2 tsp cinnamon

Using an electric mixer, cut *1/4 cup (1/2 stick) soft butter* evenly into the dry ingredients.

Sprinkle the mixture evenly over the fruit. If you like more topping, make two thin layers of fruit with two layers of topping.

Bake at 375 degrees around 40 minutes. The crisp is done when the top is lightly browned and the fruit feels tender when you stick in a toothpick. As with the **Plum Cobbler** (page 142), you can adjust the temperature and time depending on what else you are baking.

Serve warm or cool, plain or with cream, ice cream, or **Brown Cream Sauce** (page 144).

RECIPE NOTES

Fast tip: Double or triple this topping recipe and keep the extra in a glass jar in the refrigerator. Then when you want to make a crisp, all you have to do is prepare the fruit and sprinkle on the topping.

Variation: An equal volume of other fruit can be substituted for the peaches. You can start out making these crisps rather sweet, then gradually cut down on the sugar as your family develops a taste for more tart fruit. If fruit is very sour, sprinkle on a tablespoon or two of sugar per cup of fruit. Alternative fruits for this recipe could be—

Apples: Peeled or unpeeled, cored and sliced
Pears and blueberries; pears and blackberries
Fresh plums, pitted and sliced.

OLD-FASHIONED BREAD PUDDING

I said somewhere that bread pudding gives you a handy way of using up those bits and scraps of bread you have left over. Cube them and let them accumulate in a zip top bag in the freezer. Then when you get enough, make a bread pudding. This is a delicious, nutritious dessert that can double as breakfast.

Distribute the following ingredients evenly in a 9 x 13 baking pan:

6 cups cubed bread: white, whole wheat, raisin, cinnamon—whatever you have
1 1/2 cups freshly grated apple or 1/2 cup raisins or 1/2 cup Craisins or no fruit at all
1/2 cup chopped walnuts or other nuts or no nuts—your choice

Beat well together the following:

3 cups milk
3 eggs
1/2 cup brown sugar
1 tsp cinnamon

1/4 tsp nutmeg
2 tsp vanilla extract
1/4 tsp salt
1 Tbsp lemon juice

Pour the milk/egg mixture over the bread mixture. Let soak a few minutes before baking. Bake at 350 degrees for 35 minutes or until the bread pudding is lightly browned and a knife inserted near the center comes out clean.

Serve warm or cool with cream, ice cream, fresh fruit, applesauce, or nothing at all! If you were in New Orleans, you could get this with whiskey sauce. For that, you are on your own.

Variation: My variation on this recipe is to leave out the fruit, but then if I did that I would have no excuse to include it in this chapter! You can also serve it topped with fresh strawberries or raspberries, which taste wonderful.

FRUIT WITH BROWN CREAM SAUCE

Mix the following ingredients together:
1 Tbsp light brown sugar
1/2 cup low-fat or regular sour cream
1/4 tsp vanilla or other flavored extract

Pour the sauce over 3 to 4 cups of cut-up fruit:
oranges
apples
bananas
berries or nuts

PINEAPPLE UPSIDE-DOWN CAKE

This is a variation of the **Plum Cobbler** recipe (page 142).

Lay *pineapple slices* in the bottom of a 10 x 6- or 8 x 8-inch baking pan. Sprinkle with *2 tablespoons of brown sugar*, and then decrease the sugar in the recipe by 2 tablespoons. If you want to be fancy, put a *maraschino cherry* in the center of each pineapple ring.

Pour cobbler batter (page 142) over the top. If you like more fruit and less cobbler, double the fruit or halve the cobbler. Bake at 350 degrees for 40 minutes.

After baking, invert on a serving dish. Serve with ice cream.

MICROWAVE CHUNKY APPLESAUCE

Canned applesauce is good, but fresh homemade applesauce is an event! This applesauce is great as a side dish with pork, as dessert with cream or ice cream, or even with yogurt as a topping for pancakes.

Wash, quarter, and core *6 cooking apples*. Cut into bite-sized chunks. Put into a glass dish that can be covered.

Mix the following in with the apples, putting in the sugar before or after cooking:
1/4 cup water or apple juice
1/8 tsp nutmeg
3 Tbsp brown sugar

Cover and microwave on medium high for 4 minutes. Stir, and cook 3 minutes more. Check for doneness: apples will be firm but they will soften a little more as they stand. Allow to cool and serve warm or cold.

RECIPE NOTES
Variation: Peel the apples for a softer product. Before you cook the apples, add *1/2 package cranberries, halved*, or *1/2 cup Craisins*. Cranberries give the applesauce a lovely red color.

Fast tip: Cook this the night before or an hour or two ahead of time to let the apples get consistently soft and give the colors and flavors a chance to blend.

Plan for Success

- Do your meal planning in ways that are realistic and helpful and not in ways that overburden you and your family.
- Include menus that are fast and easy to prepare and keep in mind a number of "last-resort dinners" that you can easily throw together in case your plans go awry.
- Take care of yourself as well as your family. Manage your day so that you have some energy left for preparing dinner. Make sure you have eaten a decent breakfast and lunch, and take breaks when you need them.
- Manage mealtimes so that they are rewarding for you as well as for the rest of your family. Don't feel that you must wait on the rest of your family to the point that you can't attend to your own eating.
- Introduce change slowly and add new elements to your family's routine gradually. Don't try to take on everything all at once or you're likely to encounter resistance and become discouraged.
- Use the cycle menu presented in this chapter to help you plan your family's meals. Adjust as needed to make it work for you and your family.

CHAPTER

8

PLANNING
TO GET YOU
COOKING

Planning is good. You can use planning to save time, simplify feeding your family, and lower your stress level. Planning can save you from the daunting late-afternoon loss of ideas and lack of energy as you wonder, "what's for dinner?" Done kindly, planning can provide its own reward in making cooking and eating enjoyable and rewarding. However, planning can be *abused*. Unrealistic planning can cost you time and complicate feeding your family and raise your stress level. Clean tools in dirty hands can be disastrous.

You are *using* planning when you rough out a menu for the next few days, then take five minutes the night before to check the menu, put the spinach in the refrigerator to thaw, and get the canned goods lined up for the next night's dinner. You are *using* planning when you take shortcuts and use leftovers to provide PPMs (pre-prepared meals, if you recall).

But you are *abusing* planning if you let your enthusiasm or your conscience get the better of you. You are *abusing* planning when you use working ahead to make yourself into another Martha Stewart. You can decide to make everything from scratch and add super-fancy touches and do advanced preparation to turn out a meal that is so stunningly elegant that your family doesn't dare eat it. Whereupon you will be furious because you worked your fingers to the bone to make something nice for them. You are also *abusing* planning when you say, "Oh, we shouldn't eat that; it isn't good for us." Whereupon you turn out a meal that is so drab that nobody is interested in eating it.

Either way, you will get discouraged and say, "What's the use, anyway?" and take everybody out to have hamburgers with eight slices of bacon. Remember, planning is your servant, not your master.

Given today's punitive, conscience-ridden attitudes about food, many people depend on impulse in order to be able to feed themselves at all. Certainly, it is easier to eat "forbidden" food if you don't think about it too much. You'll recall from earlier chapters that in fact *there is no forbidden food*.

If you must be rigid about something, be rigid about *structure*. If you can hang on to the structure of meals and planned snacks, nutrition has a way of falling into place. For food to work well, you have to make it a priority. However, it doesn't have to be *such* a priority that it overshadows everything else. The trick is to think about food a lot when you plan it, cook it, and eat it. Then forget about it between times. If you do your planning and feed yourself well, you *will* be able to forget about it between times.

Planning Your Escape

In this chapter, we are going to get organized. That will take time and focused attention. We are going to talk about cycle menus (three weeks of menus that you use over and over again), inventories, planned shopping trips, storage, and equipment. However, because there is a lot to this topic and because I worry that you will become overwhelmed and give up—or worse, get overzealous—we will start by planning your escape. The all-important escape can be little deliberate vacations from cooking. An escape comes in handy when your planning has run amok (or was amok in the first place), when the tire went flat, the computer crashed, and you had to work late. You also need an escape when you are just so tired you can't stand to think about cooking. Make arrangements for gaps and vacations and dinners of last resort:

- Plan meals that in the past your food conscience wouldn't let you think of (assuming that your food conscience is less hyperactive after reading this book). How about hot dogs, beans, and potato chips—with ice cream for dessert? Macaroni and cheese and canned green beans? Bologna sandwiches on white bread with mayonnaise, canned peaches, and store-bought cookies for dessert? For more ideas, see chapter 6, pages 118-119.
- Order in, go out, or hit the deli for an HMR (you know, a Home Meal Replacement). You might get some ideas for meals you can make at home.
- Pull out the leftovers. Put them on the table cold. Let everyone serve his or her own plate, pile up the plates by inverting an empty plate over a full one, and nuke them in the microwave. You can still have a meal together, even if everyone is eating something different.
- Have some nutritionally worthless meals. I am hard-pressed to think of one—let's see—gum drops and Kool-Aid? Even Kool-Aid is fortified with vitamin C. I guess your toddler shouldn't have the gum drops—choking hazard. How about potato chips and soda? But even potato chips have potato nutrients. Hmmm . . .
- Have popcorn and cocoa on Sunday nights in front of the television.

Managing the Day So You Can Manage Dinner

If your planning works well, you will spend 20 to 30 minutes right before dinner preparing the meal and getting it on the table. At that time, I promise, you will be tired and touchy and your children will be the same. If you are

just home from work, you will be trying to do two things at once: connecting with your children and getting dinner on the table. If you count connecting with yourself, you have *three* priorities.

If you are a typical young woman, you will also be hungry because you will not have eaten well all day. If you are a typical young man, you may have eaten better, but all the rest will be the same. In other words, you will be feeling *stress* and *conflict*. Little wonder that 78 percent of households ate out at least once last week.

Think of the advantages of a restaurant meal: Sitting calmly, resting, giving the other family members your full attention, munching on something to keep your strength up, waiting serenely for the dinner that someone else has prepared. Ah, but think of the disadvantages. You have to get *back* in the car to go there, you have to keep the kids entertained while you wait for the meal to be served (and when they finish eating before you do). With restaurant commotion around you, it's harder to connect with other family members than at home. You have to pay two to three times more for it, and you have to settle for restaurant food. Believe it or not, you will get to the point that you enjoy what you make at home more than what you get at a restaurant.

Certainly a restaurant meal now and again is a worthwhile investment in time and money. For some guidelines on managing restaurant meals, see the box "Eating Out with Children." But, most of the time, there is a better way. Perhaps there is a way of getting the rest and nurturing you crave while you stay home to eat. How can you manage your day so you have energy for the end of the day? How can you get a little rest before you start working on dinner? How can you connect with your child so that you don't have to keep putting her off while you prepare dinner?

On the matter of energy, do think about feeding and taking care of yourself throughout the day. Have you had breakfast? A decent lunch? Have you had any breaks during the day when you could kick back and relax? Have you used lunch as time to take a break and relax? Have you had a snack in a long afternoon to tide you over from a long-ago and far-away lunch? If the answers to these questions are "no," you will pay for it at the end of the day. You will be understandably exhausted, cranky, and depleted. You will likely pay

EATING OUT WITH CHILDREN

If you eat out only rarely, you can afford to throw nutritional considerations to the winds and let your child order only what she likes. If you eat out a lot, it's worth setting up some simple guidelines to encourage nutritious eating without having her load up on fat and sugar. Here are some suggestions:

• Have at least two food groups. You'll probably find that this happens automatically anyway. A hamburger and a bun would qualify, as would pizza. By the time your child has the crust and the topping, she's covered at least two and probably three or four food groups. A salad and bread would work, so would bread and ice cream.

• Limit sweets to one per meal. If your child has a milkshake or soda for her beverage, that counts as her sweet. However, if she has milk or water to drink, she can still have a sweet.

• Keep it down to one fried food per meal. For example, if your child has French fries and a hamburger, a fried apple pie for dessert would add up to too many fried foods. To have the apple pie, she would have to skip the French fries and to fill up, she might need a second hamburger. Grilled foods like burgers don't count as fried foods because they aren't so greasy. It's the starch in French fries and the starchy coating on chicken nuggets and fish sandwiches that tend to soak up the grease.

• Keep dessert portions child-sized, just as you would at home. That might mean splitting a dessert with someone else at the table, or ordering a sundae rather than a banana split.

for it *during* the day, as well. Efficiency experts tell us that long, unrelieved work days don't pay: our productivity drops.

You won't be able to give to your child and family unless you first give to yourself. In fact, taking care of yourself teaches children an important lesson: others have needs too. A major toddler task is learning to respect others' needs. Unlike the young infant, the toddler no longer benefits from being made the center of the universe. The same, of course, is true for preschoolers and school-age children. Presumably, though, these older children have already learned to respect others' needs as well as their own. If your children have not, teach them.

How do you apply that bit of developmental psychology to the end of the day? Well, first of all, arrange to have some energy left by giving yourself food and rest during the day. Then make some choices. How do you want to use

that first half hour when you get home from work? Having some time to yourself? Connecting with your child? Cooking dinner? Put the emphasis on *want*. Any of the answers is right, as long as you work it out with your child so she knows what to expect and so she can cooperate.

Then you have to take your child's needs into account. Until she can tell you otherwise, it is safe to assume that her list is short: she wants to be with you. So how are you both going to get what you want? Talk about it. Say, "I want to spend some time with you, but first I want to change my clothes and read the mail. How would it be if I do that, and then we can play blocks for a while?" So what if she says, "I want to play blocks first"? Why not say (if you feel like it), "OK, but first I want to change clothes."

Here is a secret about playing with your child: With playing, as with eating, children like to take the lead and want you to be a supportive presence. You don't have to pile up blocks for her to knock down or make elaborate houses or teach about the laws of shapes and sizes and proportions. All you have to do is be there, pay attention, ask about what your child is doing and make little comments, like, "That's a big wall." You can even do all this in a prone position, as long as you truly pay attention and take an interest.

Playing together doesn't have to go on forever for you and your child to connect. In fact, if you really tune in, after 15 or 20 minutes you both will feel better and you can go on with what comes next. Set a timer, if it will free you to take this time. You may even feel energized enough by then that you won't need your break. But if you do, take it. A few minutes of putting your feet up could make all the difference between food preparation being pleasant and rewarding and being a real drag.

Another routine might be to get dinner started, and then sit down and play. A few of the menus will allow you to do that: the **Swiss Steak** (pages 88-89) can be warming up and the potatoes can be cooking while you rest on the floor. Not every day has to be the same. What has to happen, however, is that you deliver on your promise of time with your child. Then let her know how much it helps you when she lives up to her agreements with you as well.

Cooking together is a fine way of connecting with your child. I have made lots of suggestions in chapters 5, 6, and 7 about what your child can do to help prepare the meal. That early help will turn into real help in a few years, so be patient. Be friendly and companionable and appreciative while you cook. Don't be gushy in your praise or your clever child will decide, "She must think I am really a baby to get so excited that I can do *that*." Or, she might conclude, "If he is making such a fuss about this, it must be I'm not supposed to like it." You really can't fool a child. They may not be able to put it in words, but their feelings tell them what is going on.

What about that afternoon snack? If dinner is late, children, and probably adults, benefit from more than one afternoon snack: an early "little meal" that is satisfying for two or three hours and a later pick-me-up snack. The pick-me-up can be a small glass of juice and a couple of crackers. This is the one time I recommend putting limits on amounts. You don't want to eat enough to spoil dinner, but just to take the edge off hunger. When you start cooking, the goal is for you and your child to be hungry but not so famished that you just can't wait.

Even then, it will be hard to wait, so teach your child about distraction. "Let's just think about cutting up these mushrooms for now, and dinner will be ready before we know it." "Tell me about your day, that will make it easier to think about something else." "Let me tell you about something funny I heard on the radio today." Children can take an interest in listening to adults talk with each other, as well, as long as they know they, too, will get a turn to talk.

Manage Serving So Meals Are Rewarding

Put everything on the table at the same time (including something to mop up spills), announce the last call for table service, sit down, and don't get up until you are finished. I often work with young mothers who are trying to get a grip on their eating. Too often, they complain that they can't pay attention to their *own* meal and really enjoy it because they are running after their children.

Such attentiveness is not necessary. Children behave exactly as their adults teach them to behave. If you hover and jump up and chase after and respond to every little demand for attention, your child will ask for it all and more besides. If, however, you help your child

get served, serve yourself, and refuse to be distracted from your own meal, your child will attend to her own meal rather than try to get you to perform.

For the most part, put the food in serving bowls and let children serve themselves. Teach them to pass food to other people, and to say "yes, please" and "no, thank you." To make the presentation more interesting, have a variety of big and little serving bowls, some colorful and crazy and interesting. The bowls don't have to match. Give some thought to your serving spoons, tongs, and forks, as well. These have to work for small hands if your child is to be successful serving herself.

Master Cooking a Little at a Time

As I have written these "how to manage food" chapters, I have been aware of how much there is to learn and master. Don't try to learn it all at once. Start out by thinking about the recipes and food suggestions in chapter 5, and pick out the most familiar and appealing ones. Begin by cooking one more meal a week than you do right now and work up from there. Make this book your own by writing notes on the margins of the recipe pages. Write down how you liked it, how much you had left over, how long it took to cook or bake at what temperature in what pan.

Gradually work up to more and more foods on more and more nights. Keep your goals modest, and keep your cooking in perspective. Compare yourself not to the ideal but to the 75 percent of men and women who don't know by 4 P.M. what they will serve for dinner. Compare yourself to the average family food preparer, whose list of dinner meals consists of five dishes: baked or fried chicken, pasta, hamburgers, hot dogs, and takeout pizza. There. Feel better?

Begin by picking out your favorite recipes and recycle them a few times. For feeding children, the repetition is not all bad because familiarity enhances food acceptance. If you are one of the five-dish people, your family may resist having their dinner trifled with. They are likely to, in fact. Even though you know this new way of having dinner is better (and even though they may agree with you), the old approach is comfortable, so they will oppose the change. But if you persist, they will eventually learn to like the new menus as well.

The recipes in this book are intended to stretch your food acceptance. Begin by cooking just a few recipes that seem more familiar. Then, once you have mastered regularly cooking your familiar foods, start to experiment with some less familiar ones. In you menus, combine familiar and favorite with unfamiliar foods. If a cycle menu is your goal, it may take at least 6 months or even a year before you can use the complete, 3-week cycle menu—or a cycle menu you have adapted for yourself. A cycle menu is highly personal, so don't be afraid to make it your own. Make a copy, scratch out the foods you wouldn't cook, and figure out substitutes. But don't throw away my original suggestions.

Above all, go at your own speed. This is supposed to be a help to you, and to be satisfying and even *fun*.

The Cycle Menu

Now that we have gotten your anxiety level down a little, let's look at the big picture: the cycle menu. Here is where all those nasty jokes you made about school lunch come back to haunt you. You know, "If this is Friday these must be tacos." You said it, I didn't. I grew up in a one-room country school, and we didn't have school lunch. Actually, I am eating some words myself in these food management chapters. As a nutrition undergraduate and dietetic intern, I complained bitterly about having to take food preparation and institution management courses. What interested me was clinical nutrition. Now I am reaching into the dusty recesses of my mind for that very information!

You work the cycle menu by going all through the 3 weeks, starting with **Beef Ragout** on the first Sunday, ending with pork chops on the last Saturday, then starting all over again. Or you can start on the first Wednesday with **Mostaccioli with Spinach and Feta** and end with a pre-prepared meal: ragout on the first Tuesday. To get started, however, you might want to confine yourself to your favorite week. That works best if you start with Wednesday or after, because

THE CYCLE MENU

Sunday	Monday	Tuesday	Wednesday	Thursday	Friday	Saturday
Beef Ragout Buttered noodles Canned peaches or fruit in season Cucumber slices or bread and butter Pumpkin custard	**Tuna-Noodle Casserole** Poppyseed coleslaw Celery sticks Dill pickles Toasted bagels and butter More pumpkin custard	**PPM: Beef Ragout** Apple wedges Orange slices or fruit in season Green salad Toasted bagels and butter Ice cream	**Mostaccioli with Spinach and Feta** Scalloped corn Toasted English muffins and butter Plum dessert or fruit in season	**Hamburgers on Buns** Potato chips Celery sticks and pickles Canned fruit or fruit in season	**PPM, eat out, or** *Last-resort Dinner* Spaghetti carbonara Green salad Any appealing leftover fruits and vegetables	**Chicken & Rice** Glazed carrots or vegetables in season French bread in the oven Apple custard or fruit in season
Swiss Steak Mashed potatoes Gravy Gingered broccoli or vegetables in season Bread and butter More apple custard	**Wisconsin Fish Boil with Potatoes, Carrots, and Onions** Melted butter Bread and butter Cherry cobbler Ice cream	**PPM: Beefy Shortcut Stroganoff** Mashed potatoes or noodles Green salad Ice cream, cookies	**Lemon Chicken** Oven-fried potatoes Creamed spinach or vegetables in season Green salad Bread and butter Peach cobbler or crisp Fruit in season	**Broccoli Chowder** Homemade bread with peanut butter Fruit in season More peach cobbler or crisp	**PPM, eat out, or** *Last-resort Dinner* Frittata Fruit in season Any appealing leftover fruits and vegetables	**Meat Loaf** Boxed scalloped potatoes Carrot and celery sticks Herbed peas or vegetables in season Bread pudding with raisins or fruit in season
Savory Black Beans and Rice Corn pudding Orange rounds with parsley snips or fruit in season Ice cream	**Stir-Fry Chicken** Rice Fruit in season Bread and butter More bread pudding	**PPM: Spaghetti and Meatballs** Green salad French bread Apple and orange wedges or fruit in season	**PPM: Black Bean Soup** Variety of crackers, including oyster crackers Cheese on toast Fruit with brown cream sauce	**Herb-Baked Fish** Boxed scalloped potatoes Green salad Bread and butter Pineapple upside-down cake or fruit in season	**PPM, eat out, or** *Last-resort Dinner* Macaroni-tomato-hamburger casserole Any appealing leftover fruits and vegetables	**Braised Pork Chops with Sweet Potatoes** Microwave chunky applesauce Bread and butter Ice cream

Tuesday often uses something from Saturday or Sunday. When you get comfortable with one week, add another.

Institution food managers have known for a long time that the secret to manageable, economical feeding is having a great cycle menu. The length of the cycle varies, depending on how long-lasting (and how tolerant) the audience is. Now that hospital stays are shorter, many hospital cycle menus are down to only a week or two. School lunch and residence hall cafeterias, with customers who stay month after month, often have a 3- or 4-week cycle menu to keep people from getting tired of the food.

For a young family and a beginning cook, a 2-week cycle menu is long enough to give a lot of variety. I decided on 3 weeks to help you keep your customers from getting tired of the food. I also needed the extra week to show you how to cook a few more main dishes and side dishes and increase the chances that you would find foods that appeal to you.

The main entree dishes form the backbone of the cycle, and the vegetables, fruits, salads, and desserts provide the rest. I have filled in all the blanks by providing suggestions for quick and easy "meal accompaniments," vegetables, fruits, salads, and desserts. I hope some of these accompaniments become standbys for you. For home planning, it is typical to preplan only the main entree dishes and rely on standbys for the accompaniments. A certain salad is easy to throw together and sure to please. It is easy to send a child to the freezer to pick out the "veggie" for dinner. Put it in the microwave for 5 or 10 minutes, color on some butter, and you are done. Open a can of peaches, put it in a bowl, and dessert is served.

Some fruit or vegetable recipes are appealing enough to turn them from being an accompaniment into being the star of the menu. Examples of such special recipes for me are broccoli with Super-Quick Cheese Sauce, Gingered Broccoli, Mashed Potatoes, and Greens and Bacon. You undoubtedly have others. Seasonal fruits and vegetables can often raise your meal from ordinary to outstanding—when fresh corn and tomatoes are available, when the strawberries or cantaloupe make your mouth water, when the squash is at the roadside markets and you *have* to have some. Let the produce section provide you with inspiration.

STRATEGIES FOR PLANNING THE CYCLE MENU

Here are the strategies I used for putting together these menus:

- A variety of main dishes. I used meat, poultry and fish, cooked dried beans, cheese, and eggs. I have planned meatless meals 2 days a week, and I also used red meat 2 to 3 days per week. I have used cooked dried beans for main dishes and as salads. If you want to adapt the cycle to make it lacto-ovo-vegetarian, you will find some suggestions in the box below, "Vegetarian Menu Planning." If you want to follow a vegan diet, that is, to avoid milk, eggs, and cheese, then I am afraid you

---

VEGETARIAN MENU PLANNING

- Follow the Food Guide Pyramid and the recommendations in chapter 4 (pages 60-62) offering eggs, legumes, nuts, and seeds instead of meat, poultry, or fish. (Dried peas, dried beans, lentils, and peanuts are legumes.)
- Use vitamin D–fortified milk to provide calcium, vitamin D, and a concentrated source of high-quality protein. You can use soy formula instead of cow's milk. However, soy or nut beverages (that you buy or make yourself) don't substitute for cow's milk. They generally don't have as much calcium as cow's milk, and they don't have vitamin D.
- Keep an eye on iron nutrition. Cutting out meat, poultry, and fish makes it hard for your child (and you) to consume and assimilate enough iron without the well-absorbed heme iron and the "meat factor" from these animal protein sources. She'll absorb plant iron better if she has a good source of vitamin C (citrus fruits or juices, green leafy vegetables, green pepper, tomato) along with at least two of her meals every day.
- For children particularly, use whole grains only about half the time, enriched refined grains the rest. Your child is already getting a lot of fiber from legumes, seeds, and nuts. If she gets too much fiber, she'll fill up before she eats as much as she needs. Too much fiber can also interfere with iron, copper, and zinc nutrition.
- Make sure you include enough fat. Vegetarian diets tend to be low in fat because foods like beans, grains, fruits, and vegetables are mostly fat-free or low in fat.
- Plan meals around high-quality protein. Include some animal protein, such as milk, eggs, or cheese, or put together various plants, with their incomplete proteins, to make more complete protein.

are on your own. I don't recommend it for children.

- Flexibility. Menu planning can foster both order and flexibility. For example, with fruits and vegetables, I used fresh, canned, and frozen. For most days' menus, I have made suggestions for fruits and vegetables, but I have also reminded you to consider "seasonal fruit" and "seasonal vegetables." For a list of those seasonal foods, see chapter 9, pages 171-172. I have also planned PPM nights and last-resort dinners. The last-resort nights are generally on Fridays, when I assume you are tired and ready for a break from cooking. Those menus are especially easy.

- Time budgets. The cycle menu calls for you to cook on three weekdays; those menus can be prepared in about 30 minutes, start to finish. On weekends, I have suggested preparing meals that are equally quick to put together but take longer to cook. I am assuming you can put weekend meals in the oven or slow cooker and then peek at them from time to time. For instance, the **Chicken and Rice** on the first Saturday bakes in an hour or two, but you can get it ready to go in the oven in 10 or 15 minutes.

- Down time. On Tuesdays and Fridays you can take it easy. I have planned meals those days to let you take a little break from cooking. Tuesday is PPM day when a pre-prepared meal makes a repeat performance (as with the **Beef Ragout** in week 1) or gets a face-lift (as with **Swiss Steak's** transformation into **Beefy Shortcut Stroganoff in** week 2). Friday is "clean out the refrigerator" day. If what's left in the refrigerator is just too unthinkable, make a super-easy last-resort dinner. Or order in. You deserve it.

- Equipment use. To find the most efficient method for each meal, I have used baking, slow cooking, stewing, microwaving, stir-frying, and even—gasp!—frying. When I have used the oven, I have tried to bake an additional menu item at the same time, like potatoes or a dessert, to take advantage of the hot oven. Each cooking method has something to offer in your overall strategy for getting a meal on the table. More important, I want to give all of these cooking approaches my blessings.

- Pre-prepared ingredients. I have made heavy use of pre-prepared ingredients, like portion-cut or already-cubed meats, pre-

washed or preshredded vegetables and cheese, canned and frozen meats, fish and vegetables, sauces and broth bases. For a more detailed list of pre-prepared ingredients and suggestions for how to use them, see the box on page 154, "Grocery List of Convenient Foods and Ingredients."

Organizing Your Work Space When Children Are Around

Having children in the kitchen when you are cooking can be dangerous. The solution to the problem is not to keep children out, but rather to give some time and thought to keeping it safe for them. *You* are in the kitchen and you are doing all these intriguing things. What child wouldn't be eager to see and hear and touch and smell? Your toddler will be tugging at your pant leg, wanting to get up and see. In between times, she will sit beneath your feet. Your older children will hang around, hungry and wanting to help.

It is worth the trouble to think through your work spaces to let children be in the kitchen with you. The first and all-important safety rule? Protect children from anything that is hot or sharp. Turn the handles of pans to the back of the range so children can't grab them and pull them over. Put sharp knives at the back of the counter where children can't reach them.

Organize your kitchen into functional work areas, so you can pretty much plant your feet (or your child) and not move from there while you assemble whatever it is. Have a baking area, where you put all your measuring cups and spoons, bowls, and canisters. Have a fruit and vegetable preparation area near the sink, where you put your peelers, knives (and plastic knives for your child to use), scrubbers, and cutting boards. If you can't organize your storage in logical areas, assemble everything you need before you start to cook.

Designate an area where your child can "cook." For the toddler, this might be the sink, where she can pour water around. Let the faucet dribble and give her some measuring cups to fill and empty. Give her some sturdy vegetables, like potatoes or carrots, to "wash." Put her up to the table with a pan of rice and let her feel and measure. Whatever you give her to do, know that it won't last long. You are giving her the cooking idea, not expecting much from her except—probably—a mess. But an older child can actually be of some help. If you organize her place and equipment, an older child can open cans, wash celery, put pickles on the plate, and cube watermelon—the list can go on and on. Make use of the suggestions given with the recipes in chapters 5, 6, and 7 for how your children can help with meal preparation.

If you have counter space to spare, consider storing your most-used utensils in crocks or large jars on the countertop. Get a little crock for your measuring spoons. Have a separate crock by the stove with pancake turners, stirring spoons, and strainers. That way, you can find utensils quickly, without having to paw through a cluttered drawer. If you plan to do much baking, store your sugar, flour, and salt in canisters

that are easy to dip into. Find dippers that double as quarter- or half-cup measures and leave them in the canister so you can scoop out and measure at the same time without having to unearth the measuring cups. A pot and pan rack is great if you have the ceiling space for it.

Organizing Your Storage

The list of staples in chapter 9 includes both "staples" and "perishables." The staples are foods like flour, sugar, canned goods, and frozen foods. These are foods you can keep around awhile. The strategy I recommend is that you do a big "staples" shopping trip once every 3 weeks, and then run to the store once or twice a week for perishables, like produce

---

GROCERY LIST OF CONVENIENT FOODS AND INGREDIENTS

Grocers and food manufacturers know that your time is limited and that you want to cook at home. They cater to your needs by taking care of some of the preparation for you. Prepared foods may cost more money, but think of the extra expense as "help" cost, not as food cost. In fact, the extra cost may not be as much as you think, when you consider that what you buy is all edible. You don't have to pay for anything that gets peeled off or cut away. Prepared foods may or may not be worth the extra expense depending on what you have more of: time or money. Using them certainly is cheaper than eating out.

Meat, Poultry, Fish, Dry Beans, Eggs, and Nuts: Chicken thighs, boned chicken breasts or stir-fry, canned chicken; frozen fish fillets, canned tuna or salmon; lean ground beef; boneless pork chops, cutlets, or stir-fry; small ham roasts and slices; stew meat (needs to be cooked slowly); breakfast steaks (thin, quick-cooking steaks); prepared meat patties. Canned baked beans, cans or jars of pre-cooked navy beans, garbanzos, black beans, and refried beans. Eggs. Peanut butter. Regular and low-fat luncheon meats, sausages, and hot dogs.

Milk, Yogurt, and Cheese: Preshredded cheese, cheese slices, cheese spread in jars. Milk to drink. Instant and prepared puddings and custards. Plain and flavored yogurt. Canned cream soups to reconstitute with milk.

Vegetables: Frozen potatoes, instant mashed potatoes, boxed scalloped potatoes, canned or frozen vegetables, fresh cleaned and chopped vegetables from the produce section, preshredded coleslaw mix, peeled baby carrots, cleaned salad fixings by the pound. Vegetable juices, like tomato juice and vegetable juice cocktail. Flavored canned tomatoes, like Italian, Mexican, Cajun.

Fruits: Fresh, canned, or frozen fruits and fruit juices. Cleaned and portioned fruits from the produce section. Fruit nectars (apricot nectar is a good source of vitamin A). Dried fruits like raisins, prunes, apricots, apples, and peaches. Fig Newtons and raisin cookies.

Breads, Cereal, Rice, and Pasta: Enriched or whole grain bread. Noodles, macaroni, spaghetti. Rolls, frozen bread dough, corn bread mixes, muffin mix, Bisquick, pita bread, and tortillas. Twist-can biscuits and roll dough. Instant plain or brown rice. Pizza bread. English muffins, bagels. Pancake mix.

Convenient Ingredients: Sauces and seasonings let you put together quick and tasty meals from ready-to-go foods. Ingredients you can keep on hand include spaghetti and other sauces in jars, cream soups, seasonings to sprinkle on (like lemon pepper), to mix in (like taco mix), or to serve on the side (like picante, tartar, or cocktail sauce).

milk, and possibly bread.

Keeping staples on hand saves trips to the store for the one item missing in a recipe. It allows you to make the in-between grocery stops very quick, thus saving on time and impulse purchases. But keeping staples on hand means you need a way of storing them so you can find them.

If you have room in your kitchen for three weeks' storage, that's great. If not, build a pantry and keep only the most-used foods in the kitchen. For the backup inventory, hang a set of plastic shelves behind a door or put some shallow shelves in a closet or in the back part of the basement. To keep the canned goods as cool as possible, place the shelves away from the refrigerator and stove. Foods are easier to find if the shelves are shallow.

Having extra freezer space is great. If you have a big freezer on your refrigerator, that might be enough. Otherwise, consider buying a little chest-type freezer. These sell for under $300 and run for about the cost of a 50-watt lightbulb. In your little freezer, you can keep a 3-week inventory of meat, poultry, and fish. You can also keep on hand an assorted supply of frozen vegetables and fruits and extra bread that you can pull out as needed.

Upright freezers are easier to organize and get food into and out of, but they are generally bigger and not as energy-efficient. Because they are harder to fill up, they frost up more easily. Organization was a problem for me with my chest-type freezer until I hit on my bag method. I sort the food into cloth bags— you know, the type you get with some business name written on them or the ecology bags that you buy at the grocery store. I have a bag for red meat, one for chicken and fish, one for vegetables and fruit, and one for breads. I label the handle of the bag using a permanent marker. I pull out the bag and rummage through it for the food I want, rather than rummaging through the whole freezer.

Keeping Food Safe

When raising children, it is generally better not to get compulsive. Food safety and sanitation, however, are exceptions to that rule. Be compulsive about sanitation. Since I think you can't emphasize this topic too much, I am going to be compulsive by telling you some things I have said before. You can be compulsive by attending to some basic rules of food

handling, storage, cooking, and shopping. As long as we are both compulsive about sanitation, you have nothing to worry about.

Bacteria are always with us. By handling food properly, you keep bacteria from growing to the dangerous levels where they can do harm. Food safety experts rank food-borne disease as the greatest health risk from the food supply. Part of learning to cook is developing lifelong methods that you (and your children) can use for staying clean and handling food. Certainly food manufacturers and government regulators have an obligation to keep our food as safe as can be. However, what happens to food in the home, when it is stored and cooked and served and stored again, has a major impact on food safety. We have to do our part to ensure a safe food supply.

Because their immune systems are immature, preschool children are particularly vulnerable to food-borne diseases. Young children also bring their own hazard to the food safety issue because of their diapers, their awkward and inexperienced toileting, and their tendency to play in the dirt. When you live with children, changing their pants, helping them go to the bathroom, and pulling them out of the dirt, you have to be super careful about washing your hands. In the tragic outbreak of *Escherichia coli* 0157.H7 (*E. coli* 157) in 1993, an infant in a Washington State child care center became ill even though he hadn't eaten the contaminated ground beef that caused the outbreak. He got infected when the provider failed to wash her hands thoroughly after she changed an infected child's diapers.

HAND WASHING

Keep hands clean. To wash hands thoroughly, the International Food Safety Council says to wet your hands, soap them thoroughly, and rub them together, fronts, backs, and forearms, for 20 seconds before you rinse. This is long enough to sing "Happy Birthday" twice. Given the quick, soapless rinse that most of us give our hands, I would happily settle for "Happy Birthday" once and consider it a huge improvement. Lace your fingers together and rub them up and down to wash between them. Curl your fingers and hook your hands together to soap the fingertips. If you give them credit for good hand-washing technique, your children will take it seriously and be proud of doing a good job. Wash hands after going to the bathroom or changing diapers, before handling food, after handling any meat or fresh produce, and before eating.

Also be sure to keep clean towels around for wiping your hands, and find a place to hang the towel so it can dry. Change your towel daily—more often than that if it gets so much use that it is always damp.

Since hand cleanliness is so important, it would seem that the antibacterial hand cleaners, detergents, and soaps would be a good idea. Not so. Antibacterial cleaners tend to be antibiotic, and routine use of antibiotics leads to antibiotic-resistant bacteria. The problem with cleaners is the same as with medicine. Using antibiotics when you don't really need them can make them useless when you do. Using soap is enough to clean thoroughly, and, for really tough disinfecting jobs, chlorine-type bleach is a good choice.

PREVENTING FOOD CONTAMINATION

Keep your work area clean. Bacteria require three conditions to multiply: nutrients, heat, and moisture. That is, they need smears or quantities of food, they need moisture (dried smears don't culture germs), and they need the proper temperature to grow. Bacteria are always with us. Your task is to deprive them of any or all of their requirements for growing and thriving. You do that by keeping your tools and work surfaces clean and dry and by refrigerating foods promptly.

Keeping cutting boards clean presents a special challenge, because their grooves and slashes hide moisture and bacteria and because the boards come in such direct contact with food. Like many of the issues we have grappled with, the research and the press releases have gone back and forth about whether it is better to use wooden or synthetic cutting boards. Even though you can put synthetics in the dishwasher, they still seemed to harbor more germs than wooden boards. Or maybe not. At latest report, the recommendation is to have separate cutting boards for produce and for raw meats, poultry, and fish. I think it would be a good idea to have a third cutting board for carving cooked meats. Do what you can stand, but if you use only one cutting board, wash it thoroughly, bleach it, and let it dry after you use it for raw meats or produce.

COMMON FOOD BACTERIA

For more important ways to be compulsive about food safety, see the box on page 157,

"Food Safety." For more motivation to be compulsive, read on. Some bacteria cause infections, when they grow and multiply to levels high enough to make us sick. *Escherichia coli* and *Salmonella*, which are potentially present in all raw and fresh foods, and *Clostridium perfringens*, which is present everywhere, are examples of infective organisms. Other bacteria cause food poisoning when the bacteria produce toxins that make us sick. *Clostridium botulinum*, which causes botulism, is a toxin that grows in improperly processed, low-acid canned foods, like the cold potato soup that caused an outbreak some years back.

Although any microorganism can find its way into a kitchen, four pathogens are particularly significant when cooking for children. *Shigella* is a bacterium that causes diarrhea, fever, abdominal pain, and bloody stools. It is transmitted through fecal contamination on food or hands or through contaminated food and water.

E. coli 157 causes bloody diarrhea, severe abdominal cramps, and vomiting and is particularly dangerous because *E. coli* 157 infection can progress to kidney failure. *E coli* 157 outbreaks come from any food that has been contaminated by the feces of a ruminant animal, like a cow or deer. Outbreaks have been caused by contaminated, undercooked ground beef, raw milk, unpasteurized apple juice (made from windfalls that come in contact with cow or deer feces), contaminated water, and poorly washed lettuce.

Salmonella causes headache, abdominal pain, diarrhea, fever, and nausea, which usually begin 8 to 48 hours after eating the contaminated food. Symptoms can last from 1 to 8 days. Even though poultry-processing methods are being improved, so much poultry continues to be contaminated with *Salmonella* that we must assume that it is contaminated and handle it with care. *Salmonella* outbreaks come from raw or undercooked foods such as poultry, eggs, unpasteurized milk, and unwashed fresh fruits and vegetables. In recent years, outbreaks of *Salmonella* have been caused by the contaminated skins of cantaloupe, watermelon, and tomatoes.

Clostridium perfringens is present in all food, and given the opportunity, it will grow and cause diarrhea and gas pains which begin 6 to 24 hours after ingestion and last 24 hours. Symptoms are usually mild. *Perfringens* multiplies where there is little or no oxygen and especially likes growing in the center of casseroles, stews, and gravies that are held for extended times in the danger zone between 40 degrees and 140 degrees.

Most people know to be careful of contamination with raw meat and poultry, but not everyone thinks of bacterial contamination from the surfaces of fresh produce. Outbreaks of *E. coli* have come from lettuce, *Salmonella* from cantaloupe, watermelon, and tomatoes;

Listeria from cabbage; and *Campylobacter* from mushrooms. Reportedly, a major cause of these outbreaks is food imported from the third world, where irrigation water can be contaminated with bacteria-laden sewage. To protect yourself and your family from contaminated produce, follow the directions in the "Food Safety" box. In conclusion, let me give you a word of encouragement. Worrying about sanitation is a drag, but once mastered, these techniques will become easy and automatic.

FOOD SAFETY

- Keep hot foods hot and cold foods cold. Bacteria grow most rapidly at temperatures between 40 degrees Fahrenheit and 140 degrees Fahrenheit. Adjust your refrigerator to keep it at 40 degrees or below. When you keep food hot, maintain the temperature above 140 degrees.
- Never leave perishable food out of the refrigerator for more than 2 hours, including preparation and standing times. At room temperature, bacteria grow quickly and the food can become unsafe. If you can't go home right after you shop, take along an ice chest to keep your food cold.
- Freeze fresh meat, poultry, or fish immediately if you can't use it within a couple of days after you buy it. Freezing food doesn't destroy bacteria. If food is contaminated going into the freezer, it will be contaminated coming out.
- Thaw food in the refrigerator, not on the kitchen counter.
- Most fresh vegetables, opened canned foods, meat, eggs, and dairy products should be kept in the refrigerator. It is all right to cover the can and put it in the refrigerator. Ketchup, mayonnaise, and mustard go in the refrigerator after opening.
- Thoroughly wash your hands—and the hands of anyone who will help—before starting to prepare food. Use soap and follow the 20-second rule.
- Bacteria live in kitchen towels, sponges, and cloths. Use a clean dish towel and cloth every day, wash them in hot, soapy water. Sanitize sponges, kitchen brushes and nylon scrubbers every day by soaking them for five minutes in a solution of 1 teaspoon of chlorine bleach (like Clorox) per cup of water. Washing brushes, scrubbers, and sponges in the dishwasher doesn't sanitize them—the temperature isn't hot enough. Rinse them out with clear water. Be careful not to get bleach on your clothes or it will take out the color.

- Keep raw meat, poultry, and fish (and their juices) away from other food when you shop, store, and cook. Bag raw meats separately in an extra plastic bag. Wash your hands, cutting board, and knife in hot, soapy water after cutting up raw meat, before handling other foods. Take a clean dishcloth or sanitize your sponge after washing up from working with chicken. See page 83 for special precautions about cooking chicken.
- Cook meat, poultry, fish, and eggs thoroughly to kill bacteria. Cook ground meat to a uniform internal temperature of 160 degrees, poultry to 170 degrees, pork to 160 degrees, meats that are not ground, such as roasts, to 145 degrees, and eggs to 150 degrees (the point at which the white is set and the yolk is starting to set). When microwaving, let food stand covered for the full number of minutes recommended to finish cooking.
- Rinse all fresh fruits and vegetables thoroughly with cold water before you start working with them, even the rinds and peels you plan to throw away. You have to assume the rinds have bacteria on them and take precautions to keep from cutting the bacteria into the fruit. As a knife slices through a contaminated rind, it carries bacteria into the fruit. Wash mushrooms, even through the gourmets say not to.
- Refrigerate produce after you slice it.
- Don't use detergent to wash produce. It can soak into the produce, and detergent ingredients have not been deemed safe for consumption.
- Avoid any commercial fruit or vegetable juice that hasn't been pasteurized.
- Don't use sprouts, especially for children. The temperature and humidity necessary for sprouting seeds is also ideal for culturing bacteria, and some alfalfa sprouts have been contaminated.

Buying and Using Knives

Knives deserve special mention. Get good knives, and learn how to store them and keep them sharp. To protect both your fingers and the edges of the knives, rig up a knife block or a drawer with knife slots in it for holding your knives securely in place. Your knives don't have to be the best ones in the world, as long as you know how to use a knife sharpener and a steel. The basic four knives are the chef's knife (for vegetables), the slicing knife (for meat), the utility knife (a long paring knife or a short slicing knife), and the paring knife (for peeling and cutting small pieces of food).

While there are other variables, like the handle shape, materials, color, and type of attachment, the most important consideration in buying knives is the blade. Blades vary in method of production and in the grind on the blade. Forged knives are shaped from a single piece of steel and are heavier; stamped knives are cut out of a sheet of steel and are lighter. Relative to the cutting edge, knives can be taper, hollow, or flat grind. Pictures of these grinds, and their descriptions, are in the box "Grinds of Knife Edges." For more information about knives in general, and brand and price recommendations in particular, read *Consumer Reports*. As of this writing, the most recent article about knives was in the December 1998 issue.

For ease and safety, keep your knives sharp with a steel or a knife sharpener. It is as easy as it is flashy to give your knife a few strokes with the steel each time you use it. Ask your butcher to demonstrate. You will make a friend for life, and she will always remember you when you call up to ask for your specially cut pieces of meat. The steel doesn't actually sharpen the knife blade but only lines up the little metal burrs on the blade edge that weave around and stick out (minutely) and make the knife seem dull. Steels vary in hardness and are matched by manufacturers to their knives, so it's best to purchase the steel that is intended for your knives.

If you let your knives get so dull that a sharpening steel doesn't help, you will need to use a knife sharpener to grind off the little burrs. *Consumer Reports* recommends an electric sharpener, Chef's Choice 110 for under

GRINDS OF KNIFE EDGES

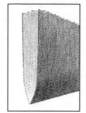

Taper grind: The most expensive knives, these are thick at the back of the blade and taper down to a fine edge. These are generally hefty, strong knives with a durable edge. They keep an edge longer, but they are also more difficult to sharpen once they lose their edge. The Henckels and Sabatier brands are generally taper-grind.

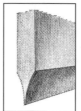

Hollow-grind: These knives are the same thickness from the back of the blade to the cutting edge. The edge is beveled down to a sharp point, and then it is hollowed out to bring it to a very sharp cutting edge. This type of blade can be very sharp because the cutting edge is quite thin. However, the hollowed-out area can be weak and vulnerable to breakage. It loses its sharpness more easily than a taper-grind knife, but the sharpness can be easily restored with a steel or sharpener. With the exception of the chef's knife, Chicago Cutlery knives are hollow ground.

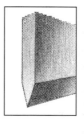

Flat-grind: These knives are like the hollow-grind, except the blade is sharpened flat rather than hollowed out. It isn't as sharp as the hollow-grind, nor does it keep an edge as long as the taper-ground. This type is the least expensive to produce, but it isn't necessarily a low-quality product.

$100, that has magnets to hold the blade at a proper angle as you guide the knife through. I use a hand sharpener that I got for $10, but the angle is up to me.

Do be mindful of your personal safety with these sharp knives. Surprisingly, sharp knives are safer than dull ones. A sharp knife cuts easily through food. Because you don't have to saw away, a sharp knife isn't as likely to slip. Use a cutting board. Don't let sharp knives lie around. After you use a knife, wipe it off and put it away. If knives need washing, put them in soapy water one at a time and wash immediately so you don't plunge your hands onto a sharp knife. Don't put knives in the dishwasher; it dulls the edge and is dangerous for whoever unloads the dishwasher. Grabbing the blade of a sharp knife is not fun.

Pots and Pans

Buy the best pans you can afford. They will be with you for life, and they hold memories. When your children start to cook more, you will say, "Take the big pan with the black handles and fill it half full of water." For the rest of your life, you will remember those young hands on those handles.

Good pans are not necessarily the most expensive. In fact, a lot of pricey gourmet pans offer improved looks more than improved function. If you like beautiful pans, and if can afford them and you find they make your cooking more enjoyable, go ahead and buy them. But you don't need to spend top dollar to get good pans. The December 1995 issue of *Consumer Reports* recommended a JCPenney cook set, at under $100, as a best buy. Do your research, and once you figure out what you want, you can go to discount stores, hardware stores, and garage sales to get the best deal on them.

The main consideration with buying pans is the cooking quality of the materials. Aluminum pans heat quickly and evenly, but bare aluminum is hard to clean. And unless they are heavyweight, aluminum pans lose their shape and develop uneven bottoms that don't sit flat on the burner. Stainless steel pans are easy to clean and are even dishwasher safe, but they get hot spots. Aluminum lined with stainless steel combines the best of both. Nonstick coatings (such as Teflon or Silverstone) are wonderful to cook with and easy to clean. However, they require plastic or wooden utensils, and they shouldn't be used with very high heat. Conventional cookware is generally better for browning and making pan sauces. There is a big variation in the durability of nonstick coatings, so if you plan to pay a lot for a nonstick pan, read the *Consumer Reports* article to find out which one will last. I find it handy to have one or two nonstick pans, but I buy less expensive ones and plan to replace them every now and again.

Enamel (also called porcelain) is pretty and heats well, but it chips. Copper heats and cools quickly and looks great if you keep it polished, but even thin solid copper cookware is expensive. Glass pans require a special little rack on an electric burner. They are heavy, and of course, they can break. Cast iron is heavy, heats evenly, and can handle high temperatures. It has to be seasoned before you use it, but that isn't hard. Just rub the pan inside and out with shortening (not butter) or cooking oil and bake it in a 350 degrees oven for an hour. Wipe off the excess oil and store. Wash it by hand using a plastic scrubber, not a scouring pad. After the initial seasoning, cooking seasons it. If it rusts or develops sticky spots, season it again. A deep-sided, covered cast iron skillet makes a great Dutch oven, and it can be used on top of the stove or in the oven.

My recommendation? If you are just starting out, get a good cook set with two frying pans, one large and one small, and four saucepan sizes: 1, 1 1/2, 3 1/2, and 4 1/2 quarts (the larger one benefits from two handles). Get a lid for each pan. Then supplement the cook set with a cast iron Dutch oven, with a lid, one or two nonstick frying pans, and an 8-quart soup pot. Casserole dishes, bread pans, and so on are listed in the box "A Starter List of Utensils and Equipment."

Utensils and Small Appliances

Utensils are highly personal and can either make or break you. I love gadgets, and I have to resist them. Looking at gadgets gives me the hopeful notion that I can buy a garlic peeler or a lemon juicer and my life will fall beautifully into place, organized and serene. I have yet to find that gadget. Some tools I use over and over again, like a potato peeler or a hand electric mixer. Other tools I use occasionally but can't get along without, like a grater. Other tools are more trouble than they are worth, like a food processor. To me, it takes more time to assemble and wash a food processor than I can save from using it. Other cooks can't get along without their food processors. They use them for everything from slicing carrots to baking bread.

Listed in the box "A Starter List of Utensils and Equipment" are the tools I have recommended in the recipes in this book. I consider this list to be adequate for a modestly well equipped kitchen.

A STARTER LIST OF UTENSILS AND EQUIPMENT

Pots and Pans
large frying pan
small frying pan
saucepans: 1-, 1 1/2-, 3 1/2-, 4 1/2-quart sizes
   with lids (The 4 1/2-quart size should have two
   handles)
one or two nonstick frying pans
Dutch oven
8-quart pan (soup pot) with lid

Baking Dishes and Bowls
covered ovenproof casseroles: 1-quart, 2-quart
9 x 13-inch glass or aluminum cake pan
10 x 6- or 8 x 8-inch baking dish
loaf pan
muffin tin
jelly roll pan (10 x 15-inch pan with 1-inch sides)
assorted glass mixing bowls
salad bowl

Small Appliances
toaster
electric hand mixer
blender
slow cooker

Utensils and Gadgets
colander
measuring cups and spoons
long-handled slotted spoon
wooden spoons
ladle
serving spoons
tongs

wire whip or whisk
plastic knives for children to help in kitchen
plastic dishwashing pan
knives: chef's knife (8- to 14-inch blade), slicing
   knife (10-inch blade), utility knife (5- to 6-inch
   blade), paring knife (3-inch blade)
10-inch butcher's steel or other sharpener
three cutting boards: one for produce, one for raw
   meat, and one for cooked meat, poultry, and fish
cheese grater
pastry brush
food thermometer (see box on page 95)
carrot peeler
potato masher
can opener
pancake turner
plastic freezer zip top bags
assorted jars with lids (for storing chopped onions,
   etc.), one fitted with shaker top
clear oven cooking bags, medium size
aluminum foil

Optional
platter
ice cream scoops: size 30 (2 Tbsp), size 60 (1 Tbsp)
salad spinner
soup tureen
wok
garlic press
roller-style pizza cutter
timer (not essential if you have a kitchen clock, but
   handy)
vegetable steaming rack

A Word of Encouragement

Getting yourself organized to cook will be time well spent. It will pay huge dividends in pleasure and achievement. You can be a good cook, and you can help your children grow up to be good and healthy eaters. You can give them—and yourself—the security they need to know they will be well and happily fed.

Shopping Strategies and Shortcuts

- Try the P&E shopping system: Every 3 to 4 weeks, go on a major shopping expedition for your major staples, like canned goods and cleaning supplies. Shop once a week for produce and dairy products, and in between do quick-stop shopping for perishables like milk and bread.
- You may decide on different grocery stores for the different kinds of shopping trips. Choose the markets that have the features that are most important to you and stick with them rather than wearing yourself out with comparison shopping.
- Use the "Staples List" box to help you determine what you need to buy when you do your staples shopping trip. Using this list will help you keep a well-stocked kitchen.

CHAPTER
9
SHOPPING
TO GET YOU
COOKING

To feed a healthy family, you have to have food in the house. To position yourself to plan and cook a meal—or to grab the ingredients to throw together a meal—you have to have tools to work with. You have to shop. It is not always fun.

As a matter of fact, it occurs to me that the amount of difficulty I am having getting to work writing this chapter is an exact reflection of the difficulty many of us have getting to writing the shopping list and going out for groceries. It is as time-consuming—and empowering—as it can be. I don't like to do it. For me, the only thing worse than conducting my grocery-shopping campaign is *not* conducting it. But my customer services manager (and tester of recipes) Clio Marsh reminds me that she *likes* shopping lists and shopping. Perhaps it is in your frame of mind. Clio is relaxed and interested in shopping and uses her shopping trips as an inspiration for her cooking. I am impatient and pragmatic. However you feel about it, it is an important chore that goes best if done carefully and thoughtfully.

Paulette Sharkey, my developmental editor, feels the way I do. Paulette says, "Even though it's painful at the time, you'll feel better later if you do it. Every weekend I just hate having to sit down and write the list and then do the shopping. But if I don't do it, I feel mad all week. I don't have the ingredients I need, and cooking is a real hassle."

Having admitted our negative feelings to ourselves and each other, Paulette and I came up with a way to *get organized*, and we offer our system to you. You may think our scheme is really nifty, or you might not like it at all. Your scheme may be totally different, and that's okay. The important point is that you *think* about it, and come up with a method that works for you. Random grocery shopping wastes time, energy, and money and defeats your cooking endeavors.

THE P&E (PAULETTE AND ELLYN) SHOPPING SYSTEM

Our strategy is to shop at three different levels:
- Every 3 to 4 weeks: Big staples shopping. This is a major shopping excursion at the grocery emporium to stock up on foods that keep, like canned, bottled, and dry foods, cleaning supplies, and paper goods.
- Weekly: Produce and dairy for the week
- Quick-stop: Milk, maybe bread

Consumer research says that on the average we make 2.2 trips per week to the grocery story. Using the P&E method, you will make about 2.2 trips per week. We hope, however, these strategies will help you make these trips *count* and cut down on time, expense, and frustration.

Do you like shopping trivia? Here is more. Consumers in general tend to shop consistently all week. Half of consumers working full-time shop on weekends. Most shopping trips are done in the morning, followed by afternoon and then evening. Only 5 percent of shopping trips are done late at night.

Picking Out the Grocery Store

You can pick out a different grocery story for each of your three levels of food shopping. For the big staples shopping, it is worth traveling a distance. For the weekly shopping and the quick-stop shopping, it will be more convenient if the stores are closer to home. It's best to pick out particular stores and stay with them. Going back to the same store time after time lets you become thoroughly familiar with the layout so you can finish your shopping and get out as quickly as possible. You can even arrange your shopping list to lead you through the store. It may be too much to ask for in today's impersonal world, but you might even get to know some of the people there, which always adds a note of comfort and connectedness.

FOOD IS CHEAP, BUT DON'T WASTE MONEY

As a nation, we don't spend that much on food. On the average we spend 12 percent of our income on food. That percentage, of course, varies enormously depending on income level. People in the lowest income bracket spend about 18 percent, those in the highest bracket spend 3 percent or less. We spend about $1,500 to $2,000 per person per year on food. Several-person households have lower per-person food costs, and single-person households have higher.

We expect ample, low-cost, safe, and wholesome food. For the most part, we get it. We are spoiled. We would benefit from appreciating and celebrating our bounty. However, that does not mean we have to throw away our food dollars. Thus, we will consider price.

It's pretty tough to do comparison pricing between grocery stores. Do try to do some price checking so you can get an idea of whether you have chosen a store that is competitive, but don't drive yourself crazy with it. It's likely that you will find that convenience and a positive shopping atmosphere dictate where you shop. Pay attention to what you value. Is price most important, or is comfort? As was evident from a Consumer Reports article on supermarket shopping in August 1997, many shoppers were prepared to pay premium prices for high-quality food sold in a pleasant environment.

Most shoppers say the quality of the produce section is their most important consideration in choosing a grocery store. Meat quality is second most important. Keep in mind that for our big staples shopping, the primary considerations are quality and variety of canned goods and staples. To get good canned goods and staples, you might have to settle for a more limited selection of produce or meat. Then you can choose a different weekly produce store, and the milk-stop store might be the gas station on the way home.

Keep in mind that the best big staples shopping store is not necessarily the biggest store. A supersized store may just wear you out. A smaller store may offer a bigger selection of the food you want. A smaller store makes for less walking and faster shopping.

Read the grocery store ads in the paper to get some idea of stores that feature price as their calling card. The ads will entice you with their appealing "loss leaders." These are foods that are priced so low that the grocer makes little or no money on them, in hopes that when you are in the store to buy the bargains, you will do the rest of your shopping as well. Loss leader foods represent savings—if you need them. Often milk, just-coming-in-season produce, or particular cuts of meat are used as loss leaders. Quick-stop stores may routinely offer low-priced milk as a loss leader.

However, be aware that sometimes food featured in grocery store ads is not bargain priced at all. Regular-priced products may be prominent in ads or on grocery store shelves because their manufacturers have paid the store to feature them.

KNOWING THE STORE SAVES MONEY

Being familiar with the grocery store can save you money. This may just be an urban rumor, but I understand there is a formula that says for every minute you spend in the store, you spend $5 on groceries. Whether it's true or not, the idea has merit. The more things you walk by, the more you'll throw in your cart. That is why many grocery stores put their "quick run-in" items like milk in the far back corner of the store, way behind all the other enticements that they hope you pick up as you go by. But that appears to be changing. Some big stores realize they have to compete with the convenience markets, and are putting their milk and bread at the front of the store, near the express checkout.

Tempting though it may be, it's generally not a good idea to run from store to store to pick up the bargain of the week. It is time-consuming and gas-consuming and will make the food buying far more complicated, laborious, and possibly more expensive than it needs to be.

However, I do not mean to say that grocers are rapacious money-grubbers who are out to spoil your food budget. They do attend to merchandising and they do keep a careful eye on what you, the consumer, want. They do not have a big profit margin. Most grocery stores hope to make about a 1 to 1.5 percent profit. That's not a lot to play around with, especially since stores work with potentially disastrous variables like food spoilage, equipment breakdown, crop failures all over the world, and the labor market. Food stores and departments that have the bigger profit margins are those that offer a lot of "value added" services (see next column) by offering Home Meal Replacements and other pre-prepared dishes.

SUPERMARKET ORGANIZATION AND MARKETING STRATEGIES

To save time and frustration in any market, it is helpful to have a general organizational plan in your head. In almost every market, the produce, meats, dairy, and—to a certain extent—frozen foods are arranged on or near the perimeter. Canned, bottled, and dry foods, cleaning supplies, and paper goods are in the aisles in the middle.

The practicalities of food storage and production dictate supermarket layout. Refrigerated and frozen foods require large coolers. Meat departments and bakeries require both refrigerated storage areas and production areas. Behind-the-scenes equipment takes up a lot of space, so putting these departments on the perimeter of the store is simply practical. Of course, these are marketing considerations as well. Smelling the aroma of fresh-baked bread when you first come into a store can't help but excite your interest in buying food!

Arrangement on the *shelf* is a marketing consideration, not a practical one. Prime retail space is the space at eye level. (Prime retail space for sugar-coated breakfast cereals is your child's eye level.) Less-prime space is that above or below eye level. Grocers tend to position the major-markup foods at eye level, the foods you will buy anyway or that have a lower profit margin are displayed above or below eye level. Think about it. Which shelf usually holds the salt? Why, the one down by your ankles, of course.

Positioning products on the end of the aisles—the endcap—and on islands in the aisles suggests bargain pricing. It doesn't follow. Check prices on those foods carefully. The endcaps might just contain products that the grocer wants to move quickly—overstocks or foods nearing their expiration dates.

Within the shelves, stockers are supposed to rotate their stock. If they don't and they have an alert boss, they don't last long. Stockers move the product already on the shelf to the front and put the products being unpacked in the back. I suppose if you wanted the freshest cans possible you could reach back and get them. However, food stays fresh in cans for a year, so fishing for the cans in back isn't really necessary.

VALUE ADDING

Earlier I mentioned *value-added* foods. Plain rice in a box is a food. Rice with flavoring and bits of herbs and seasonings is a value-added food. Something has been done in manufacturing to the rice to increase the consumer appeal. It also increases the price. I found a package of value-added rice to be eight times more expensive for a 2-cup serving than regular, converted rice. If you make your own herbed rice, the herbs and spices and extra time add to the cost. Is it worth it? You decide.

Some value-added foods are not that expensive. The boxed tuna noodle casserole, including the cost of the tuna that you have to buy separately, is only about 10 percent more expensive than the noodles, soup, and canned tuna for the tuna noodle casserole we made in chapter 5.

The value-adding chain goes all the way back to the farm. Wheat is the original food, noodles and macaroni are value-added products, boxed tuna noodle casserole is value-added again. The farmer doesn't get much of the money for a food. The value adding comes later. The North Dakota farmers got tired of settling for their small portion of the food dollar, so they built a noodle manufacturing plant, Dakota Growers Pasta Company. They now process their own fine semolina wheat into pasta and keep the value-added profits closer to the grower.

The value-added issue has an impact on how shelf space is assigned in stores. High markup items tend to be assigned more shelf space. Both my supermarkets devote a full aisle to chips and snacks, another aisle, or even two, to soft drinks. All supermarkets have *lots* of breakfast cereals, most of them featuring value-added gimmicks like flavoring, sugar, shapes, or large amounts of added nutrients. Before you spend extra for a cereal with "100 percent of your total daily requirement," consider that you don't need cereal to contribute that much. Each food contributes something to the diet. You count on cereal to give you B vitamins and iron. Added together with all the other bread and cereal choices you eat in a day, it will give you what you need. If it is whole grain, you also get a wide range of other vitamins and minerals in moderate quantities. To pay extra for all those vitamins and minerals is unnecessary.

My staples market has a full aisle of canned fruits and vegetables, my produce market only about a fourth of an aisle. My produce market has a full aisle of candy and two full aisles of cleaning products. Very strange. If they didn't have such good produce, I wouldn't bother.

Manufacturers compete for prime positioning in supermarkets—or for any position at all. If an item doesn't sell, it loses its space on the shelf. Many new products come on the market every year, are test marketed regionally, and then are sold nationwide. To make it, a new product has to sell fast and sell consistently. Products that don't sell are discontinued. Even old, favorite regional products can be discontinued if they don't sell well nationally.

The folks in the northeast were stunned when Nabisco discontinued Pilot crackers, a plain, unleavened cracker that is often referred to as "hard tack" or "ship's biscuit." The northeasterners thought that took a lot of nerve, especially since the Nabisco Baking Company was started by a Massachusetts baker who created "pilot bread" and sold it to sailors for long sea voyages. New Englanders quickly made the crackers a staple, putting them in stew and chowders, spread with jam, soaked in milk, and even giving them to their babies for teething biscuits.*

The northeasterners didn't know how they were going to eat their clam chowder without

Pilot crackers, and they begged the company to reconsider. Eight months and 3,500 passionate letters, calls, and e-mails later, Nabisco reconsidered and reintroduced them regionally. If you want Crown Pilot Crackers for your clam chowder, you have to go to the northeast to get them. Alternatively, you can call Nabisco and order a case. Get on the Web and look up Nabisco's Web site (www.nabisco.com) to get the recipe for Crown Pilot Fish Chowder.

The Big Staples Shopping Trip

I assume that when you do the big, occasional staples shopping you will pick up your produce and meat for the week and your dairy for the next few days. The staples shopping trip is serious shopping. It is on the order of a campaign. To make a list that is as complete as possible, check your menu, consider anything special or extra you want to make, unearth your running list of "things we need," and get the master list ready. Then check the inventory to see what you have on hand and what you have to restock, and get your money lined up. Don't forget the money! It is darned aggravating to have all the groceries gathered and checked out, only to find that the checkbook is empty and the debit card is at home on the counter.

THE STAPLES LIST
The "Staples List" at the end of this chapter is a roll call of all the foods I used in all the recipes on the 3-week cycle menu. Some foods on the list (like salsa) I didn't use, but I've included them to give you a well-stocked kitchen. Still other foods are on the list to help you get ideas of nutritious foods you might enjoy, like the list of canned juices or the partial list of breakfast cereals that are nutritious and moderate in sugar. To help you when you get to the store, I have grouped the staples list the way foods are often grouped in grocery stores.

Like a lot of the issues we deal with on this project, the staples list is daunting but manageable. Make some photocopies of the list and highlight the items you need for the recipes you plan to make. I leave it to you to trim down the list to fit the way you plan to shop and cook. I thought it would be easier for you to *eliminate* foods than to try to remember to include them. You may already have many of

---

*I can't help throwing in the caveat that it is best if babies are 9 months old before they are introduced to wheat-containing Pilot Crackers to avoid developing wheat allergies.

these foods on hand. Other foods are very occasional purchases, like spices and baking powder. Still other items on the list aren't foods at all, but you still need to remember to buy them, like paper products, cleaning supplies, and plastic bags.

The staples list works as an inventory list, as well. After you decide what to cook and highlight those ingredients on the staples list, check the pantry and all the hiding places to see what you have. Go on an excavation through the refrigerator and throw out anything questionable. Make a mental note that you really *didn't* use the eggplant you bought last time.

ORGANIZING THE STAPLES LIST
I take my staples shopping one step further. I hesitate to recommend it to you for fear it will make you tear your hair. But it helps me so much that I will tell you. I keep printed copies of my staples list, arranged to match the path I follow through my favorite grocery store. I type my inventory on the computer, arrange it, and print copies. Then when I get ready for my monthly shopping, I take a copy of my staples list and highlight what I need. I keep a running list of things I need on a handy scrap of paper, and then transfer it to the staples list when I get ready to go shopping.

I map my path through the grocery story so I can end up with produce near the end and refrigerated and frozen foods last. That shortens up as much as possible the time cold or frozen foods have to sit in my cart at room temperature. (On my better days, I pick up extra plastic bags in the produce section for bagging the meat.) I move through the aisles in the order I want to pick up foods. If I followed the order in which the store is arranged, I would be picking up the perishable foods first and the canned and dried foods and cleaning products last.

But you know, being compulsive is not all bad. It lets me organize and write books and even keeps me going when the task is writing a chapter on shopping. Like with planning, being compulsive is bad only when it becomes your master rather than your servant.

TAKE CARE OF YOURSELF
Get all the help you can. If you are organized, it will be easier for other people to take on part of the chores of food shopping and preparation. Taking a tip from Tom Sawyer, maybe you could interest your school-age child in

taking your well-organized list and conducting the food inventory. In fact, he might even *like* doing it, especially if you make sure to say how much it helps you.

The staples trip is big. Try to be rested for it, and don't be hungry. Consider whether you really want your children along for this trip. It will take a lot of energy to tend children and shop as well. Not only that, but you will have to unpack and put away the groceries once you get home, so preserving yourself is your first priority. Do recruit other family members to help carry in groceries and put them away once you get home. It will help a lot, and if they know what comes in, they will feel more capable of helping to cook it.

You might find that another family member would do the shopping, at least on an occasional basis. With a complete shopping list, having someone else take over is much easier.

COUPONS
I do not use coupons, although I have found that reading the coupon fliers gives me an idea of what is new, weird, and wonderful on the market. If you make good use of coupons, I congratulate you. Shoppers who make a science of coupons and don't let coupons entice them into buying food they don't need can save money. Shoppers who don't use coupons usually can't stand the fussing and the time it takes, no matter *what* it saves them. It seems to me that it comes down to whatever you have more of: time or money. If you have more time, you can use it to good purpose by clipping and organizing coupons. If you have more money, you can afford *not* to do that.

My cousin Arda had lots of time, and she *loved* coupons. She made a *career* out of coupons. You may have heard of the Iowa housewife refunding ring that was busted by federal prosecutors a while back. Arda was lucky not to be one of them. Arda clipped every cents-off coupon she could find, but her antenna really went up at the money-back offers. Of course, cash-refund offers were more complicated because they required a cash register receipt and a bar code from the package. But Arda was a good organizer—she had everyone in our large family collecting receipts and bar codes for her. The extra bathtub in her trailer house was always full of boxes and packages waiting to be processed.

Eventually, Arda's needs outgrew the family. She went to refunding conventions, where she traded coupons and bar codes and cash register receipts with other conventioneers who were as committed as she was. Arda's favorite pastime was searching through a certain small-town dump with her friend Virginia, rummaging through the refuse with the eyes of connoisseurs, looking for just the bar code they needed to complete their money-back offers.

Arda loved to tell about her neighbors catching her in the dumpster when she crawled in to get a bar code. Arda was a good storyteller, so I laughed when she told it, even though I didn't believe her. But then, I didn't believe her when she said she bought her own cash register, either. That was before I saw it on her kitchen counter.

Just for the record, I don't recommend Arda's methods. I admired my cousin—she was one of the great survivors—but I do know that some parts of what she was doing were illegal, and I don't believe in sending my readers off on a life of crime.

So make up your own mind about coupons. Feeling obligated to use coupons can complicate your shopping so much you can't do it, just as counterproductive feelings of obligation can backfire when you're trying to feed yourself and your family. Arda didn't have a paying job and her kids were grown. She had time. You may not.

IN-STORE SHOPPER'S CLUBS

As a member of an in-store shopper's club, you receive a card that entitles you to automatic discounts on products without having to clip coupons. You may also receive access to unadvertised specials. Stores may also use the information they receive when you use their card to target you for particular promotions. For instance, new parents who buy disposable diapers may be mailed coupons for baby food. At this point, supermarkets' selling personal information doesn't seem to be a big problem. If it bothers you, check off the box on the application form that asks for privacy for your name and address.

SHOPPING FOR CANNED GOODS

Choose clean cans without bulges, rust, or gouges. Pick out cans that are not dented to decrease the chances that the seal on the can will have been damaged. A broken seal allows spoilage. However, if you get home with a dented can, it's still likely to be all right as long as the seal is intact. If you can't tell by looking, you will be able to tell when you open it. If a can is intact and still properly sealed, when you cut into it with the can opener it will make a whooshing or spitting sound. Never buy—or use—a can that bulges.

Canned goods have packing dates and even times on them, but the dates are written in codes that most of us can't figure out. The grocer can figure it out and uses the pack dates for tracking inventory, rotating food on shelves, and locating items in case of recall.

Make use of unit pricing. The unit price label on the shelf shows both the retail price (the total price you pay) and the price per pound, ounce, quart, or other unit. The unit price will tell you that the biggest package is not necessarily the best buy, especially if you don't use it all. Keep in mind the use you are making of the product. You don't need premium tomatoes to make macaroni-tomato-hamburger casserole and you don't need fancy peaches to make peach crisp.

BAKED GOODS

You can buy bread periodically and freeze it, get it once a week on your produce-shopping trips, or pick it up at the quick-trip store. It depends on where you can buy the bread that you and your family like. Some communities have great bakeries, and it may be worthwhile for you to make a special trip to stock up—and to pay the extra price those breads command. They are no more nutritious than other breads, just more interesting.

You don't have to eat whole grain unless you like it. Most white bread is made with enriched flour, but do check the label to be sure that is what you are getting. White flour still has a variety of nutrients, at about 10 to 25 percent the level of that in the original whole grain. Enriched flour has some of the nutrients added back that are removed along with the brown outer coating during the milling process. Enrichment brings iron and niacin to levels found in whole wheat, and thiamin and riboflavin to even higher levels. Since January 1998, folic acid is also added to enriched flour to triple the level found in whole wheat flour. This change was made in response to the discovery that folic acid deficiency during pregnancy is associated with neural tube defects in infants. Spina bifida is a neural tube defect.

Use whole grain about half the time. Whole grain contains more fiber and more of a wide range of vitamins and minerals than are left in white, refined breads and cereals. Ironically, however, the level of natural folic acid in whole grain flour is lower than the supplemented level in enriched flour. This provides another argument for not using whole grain bread exclusively. Furthermore, if children get too much fiber in their diets, it can fill them up and not leave room for other food.

If you want whole grain, read the ingredients label to be sure that is what you are really getting. For whole wheat bread, the first listed ingredient should be *whole wheat flour*. If the label simply says "wheat flour," it doesn't tell you anything. It might be whole wheat or it might be white—which is "wheat flour" as well. The key word to look for on the ingredients list is *whole*.

Sometimes breads are made to look like whole grain with the addition of caramel coloring or flecks of bran. Those breads can taste good and be interesting, but they are not whole grain.

RICE, BARLEY, BULGUR, COUSCOUS, OTHER CEREAL GRAINS

Other cereal grains add interest and variety to the menu, and when you feel like experimenting, this is a good place to start. You can buy other grains prepackaged or in bulk. Many times the more unusual grains are available only in bulk, often called the "organic" section. I have only been able to find short-grain brown rice in bulk. This rice takes longer to cook than the other type—about 45 minutes— but it is delicious. You may be able to find other types of rice as well. In my most recent swing through the natural food stores, I found *wehani rice* and *basmati rice*.

Barley is a wonderful grain to include in beef vegetable soup. Bulgur is a coarsely cracked and toasted whole wheat product used mostly in the Middle East. Tabbouli, a salad-side dish that you are likely to find at Middle Eastern restaurants, uses bulgur. Couscous is another Middle Eastern grain that you can use instead of rice as a side dish. Couscous cooks fast and easily: just pour an equal volume of boiling water over the couscous, let it stand five minutes, fluff, and serve.

From time to time other cereal grains are touted by "health foods" people as being particularly nutritious. Quinoa (keen-wah) comes to mind. This is presumably a highly nutritious grain used by the Incas. Quinoa adds an interesting flavor and texture to soups, and I recently tasted a wonderful salad with quinoa, chickpeas, vegetables, and balsamic vinegar. However, when I made a nutritional comparison of quinoa to whole wheat, whole wheat came out ahead except for vitamin E and iron. While quinoa has something to offer, being exotic doesn't give it any unique nutritional properties.

Storage of staples: In chapter 8, I suggested supplementing kitchen storage space with a pantry in the basement or an out-of-the-way closet. This storage space should be clean and dry, with shelves that keep food and supplies up off the floor.

Plan to keep whole grains just a month or two before you use them, or put them in the refrigerator to keep them from getting stale. For other dry products and canned goods, plan to use your stock within 6 months. While canned goods and packaged and bottled products keep up to a year, unless you are canning annually or buying in bulk from a canner, there is nothing to be gained from letting your inventory sit there so long. Move the older foods to the front of the shelf and put the newer ones behind.

Fish, Poultry, and Meat

For a list of cuts of meat, poultry, and fish categorized by fat content, see the "Fat in Meat" box.

BUYING BEEF, LAMB, AND PORK

In the past, pork was high in fat and often contaminated with a parasite called *trichina*. Today's pork is far lower in fat and is free of *trichina*. Pork makes an enjoyable and worthwhile addition to your cycle menus because of its distinctive and enjoyable taste. Pork is high in B vitamins, especially thiamin, which is necessary for nerve health.

BUYING CHICKEN

To make chicken preparation easier, purchase the individually frozen chicken breasts in zip top bags. Because they don't stick together, you can take out as many or as few as you want at a time. You can get them bone-in or boneless, with or without skin. I have figured the boneless, skinless breasts for the recipes in this book because they are easy to store, and

FAT IN MEAT, POULTRY, AND FISH

Lean Choices: Lean meat has about 3 grams of fat per ounce. With the exception of top sirloin and tenderloin, beef cuts on this list need to be tenderized or cooked with moist heat. The pork, poultry, and fish are tender because they don't have much connective tissue. If you are careful not to dry them out with too much cooking, they will be tasty using any method of cooking.
Beef: round, sirloin, chuck arm, tenderloin, and flank steaks. Ground round and chuck.
Pork: boneless center loin roast or chops, tenderloin, Canadian bacon, and ham
Chicken and turkey cooked without skin
Wild game
All veal cuts except ground or cubed cutlets
All fresh and frozen fish (even "fatty" fish like salmon) and fish canned in water

Not-Quite-So Lean Choices: Not-quite-so lean meat meats have about 5 grams fat per ounce, still a modest amount. Fresh meat cuts on this list are tender and good for grilling and roasting.
Beef: rib roast and steak, chuck blade, regular ground beef
Pork: shoulder roast and steak, loin rib chop
Veal cutlets
Chicken and turkey with skin
Duck, goose
Fish canned in oil
86 percent fat-free lunch meats

Higher-Fat Choices: Higher-fat meats have 6 or 7 grams fat per ounce.
Beef: short ribs
Pork: sausage
Regular luncheon meats

they let you take out only as much as you need without having to thaw what you don't need.

You pay for your convenience, but you don't have to mess with cutting up the chicken and discarding extra fat and pieces you don't use. When you buy a whole chicken or a quartered chicken, you have to do some dissecting, and you may or may not know how to do that. It is also messy, and you have to be excruciatingly careful about contamination.

BUYING FISH
Your butcher may be able to help you learn what fresh fish really looks like, or you may get better information by going to a fish shop to do your learning. Such places generally pride themselves on *really* fresh fish, and they go to special trouble to buy it fresh, ship it fast

and store it properly.

When you buy frozen fish, look for the freshness date. Make sure the packages are undamaged. Be sure the fish does not have freezer burn (off-color patches and dried-out edges) and is not partially thawed or covered with ice crystals. Ice crystals mean the fish was thawed and refrozen, so the quality and bacterial safety will be lower. Use frozen fish within 3 to 6 months. The longer you keep it, the more likely it will be to develop off color, texture, and odor.

Weekly Shopping: Produce and Dairy Products

For the produce and dairy trip, you can shop the perimeter of the grocery store. As you recall from the organizational section in this chapter, produce and dairy cases tend to be on the outside border of the market primarily for the grocer's convenience. Now you can capitalize on that bit of information to cut down on time, distraction, and money.

Having a weekly produce and dairy shopping trip gives you the flexibility of buying perishable foods and filling in the blanks from the big staples trip. This weekly produce and dairy venture might also help keep you from doing the time- and gas-consuming last-minute run to buy one or two items to finish a recipe. If you know the produce and dairy trip is coming up, you can save the recipe for a day or two. This shopping trip is manageable enough that it can become an outing in which you include the children. You can explore the vegetables together and see what takes your fancy, and you can keep them out of the cereals aisle.

This trip also helps you make productive use of the farmers' market, if you are lucky enough to have one. Our cycle menu has plenty of places where seasonal fruits and vegetables are suggested. At the farmers' market, you can fill in those gaps and have a good time besides. But stay realistic about when you will *use* all of that luscious food, or your budget will suffer.

AVOID WASTING PRODUCE
Almost everybody throws away fresh fruits and vegetables that get spoiled before they can

use them. I do it. Alison Lockridge, another of my helpers, jokes with herself by saying, "I can have fresh produce when I become more responsible." Alison says she may buy only one or two fresh fruits or vegetables, and then only when she has specific plans for when she is going to use them. Even though you have such good company in this bad habit, try not to do it. Waste of this sort is the enemy of the family food budget. Some kinds of waste can't be helped, like plate waste when kids are around or having to throw away the rest of the casserole that's already been reheated once. But it's best to avoid wasting fresh produce if you can.

How can you avoid it? Don't buy impulsively. Buy produce only when you have an idea of when you are going to use it. Since fresh fruits and vegetables deteriorate in quality and nutritional value the longer you store them, use them early in the week; don't save them. Clean salad greens before you store them, so it is easy to throw together a salad at the last minute.

CHOOSING PRODUCE
You choose most produce by color, shape, and size. Choose oranges and grapefruit by hefting them. A relatively light fruit means that a lot of the volume is skin. Press the blossom end of a cantaloupe. It should give slightly, indicating it is ripe. Nobody really knows how to tell if a watermelon is ripe, short of cutting into it. Smelling it may be the most accurate method, but then you have to know what a ripe watermelon smells like. Honeydews are mystery to most everyone—good luck!

Pears and bananas are generally picked and sold green, then you ripen them on the counter. Someone said you had to sit up all night waiting for a pear to get to just the correct ripeness so you can eat it! Pineapples are picked and shipped ripe. Look for the wonderful "gold" pineapples. They are very tender and sweet; the flesh has an yellow-orange color to it. Pineapple experts say to put a pineapple upside-down for a couple of hours before you slice it to distribute the sweetness. Is this true? I do not know. Try it and see what you think.

KEEPING SALAD GREENS FRESH
To keep delicate produce like salad greens very crisp, you must keep it moist but avoid having water on the surface, which can make it rot. Make sure the cells of greens are filled with water before you store them. Soak the salad greens in very cold water for a few minutes, shake or spin off the moisture, wrap in a moist towel, place in a zip top plastic bag, squeeze out the air, seal (to limit oxygen exposure), and refrigerate. If you want to keep your greens longer than a day or two, make sure the paper towels are dry.

You will be justified in decreasing your salad complications by using prepackaged, prewashed greens. These last longer in the refrigerator because manufacturers know the secrets of hydrating fresh greens, then removing the surface water. I have wondered how to get greens dry, so I have been doing my own little survey of the vendors at the farmers' market. One vendor said she simply washed and drained her greens, then spread them out to dry for a while. She recommended putting a paper towel or two in the plastic bag to wick off the moisture. Another didn't have much to offer—he said he simply drained his greens in strainers. But I knew still another would be my favorite from the sheepish expression he got on his face when I asked. He told me he used net bags and an old washing machine. He hand-washed the greens in the bags in a tub, put bags and all into the washing machine, and then spun them dry!

It makes sense to me. However, most of us don't have an old washing machine sitting around to use for spinning out salads. You might prefer a salad spinner, and I certainly recommend one. Or put the greens in a net bag to wash them, and then send one of the children outside with the bag on a string and have him spin them dry for you. He'll think it's a hoot! In years to come when he learns about centrifugal force, he will have his own, odd little mental example to think about.

SEASONAL FRUITS AND VEGETABLES
In years past, the availability of fresh fruits and vegetables in grocery stores was limited to what was grown seasonally and locally. With modern systems of storing and shipping, you can buy almost any fresh fruit or vegetable at any time of the year.

For those of us living in the north, buying nationally or globally is the only way we get some fruits and vegetables, like bananas, oranges, pineapple, and artichokes. Wherever we live, most us of eat summertime crops year round, like apples, squash, or potatoes. The price and quality of these foods, and others like them, are generally good because they are sturdy and store and travel well.

There are still seasons for fresh produce, and quality and price will reflect those seasons. Apples and squash are best and lowest priced in the fall. New potatoes are harvested when the vines are still growing and green. They come on the market in mid- to late summer, and they are delicious. Citrus is best and lowest priced in the early months of the year, when the Florida and California trees are producing. Pineapple is best in late summer.

For other out-of-season fruits and vegetables, like raspberries and tomatoes, you will pay a premium, and the quality won't be as good as when they are in season. Raspberries that are grown in the South American summer, for instance, are flown to us to be available during our North American winter. However, to make them more durable during shipping, raspberries are picked relatively unripe. They soften during transit, but they don't really ripen. As a consequence, they lack the flavor and texture of locally grown raspberries that ripen on the bush.

For your own region, the best way to know when vegetables and fruits are in season is by watching the produce section: they will be plentiful, reasonably priced, and of good quality. Asparagus, and rhubarb are spring produce. Cherries and berries appear early to mid-summer. Melons, tomatoes, corn on the cob, green beans, cucumbers, peaches, nectarines, plums, and grapes are mid- to late summer crops.

The truth is, if you are willing to pay for it, you can have what you want at any time of the year. However, eating locally and respecting the local rhythms of crop production tastes better and costs less.

BUYING LOCALLY

Many fine restaurants are making their calling card featuring fresh, locally grown meats and produce. Madison's own Odessa Piper, who runs a very fine restaurant, *L'Etoile*, features locally grown seasonal food. Further, she favors food that has been raised with respect for the land. The concept of *sustainability* in food production is important to her, and she enacts her conviction by patronizing local growers who use minimally invasive methods of food production. Many areas now have community-supported agriculture programs,

where you can contract seasonally with growers for produce in season.* Many of these programs also emphasize sustainable agriculture.

Whether you buy it in the supermarket or at the farmers' market, fresh, recently picked produce *does* taste better. Depending on how it is handled and stored, it may or may not be more nutritious than what you buy frozen or in cans. Holding produce in the fresh state makes it vulnerable to losses in nutrients and quality. However, there is a certain grounding (no pun intended) that comes from honoring agriculture as part of eating. Making a connection with the land on which food is grown and with the people who grow it dignifies and enriches shopping, cooking, and eating.

You may or may not want to get that involved. If you do, you may not want to be slavish about it. You can still make some trips to the farmers' market or to local farms. There is certainly an excitement of discovery and a broadening, for parents as well as for children, in discovering how food is grown and how it gets to your table. Odessa Piper is excited about farmers' markets and says a trip to such a place is an "inspiration for the cook."

DAIRY AND EGGS

Buy the biggest container of milk that you will use by the end date on the package. Buy plain yogurt and add your own sugar and fruit: you will be nutrients ahead. Choose ultra-pasteurized half-and-half. Unopened ultra-pasteurized dairy products keep a long time; the end date on packages usually gives you a month or two. After you open the package, ultra-pasteurized dairy products have about the same shelf life as regularly pasteurized products.

Open the package of eggs in the store and examine them to see if they are cracked or broken. Shift each one around to see if any are cracked and stuck to the carton.

Check the date on packages and buy dairy products and eggs with the latest dates possible. The "sell by" date is often used on milk. This indicates the last day the product should appear on a supermarket shelf. Depending on how well it is stored, most milk is safe to drink

---

*The Madison Area Community Supported Agriculture Coalition puts out a *great* cookbook, *From Asparagus to Zucchini: A Guide to Farm-Fresh, Seasonal Produce*. To have a copy of *From Asparagus to Zucchini* mailed to you, send $18.50 to the Michael Fields Agricultural Institute. W2943 County Rd ES, East Troy, WI 53120.

for about a week after the "sell by" date.

Eggs, yogurt and cottage cheese generally have a "use by" or expiration date, which indicates when the quality of the product will have deteriorated. Don't buy eggs, yogurt, and cottage cheese that are past their "use by" dates.

Get grade AA eggs if you can. Many markets have only grade A eggs, which are all right but of somewhat lower quality, although equally as nutritious as grade AA eggs. Even when the "use by" date is okay, the only way you can tell how fresh eggs *really* are is by the way they behave when you fry or poach them. A fresh egg stands up. The yolk makes a high, rounded dome and so does the white. The white surrounds the yolk and keeps it well centered. There is only a small amount of watery white around the outside edge. A not-so-fresh egg flattens out and a *really* less-than-fresh egg lets the yolk wander off to the side and even break. In my experience, some markets have fresher-performing eggs than others.

STORAGE OF PRODUCE AND DAIRY

Generally, fresh produce has to be refrigerated, although there are exceptions. For example, one of the critical flavor components of tomatoes disappears when tomatoes are chilled. Tomatoes taste best when they are stored on the counter and eaten at room temperature. Bananas have to be stored at room temperature or they get black. To ripen fruit, put it in a loosely closed paper bag on the counter until it is as ripe as you want, then refrigerate dry. To ripen faster, put an apple in with the fruit. The apple gives off ethylene, which aids the ripening process. Wash fruit just before you use it.

Store celery, carrots, and greens in waterproof bags so they don't get wilted. Keep strawberries and mushrooms dry and in the refrigerator until you are ready to wash and use them.

Store dairy products covered, and use the oldest supplies first. If you are willing to risk dumping the contents, turn opened cottage cheese and yogurt containers upside down to store them. That makes a tighter air seal so they keep fresher longer.

To keep produce and dairy products fresh as long as possible, maintain your refrigerator temperature somewhere between 35 and 40 degrees. Don't store eggs and dairy products in the door of the refrigerator, because the temperature varies and can cut down significantly on the shelf life. Put your ketchup, mustard, and jellies in the door.

Quick-Stop Shopping

Convenience stores that sell gasoline have become our neighborhood grocery stores. They provide a great service and deserve to be patronized. The economics of convenience stores means that selection is limited, most food costs more, and package sizes are small. However, it is worth paying for the convenience of the regular milk stop and for the occasional purchase of other items. Actually, many convenience stores have milk prices that are often quite competitive, which makes convenience stores even better for milk stops. Milk sells quickly and is likely to be fresh. But since convenience stores are generally gas stations, not grocery stores, standards of cleanliness may be a little spotty. Take a look at sanitation. Are the floors and shelves clean? Are food spills wiped up promptly? Are the end-dates on cartons and packages current?

Summary

That does it. If you have more ideas for shopping, let me know. I wish you the best on your shopping campaign. I hope you find a way to make it gratifying and rewarding. If you don't, I can only tell you that the *product* is well worth the effort. Being orderly and planning carefully about your shopping can improve the quality of your mealtimes and can save you a *lot* of time, money, and frustration.

STAPLES LIST

With this list, you can make all the recipes in this book—and be ready for quick cooking on many other occasions.

Baking Supplies

Baking powder
Baking soda
Bisquick
Bread crumbs
Buttermilk powder
Cake mixes
Chocolate chips
Corn meal
Cracker crumbs
Dried fruit: dates, pitted prunes, raisins,
    Craisins, etc.

Flour: white, wheat, quick-mixing (e.g., Wondra)
Muffin mix
Nuts: almonds, pecans, walnuts, etc.
Pudding mix
Canned pumpkin
Sugar: white, brown
Vanilla extract
Yeast

Crackers

Oyster
Saltines
Wheat Thins

Triscuts
Sociables
Your Choice

Cereal

Oatmeal
Cheerios
Kix
Rice Chex

Rice Krispies
Wheat Chex
Wheaties

Condiments and Seasonings

(In addition to the ones here, stock what you like)

Chiles: canned, dried
Herbs and spices
basil, chives, cinnamon, cloves, dill weed, garlic
    powder, ginger, Italian seasoning, lemon pep-
    per, mint, mustard (dry),
    nutmeg, onion flakes, onion powder, oregano,
    paprika, parsley, pepper,
    poppyseeds, rosemary, sage, salt, thyme
Jam or jelly
Ketchup
Mayonnaise
Miracle Whip
Mustard: yellow and Dijon

Oil: olive, peanut or canola, toasted sesame
Olives: black, green
Peanut butter
Pickle relish
Pickles
Salad dressing
Salsa
Sauce mixes
Soy sauce
Taco seasoning mix
Vinegar: white, balsamic, rice, wine, flavored
    (e.g., raspberry)
Worcestershire sauce

Pasta, Rice, and Other Boxed Grains

Barley
Bulgur
Couscous
Egg Noodles
Macaroni
Macaroni and cheese (boxed mix)

Mostaccioli (or penne)
Potatoes: instant mashed, boxed scalloped
Rice: brown, white, seasoned
Spaghetti, fettuccini, etc.
Stuffing mix, dried

STAPLES LIST (*Continued*)

Soup

Bouillon: crystals or cubes
Broth (stock): canned chicken broth, beef broth
    concentrate
Chicken rice
Cream of mushroom
Cream of potato

Golden mushroom
"Hearty" style (with at least 5–7 grams of protein
    per serving)
Onion soup mix, dried
Tomato
Vegetable soup mix, dried

Canned Vegetables and Sauces

Artichoke hearts, marinated
Green beans
Corn (whole kernel and cream style)
Mixed vegetables
Mushrooms
Peas
Potatoes, small whole

Spaghetti sauce
Three-bean salad
Tomato paste
Tomato sauce
Tomatoes: stewed, diced (with and without
    seasonings)

Beans, Mexican

Canned or dried beans: black, garbanzo,
    kidney

Pork and beans
Refried beans: instant or canned

Canned Meat and Fish

Beef stew
Chicken, canned deboned

Salmon
Tuna

Canned Fruit and Juices

Apple juice
Apricots
Apricot nectar
Cherries
Cranberry juice
Mandarin oranges

Maraschino cherries
Peach nectar
Peaches
Pears
Pineapple rings
Tomato juice

Cleaning Supplies and Paper Products

Aluminum foil
Bar soap
Dish washing detergent
Fabric softener
Garbage bags
Laundry detergent

Napkins
Oven cooking bags
Paper towels
Plastic wrap
Freezer zip top bags

Baked Goods

Bread
Croutons
English muffins
Hamburger buns

Pita bread
Soft taco shells
Crisp taco shells

STAPLES LIST (*Continued*)

Fresh Produce
(Fresh produce will vary a lot depending on meals planned and family preferences)

Apples
Bananas
Basil
Bean sprouts
Berries: blueberries, strawberries,
    raspberries, etc.
Broccoli
Brussels sprouts
Cabbage: preshedded (also consider
    already-shredded coleslaw mix, broccoli
    slaw mix)
Carrots: baby peeled, preshredded, whole
Cauliflower
Celery
Chard
Chives
Cranberries
Cucumbers
Dill
Eggplant
Garlic (buy fresh bulbs or bottled minced
    garlic)

Ginger (buy fresh ginger root or bottled
    chopped ginger)
Green beans
Lemons (or lemon juice)
Lettuce and other salad greens: romaine, spinach
    (consider prewashed greens)
Mushrooms
Onions: green, white, red
Oranges
Parsley
Peaches
Pears
Peppers: green, red, yellow
Plums
Potatoes
Snow peas
Summer squash
Tomatoes
Yellow squash
Zucchini

Meat and Fish

Bacon
Chuck beef roast
Ground beef
Round steak
Stew beef

Chicken: boneless breasts
Fish: cod, halibut, etc.
Ham
Pork: boneless chops
Breakfast sausage

Frozen Food

Breads:
    Bagels
    Bread dough
    Waffles
Main dishes:
    Pizza
Fruits:
    Cherries
    Juice concentrate
    Raspberries, strawberries, etc.
Desserts:
    Ice cream

Vegetables:
    Broccoli
    Brussels sprouts
Greens:
    mustard, turnip, beet, etc.
Hash browns
Onions, chopped
Pearl onions
Peas
Spinach
Stir-fry vegetables
Snow peas

STAPLES LIST (*Continued*)

Dairy and Other Refrigerated Foods

Dairy:
    Butter (or margarine)
    Cheese:
        Blue
        Cottage
        Cream (or Neufchâtel)
        Feta
        Parmesan (or Asiago)
        Ricotta
        Sharp Cheddar
        Swiss

Half-and-half
Milk
Sour cream
Yogurt
Other:
    Eggs
    Fresh pasta
    Juice
    Refrigerated biscuits
    Tortillas

Enlightened Nutrition Education

- The best nutrition education helps children support and extend their intuitive eating capabilities.
- Children aren't able to apply nutrition rules and may find them confusing and even frightening.
- Children benefit from opportunities to learn but not from pressure.
- Don't try to get children to change their food acceptance or their eating behavior. Trust them to make the most of what parents and other adults make available.
- Avoid pressure. Even playful and positive outside pressure does not help and may hinder a child's progress with respect to food acceptance.
- When evaluating a nutrition education program, consider the extent to which children are simply exposed to new foods rather than being pressured to eat new foods.
- Use the lesson plans presented in this chapter to teach children food acceptance skills, regulation of food intake, and respect for diversity in body size and shape.

CHAPTER
10
RAISING A HEALTHY EATER IN YOUR COMMUNITY

So we end at the beginning. As I said quite a few pages back, the secret of feeding a healthy family is threefold: love good food, trust yourself, and teach your children to do the same. If you have been able to maintain a division of responsibility in feeding, doing your job and trusting your child to do hers, chances are your child will enjoy eating and will feel good about it. Furthermore, she will *feel* good about enjoying eating. She'll like many different foods and, she'll assume she can eat as much or as little as her body needs, even when she eats more or less than usual. She'll be comfortable with feeling hungry because she knows that she can eat enough to satisfy her hunger. She'll be comfortable with feeling full because she knows that it's natural; she'll empty out, and she'll get hungry again. She'll know how to behave around food and in social eating situations. She'll be secure in her expectation that others won't criticize her eating or try to control it. Finally, as a result of all these positive feelings, attitudes, and capabilities, she'll be confident and unselfconscious about eating. For a fun little test to check how both you and your child are doing, take a look at the "What Is a Good Eater?" box.

The problem is that you have raised a healthy eater, and now she's going out into a food- and body-crazed world. What will happen to your child's comfort and confidence with her eating and body when she goes to school? When she watches television? When she goes to the doctor's office? Girl Scouts? 4H? How do the nutrition lessons that your child learns elsewhere support or undermine what she is learning at home?

What can you do to help and protect her? You have discovered in this book how you can swim against the tide of prevailing thought about eating, nutrition, and food selection by the way you feed yourself and your family in your home. Now we need to consider how you can help your child swim against the tide—or how you can work to *turn* the tide—*outside* your home. Your child will hear about nutri-

---

WHAT IS A GOOD EATER?

A "good eater" is someone who . . .
- Likes eating.
- Is interested in food.
- Feels good about eating.
- Likes being at the table.
- Can wait a few minutes to eat when hungry.
- Can try new food and learn to like it.
- Likes a lot of different foods.
- Can eat until full.
- Can stop when full.
- Can eat in other places besides home.
- Can say "no" politely when she doesn't want to eat.
- Can be around new or strange food without getting upset.
- Has pretty good table manners.
- Can make do with less-favorite food.

Copyright © 1995 by Ellyn Satter. May be reproduced only by registered purchasers of *Ellyn Satter's Feeding with Love and Good Sense: Reproducible Masters.* For purchase information see www.ellynsatter.com or call 800-808-7976.

tion and eating from teachers, coaches, health professionals, volunteer leaders, and other people. They all do the best they can.

They are, however, grappling with the same distorted set of ideas that have made it hard for us, and they are giving the standard negative nutrition messages. As a consequence, kids are being taught *avoidance*, they are being given directions they can't follow, and they are being taught information that they can't compute. Although most of the teaching is direct, much of it is attitudinal, as when organizers who don't make family meals a priority schedule sporting or school events at family dinnertime. The message to children? Eating with your family isn't important.

The Division of Responsibility in Nutrition Education

In chapter 3, you learned about dividing responsibilities between the parents' tasks and children's capabilities. The parent's job is feeding; the child's job is eating. The parent's job is to understand nutrition and to choose food for his or her child. The child's job is to decide whether or not to eat what is put in front of her. In child care and at school, the division of responsibility applies to adults who take on the role of parents. Adults make the nutrition decisions and provide the food. Children eat—or don't eat.

FOCUS ON CHILDREN'S CAPABILITIES

As your child has grown up at your table, and as you have executed your tasks with feeding and let your child develop her capabilities with eating, she has received *intuitive* nutrition education. She has learned about food selection and regulation with her *body*. The best nutrition education at school helps children support and extend their intuitive eating capabilities. It reinforces their trust in instinctive capabilities, and for older children, it adds an understanding of those capabilities. That understanding needs to be positive and to build on the competencies your child has developed at home. Just as at home, good nutrition education exposes children to the possibilities, lets them learn through experience, supports their love of all kinds of food, reminds them that they know how much to

eat, and helps them to remember that they have good and trustworthy bodies. For a list of children's books that support positive attitudes about food and eating, see the box called "Great Food Books for Children."

In kindergarten and possibly in first and second grades, children are allowed to have fun with food. Then, too often, the nutrition lessons start. Current nutrition education teaches children jobs that belong to adults. Children are taught avoidance of high-fat foods, instructed in the Food Guide Pyramid, and expected to be able to apply the pyramid in choosing types and amounts of food to eat. Children can't make use of such lessons. In

---

GREAT FOOD BOOKS FOR CHILDREN
In preparing this list, I had the fun of reading many children's books about food and eating. Most of the books emphasize exploring and learning about food and stress the joy of eating delicious food. Some talk about cooking and even growing food. With regret, I had to exclude some beautiful books because they had lines—or even words—that talked about restricting or avoiding food or eating certain foods in order to manage body size and shape. With even more regret, I found I could not endorse some very popular children's books because feeding dynamics were distorted.

For Preschoolers:
Caseley, Judith. *Grandpa's Garden Lunch*. New York: Greenwillow, 1990.
Ehlert, Lois. *Eating the Alphabet: Fruits and Vegetables from A to Z*. New York: Harcourt Brace Jovanovich, 1989.
Ehlert, Lois. *Growing Vegetable Soup*. New York: Harcourt Brace Jovanovich, 1987.
Falwell, Cathryn. *Feast for 10*. New York: Clarion, 1993.
Goldstone, Bruce. *The Beastly Feast*. New York: Holt, 1998.
Katzen, Mollie, and Ann Henderson. *Pretend Soup and Other Real Recipes: A Cookbook for Preschoolers and Up*. Berkeley: Tricycle Press, 1994.
Modesitt, Jeanne. *Vegetable Soup*. New York: Macmillan, 1988.
Morris, Ann. *Bread, Bread, Bread*. New York: Lothrop, Lee, and Shepard, 1989.
Shelby, Anne. *Potluck*. New York: Orchard, 1991.

For School-Age Children:
Dooley, Norah. *Everybody Cooks Rice*. Minneapolis: Carolrhoda, 1991.
Creasy, Rosalind. *Blue Potatoes, Orange Tomatoes: How to Grow a Rainbow Garden*. San Francisco: Sierra Club, 1994.

fact, they are confused and overwhelmed by them. Such teaching is beyond their ability to understand.

To a lesser extent, dealing with size and shape issues follows a similar pattern. The learning is exploratory and benign in the younger grades and becomes more controlling and critical as time goes on. Along with the control and criticism, children learn to feel bad about their eating and weight. Subjectively or objectively, weight standards and body comments start to creep in as health curricula, classroom and physical education teachers, school nurses, coaches, dance teachers, den leaders, and others begin to take it upon themselves to intervene with children's size and shape. Too often, educators weigh children, and even evaluate their weights using tables or other external standards. Some schools even offer size and shape interventions by putting children in special physical education and nutrition classes for the express purpose of slimming them down. In my view, such evaluations and interventions belong only in a medical setting.

DON'T TEACH CHILDREN ADULTS' TASKS

My friend Libby Jackson, a registered dietitian who is in the process of raising three healthy eaters, was mad.

"When I offered ice cream for dessert last night, Zoe [her 4-year-old] announced to me that ice cream is bad food," fumed Libby. "Bad food," said Libby, trying not to blow up or be critical. "Where did you learn that?"

"From my teachers," Zoe said.

"Oh," said Libby, in what she hoped was a neutral tone, "then what is good food?"

"I guess an apple," responded Zoe.

"I can't believe it," Libby sputtered. "Giving a child that age a message like that."

While I was concerned about the message, I was still preoccupied with dessert. "Well, what did Zoe do about her ice cream?" I asked.

"She ate it," said Libby.

It didn't seem that the message had damaged Zoe's ice cream eating. Hard to know, however, if it damaged her attitude about ice cream—or about herself for eating it. Children, like adults, don't always do what they *should* do. But they do feel bad about themselves when they don't live up to the expectations of adults who are important to them.

Zoe could parrot the doubtful wisdom about ice cream, but she couldn't make use of it. It was beyond her mental ability to understand or apply it. So what if ice cream was bad for her? What did that mean? That it would make her clothes dirty? That it would make her wet the bed? That it would give her heart disease? What is a heart anyway, and what does disease mean? Not only that, but here was her mother, giving her something the teacher said was bad. What did that say about her mother?

Zoe isn't the only child who can't follow such directions. In Minneapolis, researchers found that students in kindergarten through the sixth grade had difficulty using the Food Guide Pyramid and other standard nutrition guidelines to evaluate the acceptability of foods. Younger children freely used terms such as "low-fat" or "low-sugar," but they had trouble naming foods in those categories. Children in the third through sixth grade still had difficulty understanding concepts like "avoid high-fat food," "eat a variety of food," and "maintain a healthy weight."[1]

Why would children want to learn these rules? Provided they are being offered regular and nutritious meals and snacks in a positive environment, children have within them far more sophisticated mechanisms for achieving nutritional adequacy, regulating food intake, and maintaining a healthy weight. For a child, learning how to manage eating is like learning how to breathe. It doesn't arise. It's there, and you take it in. Children don't need "shoulds" and "oughts" to help them with their eating. They eat a food if they like it, and they like it partly because they felt comfortable and satisfied when they ate it last. Children can't plan menus or select from the wide array of available food to put together a healthy diet. They don't have to. It's not their job. It's the job of their adults to do that for them.

Rule- and avoidance-based nutrition lessons stress negativity and restraint. Such strategies are not only destructive, but they are frightening for children and absolutely contradictory to a child's approach to the world. In contrast, optimism, self-trust, and adventure are in concert with a child's way of being and doing. For children, as for adults, these seeking and exploring attitudes are good motivators.

Let me be even more blunt: We have no business teaching the Food Guide Pyramid to children. In chapter 4, we had to work *hard* with the Food Guide Pyramid to keep it from getting negative and medical *for adults*. Even making positive use of it involves thinking abstractly, making value judgments, and keeping the rules in perspective. These ways of thinking are all completely beyond the capability of children under the age of 11 and, for many children, even ages 12 or 13.

CHILDREN AREN'T ABLE TO APPLY NUTRITION RULES

Even if children do want to learn nutrition rules, they don't have the ability. When children are under age 7 years, they can describe foods, but food only has meaning through its effect on them. Ice cream is for eating. They can't think of some far-distant effect on them from eating a food. Stringing together logical consequences like "Ice cream is high in fat and fat is bad for you and you shouldn't eat fat and you shouldn't eat ice cream either" is beyond the understanding of a child under the age of 7. Fortunately.

Such logic is even beyond the grasp of children ages 7 to 11. Second- to fifth-graders can classify. They can sort foods into the right places on the Food Guide Pyramid. However, they can't apply the classifications to choosing what they eat during the day because that involves thinking abstractly: "Eat moderately from the high-fat foods at the top of the pyramid" is meaningless to them because it involves identifying high-fat food *and* making a judgment about where ice cream fits and understanding what "moderately" means. Children in the Minnesota study couldn't name high-fat foods after a *lesson* in high-fat foods. School-age children *can* think in terms of cause and effect. However, the correlation between cause and effect has to be concrete: "If I eat ice cream it will taste good." "High in fat" and "bad for you" are not concrete issues.

At age 11, *some* children begin to think more abstractly and can apply value judgments that are beyond younger children. I have trouble understanding the concept of abstract thinking, so maybe this example will help us both. When I was a sophisticated 13-year-old, I decided to teach Doug, my 5-year-old cousin, the laws of mathematics. "I will teach you how to add," I said grandly, picking up the salt shaker and the pepper shaker. "Here is the salt shaker, that is one. How many salt shakers are there? (He answered me correctly on the first try, but I was being so patronizing, it's funny he didn't hit me.) Here is the pepper shaker, that is one. How many is that?" (Doug gave me the right answer again—this kid was *willing*.)

"Now, if you put them both together, how many would that be?"

"A salt shaker and a pepper shaker," he responded.

"No, *no*," I corrected. It is *two*. Let's try it again. What happens if you put them together?"

He looked very puzzled. He looked at them and looked at me. A disgusted expression crossed his face. "Why do you want to do that?" he asked.

At 13, I could think abstractly enough to classify a pepper shaker as a "one" and I could think about adding this "one" to another "one" that was equally abstract to make a third abstract classification of "two." In fact, it may have been my own discovery of abstract thinking that led me to victimize my cousin! If I had asked Doug to give me two things off the table, he could have done it because that would be concrete. But his prelogical, literal, egocentric mind couldn't make the leap to classifying and then adding. Furthermore, he couldn't figure out why I would want to do that if it didn't have any impact on me.

Asking children to classify vegetables in a list and get those vegetables to add up to a certain number of vegetables in a day is like my failed mathematics lesson with Doug. They can't do it and they don't know why they would want to. Doug asked the right question: "Why do you want to do that?" I can ask the same about learning nutrition rules. Even the 11-year-old is much better served by the intuitive eating capabilities she grew up with than by learning the rules.

NEGATIVE LESSONS SCARE CHILDREN ABOUT THEIR BODIES

Let me give you another example of how the nutrition lessons go awry. Martha, a lovely, very slender fourth-grader, was distraught. "I'm fat!" she announced to her mother the moment she arrived home from school. "I can't eat that!" she wailed when she saw the peanut butter and crackers her mother was getting out for her snack.

Little wonder that her mother was alarmed. Like other parents of preadolescents, she was all too aware of dieting behavior in girls her daughter's age, and afraid that early preoccupation with being fat could forecast an eating disorder. Her alarm sent her for help to a fortunately enlightened dietitian—Libby Jackson, again—for a professional consultation.

Everything at home checked out. The mother was observing a good division of responsibility with feeding, doing her job and letting her daughter do hers. Martha was comfortable with eating and had always grown in a consistent fashion. The problem was at school. The class had been given a nutrition lesson, one that stressed to the 10- and 11-year-olds the dangers of eating fat.

Martha had made the connection that fat was bad and that when she ate fat it went right onto her body, and fat on her body was bad too, and since she ate fat, that made *her* fat. This progression doesn't make sense to us because we don't think like a 10-year-old does. But to Martha, who filtered her information through its immediate impact on *her*, it made all kinds of sense. Once she was able to understand where the distorted idea had come from, Martha's mother straightened her out. She also reassured her.

Martha's mother explained to her that all foods were good for her, including foods with fat in them. She reassured Martha that she would take care of choosing foods for her that are nutritious and have the right amount of fat. All Martha had to do was eat as much as she was hungry for.

Information about food avoidance only scares and overwhelms children; it gives them bad feelings about food and may even carry over into bad feelings about their bodies. It is frightening for children to try to carry out instructions that are beyond them. To cope, they either become rigid and try to live by illogical rules, or they give up and become rebellious. Either way, they lose. As Martha's mother demonstrated, there is something you can do about early dieting behavior. Most children who worry about their weight are doing the best they can to manage something that can't be managed without adult help. Adults can help by taking care of the what, when, and where of feeding and by reassuring children that dieting—and worrying about fat in food— isn't necessary.

Body- and food-friendly attitudes by people important to children can go a long way toward inoculating children against feeling bad about their bodies. Laid-back, positive leaders have an enormous impact on children when they help them to be successful and to develop their unique physical capability. In contrast, few adults would deliberately make a child feel bad about her body. However, casual observations to a child linking size and shape to performance can be devastating. Medical clinics and fitness programs absolutely must not use a child's weight or percentage of body fat as a fitness indicator. Children can't choose their weight and body composition, and they must not be asked to try. But they can do something about other fitness indicators, such as endurance, strength, agility, and speed. Comparing a child to herself with respect to these indicators—and *only* to herself—allows her to experience her body as positive and capable.

Respect for the Family Unit

Most teachers of nutrition are not nutritionists—they are committed amateurs. To give them their due, people who go to the trouble of teaching nutrition to children are those who assign value to eating well. They do the best they can to act on children's behalf, and they teach from the usual understanding of nutrition.

There are, however, people who make a profession of nutrition education. The *Society for Nutrition Education* (to which I belong) publishes a journal, called—not surprisingly—the *Journal of Nutrition Education*. Nutrition educators take their work seriously and, like the amateurs, are genuinely out to improve the nutritional lives of our children.

These professionals evaluate the quality and efficacy of nutrition education programs. After an enormous review of such programs, university specialists found that the few programs that were successful in increasing children's food acceptance were programs that took significant time with nutrition education, that let children *eat or work with food*, and that involved families, schools, and communities.[2] After a thorough review of environmental influences on children's eating, other nutrition educators reminded readers that basic respect for the family unit was the essential means of ensuring children's health and well-being.[3]

Basic respect for the family unit means respecting what the family *eats* and is able to *provide*. Nutrition lessons can introduce children to new and different food. Children can go home and talk about that food with their parents, and some parents may choose to include that new food on the menu. If nutrition messages are kept neutral, the family is involved without being criticized. But if nutrition lessons say "ice cream is bad" or "fat is bad" (or *broccoli* is bad, for that matter), it undermines the family, and the child as well.

Teaching Eating Capability

Now it's my turn to offer alternatives to the current approaches. What approaches to nutrition education help children enhance their eating capabilities while staying away from teaching them adult tasks? To demonstrate my answers, I have chosen three topic areas: food acceptance, regulation of food intake, and respect for diversity.

For the food acceptance topic, I have written a unit that teaches the process of food acceptance. It can function as an introduction to any of the good food-exploration lesson plans available (see page 185). However, in most cases those lessons don't give children any help with the actual process of food acceptance. Instead, they may feature methods of "motivating" children to taste and eat.

The box "Learning about New Food" gives examples of teaching food acceptance. My experience tells me that children will push themselves along to become familiar with and learn to eat new food. Children do poorly with food acceptance for two reasons: Too much pressure and too little opportunity to explore. Either way, they are likely to have negative feelings to overcome before they can feel comfortable with unfamiliar or disliked foods. The intent is to help children learn to tolerate their negative feelings and perhaps even overcome them.

With *food regulation* I have given more complete teaching guidelines because the topic is less familiar and concrete. The boxes "Tuning In on Eating" and "Hunger, Appetite, and Satiety" can stand alone as lesson plans. Like my food acceptance suggestions, these plans are based on experience: helping children become more aware and trusting of what goes on inside of them.

The "Respect for Diversity" lesson plan is complete but brief. I think when you get the basic idea—respect for individual differences in size, shape, and physical aptitude—you will have lots of lessons and applications of your

own. Cultural diversity lessons can be expanded to include these individual physical differences. As with cultural diversity lessons, the idea is *trust*, not *control*. This is a tough one to grapple with because of deeply embedded ideas that size and shape are voluntary. The perspective of cultural diversity will be helpful in making the shift to thinking of size, shape, and physical aptitude as *givens*, not *options*. Everybody's different. Everybody's okay the way they are. We aren't trying to make anyone over; we're simply helping them to understand and accept themselves and each other just the way they are. The idea is to make the lessons accepting and child-centered rather than setting standards and trying to make children over.

The bottom line with all the lessons is to make them positive, based on experience and free of any tactics that impose outside expectations on children. I hope these child-centered approaches, or ones like them, find their way into the hands of people who are able to take the time and energy to grapple with them. In this section, I talk with "you," but I quite realize that you have a life. You might get an opportunity to teach positive nutrition lessons at school or Scouts. You can pass the ideas along to your child's teacher and suggest them as possibilities. In my wildest dreams, the adaptations could even find their way into teacher curricula!

Here is a message for whoever does the lessons: have fun, hang loose, and prepare to be surprised. It is alarming to face a room full of fourth-graders or kindergartners, but I think you will find the rewards are worth it. Children are interested in food and their bodies, and the topic carries the lesson. The goals of the lessons are to *slightly* increase children's awareness and comfort with food, eating, and their bodies. Accept what children say, be interested, and say "uhm-hmm." But stay away from being a cheerleader. Cheerleading is, well, cheery and energetic and seemingly positive, but it is pressure nonetheless.

Above all, don't try to get children to change their food acceptance or their eating behavior. You don't have to get children to eat more vegetables, and if you try you will take away their joy and initiative in learning about new food. If you are one of these wonderfully charismatic and cheerful people who is full of ideas and praise, with stickers and posters and rewards, take it easy. Use them to have fun, but don't let the fun turn into pressure. In some ways, such positive pressure is harder to deal with than negative pressure because it is harder to identify and defend against.

If you give children opportunities to explore, the insights will emerge from the children themselves. Set up a safe environment in which children will not be shamed or challenged about their points of view. Teach children to respectfully accept whatever another person says. Nobody criticizes, nobody snickers, nobody corrects.

Food Acceptance

The best food acceptance lessons expose children to the possibilities and encourage them to explore. Children learn about food from experience. Your goal is to help children develop their familiarity and comfort with a variety of foods. It is not to get them to change or to eat five-a-day or even to discover a new favorite food. If you try, you will spoil the lesson. To review the research on food acceptance, see appendix F.

Children benefit from touching, cooking, and tasting food. They love finding out how it is grown or having a garden, discovering what different people eat, reading a book about people or animals, what they eat, and why they eat it. These lessons teach children about *food*, and they teach them about *themselves* as well. Children assume that they will learn to like the food that is put before them. You don't have to *motivate* children to learn to eat new food. You only have to support their natural inclination to learn and grow.

Help children learn food acceptance skills. See the box on the next page, "Learning about New Food."
Expose children to a wide range of foods (but leave it up to them to decide whether they eat them).
• Let them touch, smell, and work with the food.
• Help them learn where foods come from and how they are grown.
• Help them discover what people in other homes and cultures eat.
• Let them experiment with different ways of preparing food.

TEACHING FOOD ACCEPTANCE LESSONS
If you love good food, enjoy eating, and trust children to explore and learn, you will be a good teacher. For some children, it may be a novel idea to feel positive and relaxed about food and eating. To become comfortable with new foods, children need to be exposed to them without being traumatized by the exposure. As you work with different foods and react to children's comments, be careful not to say or imply that some food is healthier or better than other food. Such value judgments merely confuse children and put a barrier between them and their eating. You made the value judgment when you chose the food. Children don't have to make a value judgment when they eat it.

As we said in chapter 3, children are capable of learning to accept new kinds of food. When presented with something unfamiliar to eat, most are both curious and dubious. They will explore it—in their own way—but they probably won't like a food the first time they taste it. Beyond the initial exposure, given the proper support, they make it their business to learn to like new foods. The proper support is an adult to offer the food to them, time after time, with no praise or pressure. Given this positive opportunity, children learn at their own pace to like the food. Children who are bold and inquisitive will be more likely to taste and experiment. Others who are more cautious or indifferent may limit themselves at first to looking and touching. But even cautious children will move themselves along if they are given repeated neutral access to the food (again, no pressure or praise).

CHILDREN MAY HAVE DIFFICULTY WITH FOOD ACCEPTANCE
When a child is *really* cautious or put off by trying new food, it is usually because of past experience. She may have been forced to eat more or different food than she wanted to, or she may have been sheltered from unfamiliar foods by family menus that were limited to foods that she could readily accept. Sometimes a child has been both sheltered and forced: the cook catered to the child, then made her eat the special food whether she wanted to or not. Families who have tight food budgets sometimes limit menus to what a child can readily accept, feeling they can't afford to serve foods that she doesn't eat.

Parents of a very cautious child may have given up on offering new food experiences. It isn't very rewarding to introduce anything new to a cautious child. Often, adults working with cautious children resort to pushing them along, which is a mistake because it makes the child feel both controlled and cautious. Children always do more and dare more if they feel they have control. The cautious child benefits from learning to cope with herself. You can help by both challenging and reassuring her: "When you are ready, you may like to eat this. For now, you might just like to taste it and then take it back out of your mouth. But you don't have to do that, either."

Bold or cautious, children learning food acceptance need tools for approaching food, and they need an escape hatch. Establish the ground rules: Children have to be polite about accepting and refusing food, and they can't make negative remarks about the food. From there on, children benefit from receiving both encouragement that they can manage and reassurance that they don't have to eat. The suggestions made earlier for how to teach children to approach new foods incorporate both tools and an escape. When children (and adults) are comfortable in their eating envi-

---

LEARNING ABOUT NEW FOOD

Everybody has favorite foods and some foods they don't like at all. Some people enjoy tasting new food and learning to like it; others can't imagine feeling that way and stay away from eating new food whenever they can. Most people are somewhere in between. In our food lessons, you don't have to eat anything you don't want to eat. There are lots of ways for you to take part in the lessons without having to eat. You can have fun learning where foods come from, how they are grown, and what children in other homes and cultures eat, and you can even help prepare foods.

Before you can feel comfortable working with and learning about food, you need to know how to refuse to eat the food. Whether or not you like to taste new foods, sooner or later someone is going to offer you a food that you do not want to eat. You don't have to eat it, but you do have to figure out how to be firm and polite about saying no. In these lessons, you can say "no, thank you" and expect that your teacher and classmates will take "no" for an answer.

Learn to Say "No, Thank You"

Pair off in twos and have one child be a pushy host and the other one be the guest who doesn't want to eat what is offered. Then have the children trade places. The host can run through all the statements, and the guest can practice being polite but firm and not yelling or getting mad.

What the host can say:
"Have some of this wonderful _____."
"I made it especially for you!"
"You should eat it—it's very good for you."
"I can't understand why you don't like it—I like it a lot."

(Kids will have their own ideas and experiences of what people have said to them to get them to eat.)

What the guest can say:
"No, thank you. I don't care for any."
"No, thank you. I don't care for any."

(The guest says the same thing over and over again. Teach the kids that this is the "stuck CD" approach, where the answer is always the same, no matter what the host says.)

Having Fun with Food

What are some of the pleasures of working with food? Practice working with the food without feeling you have to eat it or even taste it.

Look at the food and touch it. You don't have to put it in your mouth.

What are some of the ways you can have fun with food? You can learn about the color, shape, and texture of the food and the designs it makes when it is cut and arranged on a serving plate.

Join in with the cooking lesson. This might make you curious about the food and feel like you want to taste it. But you don't have to.

Learning to Eat New Food

Everybody's different with what they like to eat. Foods taste different to different people. It takes time to learn to like new foods. Some of the foods we make in school will be foods your family eats; others will be new to you. Usually familiar foods taste best to us, but you can also learn to like new foods. It helps to like a lot of different foods because that can give you pleasure and let you eat in lots of different places with lots of different people. If you feel you want to taste a new food, take it slowly. Here are some ways you can sneak up on a new food.

Look at the food; smell it. Do you still feel like tasting it? You don't have to if you don't want to. Every time you get a chance, look at and smell the food, but don't taste it until you're ready.

Put a small amount in your mouth. Taste it, feel it in your mouth, and maybe chew it. Do you feel like swallowing it? You don't have to if you don't want to. Don't make a fuss about it. Just keep a paper napkin handy and quietly spit it out.

Swallow that first bite, and then decide what to do next. You might find you like the food and want to eat more. You might find that one bite is all you want.

ronment and have the conviction that they don't have to eat if they don't want to, they become interested in learning to like new foods. It is natural for children—and adults—to seek diversity with food, just as they do in other areas of life.

Keep in mind that the goal of this lesson is to introduce children to the possibilities, not to have them learn a new behavior or change their eating habits. Learning to like a new food takes 10 or 15 or more neutral exposures, and it's unlikely that children will get that many exposures in the classroom. However, if the classroom teams up with the school lunchroom, magic can happen. A friendly and interested school nutrition provider can plan menus in tandem with classroom food acceptance lessons. Or foods for classroom lessons can be chosen from the school lunch menu. Either way, foods children work with in the classroom can appear again and again on the school lunch menu. Eventually, most children will learn to like most foods.

DEALING WITH CULTURAL ISSUES IN FOOD ACCEPTANCE

It is essential to cultivate an attitude of acceptance of differences in food selection and eating patterns. If a child learns to say "How can you eat that?" to another child, it means "I don't respect you or your family." In the chapter 4, you learned the *Mother Principle* for planning meals. Every culture and family has its own Mother Principle that governs what goes on the table to make up a meal. It is not good to criticize someone else's mother.

People eat what they can. Parents of different cultures and economic circumstances feed their children the best they can. Unfortunately, in our nutrition-deranged society, it is socially acceptable to criticize politically incorrect, unsophisticated, or even unfamiliar food. Such snobbishness isn't acceptable to me, and it doesn't have to be acceptable to you.

It is needlessly unkind to ridicule the food preferences of other times, places, or people. Whatever the reason for sneering at someone's food, it isn't valid. Deriding someone's food scorns their culture and their family and their history. All people have used considerable ingenuity to make do with what they have, to survive on it and even to create valued food traditions. Look at tripe. Look at duck's feet. Look at caviar. The respectful study of food and food traditions offers children a vivid understanding

of what people of other cultures and eras were up against and how they managed.

Look at fry bread. American Indian fry bread is a delicious, filling, greasy, and therefore politically incorrect staple of native American people across the country. If you scout around in your local food emporium, you might even find WoodenKnife Indian Fry Bread Mix,* a South Dakota product that contains prairie turnips, one of the most important wild foods that was gathered by Lakota Indians. Rent the video *Smoke Signals* if you want to see what fry bread looks like. This simple food commemorates a people's joyous coping with difficult circumstances. In the late 1800s, Indian mothers forced to live on reservations learned to use their government food commodities to make fry bread for their hungry families.

CURRICULA ON FOOD ACCEPTANCE

Are there some good food acceptance curricula available? Possibly. In the two-year 5-a-Day Power Plus Study done in St. Paul, Minnesota, children significantly increased their fruit and vegetable consumption both at school and at home. The intervention consisted of 28 lessons or classroom curricula over two years, 10 take-home activity packets, and exposure to additional vegetable and fruit choices in the School Nutrition Program. The National Cancer Institute (NCI) has sponsored 5-a-Day school intervention programs that appear to do equally well with increasing fruit and vegetable consumption. Unfortunately, the NCI program also emphasizes fat restriction.[4]

How do these results square up, asks Mary Ray Worley, my extremely perceptive editor, with my earlier statements that adults shouldn't try to alter what and how much children eat? Most children don't eat enough fruits and vegetables, so increasing consumption is a legitimate outcome of nutrition education. The important distinction is in how you arrive at that outcome. Is it by offering children opportunities to learn, or is it by putting pressure on them to change? Nutrition lessons that pressure children to eat fruits and vegetables (by teaching them that they are healthful foods and telling them how many they "should" eat) don't work in the long run. Like similar lessons for adults, they make children feel guilty or wary but don't alter children's food consump-

---

*If you can't find it, write to WoodenKnife Co. Mfg., Box 104, Interior, SD 57750; or call 605-433-5463.

tion. In contrast, curricula like the ones above that include family and school nutrition components increase children's exposure to fruits and vegetables. Such exposure boosts their long-term food acceptance, provided that exposure isn't accompanied by pressure to eat. Otherwise, when the pressure is off, children stop eating fruits and vegetables.

In contrast, the CATCH (Child and Adolescent Trial for Cardiovascular Health) Eat Smart curriculum, funded by the National Heart, Lung, and Blood Institute, invested 25 percent more teaching time than the Power Plus curriculum and showed no change in fruit and vegetable consumption. The CATCH study emphasized fat and sodium avoidance, encouraged increasing physical activity, and recommended that children eat more fruits and vegetables. The trial lowered fat consumption and increased regular physical activity.

When evaluating any nutrition education curriculum, including the Power Plus and NCI curricula, it is vitally important to consider the extent to which children are simply *exposed* to new foods, in contrast to their being "motivated" to eat new foods. I don't feel comfortable with "motivating" other people to do anything because I consider it paternalistic and controlling. Exposing children to the possibilities and teaching them to cope is fine. Motivating them is not. Pushing from the outside—even positive pushing—makes children feel bad and slows their learning and growth. If you cheer, reward, monitor, and motivate children to eat fruits and vegetables, they will eat vegetables while you keep up the outside encouragement and stop once the pressure stops. The goal is not to get children to eat fruits and vegetables today, it is to help them master eating fruits and vegetables for a lifetime. To do that, children have to make use of their own drive for mastery to push them along, without pressure from the outside.

Regulation of Food Intake

The goal of lessons about food regulation is to reinforce children's intuitive understanding that their bodies know how to eat and grow. The lessons make conscious the unconscious mechanisms that children (and the rest of us) use to manage the amount of food they eat: their feelings of hunger, appetite, and satiety. Food regulation lessons support children in trusting their internal regulators. Teaching food regulation is a consciousness-raising activity, and that's *all*. There are no rules or guidelines attached to how much children *should* eat.

Teach children about their internal regulators of hunger, appetite, and satiety.
- Teach "your body will tell you how much is enough"
- Define hunger, appetite, and satiety in neutral terms (see the box "Hunger, Appetite, and Satiety").
- Have children talk about their experience of hunger, appetite, and satiety.
- Do an eating exercise (see the box "Tuning In on Eating") to give children experience with paying attention to how they feel inside when they eat.
- Have children talk about what they can do to help themselves become aware of their internal regulators. Ideas might be to slow down, to avoid doing other things while they eat, to talk with friends about the food, or to shut their eyes when they taste.

TEACHING FOOD REGULATION LESSONS
If you know and trust your own internal regulators of hunger, appetite, and satiety, you will be able to help children with theirs. Your task is to help children learn about, explore, and trust their own capabilities. Set up the activity, take an interest, and say, "uhm-hmm." Reiterate the expectation that children be accepting and noncritical with themselves and each other. Children need a safe environment so they can learn and grow, and they need not to be traumatized by new experience.

The internal cues that regulate food intake, hunger, appetite, and satiety are hard to teach because they are so subjective. For younger children, just giving the message "Your body knows how much you need to eat" is enough. You can take it a little further if you want to and have them do a little self-awareness exercise: "How does it feel inside when you are empty and when you are full?" "Do you feel like it is all right to be hungry?" "Do you feel like it is all right to be full?" No matter what a child says, you can say, "Sometimes people feel like that. When they aren't sure they are going to get enough to eat, it can be scary to be hungry." Or, "Sometimes people feel upset when they get too full. It is okay to feel full after you eat. You will empty out and get hungry again."

For older children, experiment with the

HUNGER, APPETITE, AND SATIETY

When you are hungry, you might feel like something is gnawing on your stomach or like your stomach is growling. You might feel weak, or grouchy, or like you can't sit still. You might get a headache or have a hard time paying attention to your teacher.

Appetite is when you want food that you like. Your appetite tells you when something will taste good to you. It also makes you eat a lot of different foods, and it lets you enjoy your eating.

Satiety is when you feel ready to quit eating. It is when all those body feelings that say you want to eat go away and you feel better. Usually food still tastes good even after you stop being hungry. But then your appetite goes away, too, and food doesn't taste so good anymore. Pay attention, but keep eating until you feel like quitting. Your body know it needs enough food to satisfy both hunger and appetite.

Sometimes people keep eating until they feel full. That's all right. Most people like being full sometimes. When you are growing fast or being really active, a lot of times you might eat until you feel full because you need more to eat. Sometimes meals are so good that you just want to be full. Sometimes being full helps you to relax or to fall asleep. Other times it just keeps you awake.

If you keep on eating past being full, you will begin to feel stuffed. Stuffed is when you can't eat another bite. Most people find they don't like that feeling because it is uncomfortable. Maybe you have eaten until you were stuffed by mistake, like on Thanksgiving Day. The food tasted so good that you kept right on eating. Then it caught up with you, and you felt like you couldn't move. Sometimes people eat until they are stuffed because they don't know when they are going to get to eat again. Have you ever been hungry and unsure about when you were going to get to eat? It's a scary feeling, isn't it?

People who aren't sure they will get enough to eat feel they have to eat as much as they can while they have food available. In between times, they don't just get hungry, they become famished. It doesn't feel good to be too hungry, especially if you don't know that you can make the hunger go away. When people are famished, lots of times they eat fast and eat until they are stuffed because it feels so bad to be famished.

There is no right or wrong way to eat. There are just choices. Most people do best with eating when they have meals and snacks at about the same times every day. Then they can go to the table hungry, but not famished, and they can eat until they are satisfied but not stuffed.

---

focused eating exercise in the box "Tuning In on Eating." Have children pay attention to how they feel while they eat a simple food. Making a special effort to be aware while they eat begins to make conscious the processes that, for most children and adults, are unconscious. Doing a focused eating exercise in a classroom setting is fun and full of surprises. Children often giggle and act silly, but they get something out of it nonetheless.

Let me stress again that the goal of the food regulation work is not to try to change the way a child eats. The focused eating exercise is not a technique to slim down the fat child or fatten up the skinny child. It is a way to help children become more aware of what goes on inside of them. If you can be accepting and interested in what they say about their own experience, you will help them be more comfortable and accepting about who they are and how they eat. Paradoxically, once children (and other people) feel more comfortable with themselves and their eating, they are able to change and grow. But your task isn't to change them—it is to understand and accept them. Your understanding and acceptance will help them to understand and accept themselves.

CHILDREN MAY HAVE TROUBLE WITH FOOD REGULATION

As with food acceptance, you may encounter some children who don't seem to have intuitive capabilities with food regulation. Such children may be puzzled about the idea that they can experience hunger and satiety and may say, "I don't feel anything" or "I just eat as much as my mom tells me." All you have to do is respond, "That's all right. Those sensations are there, even if you can't feel them right now. I think if you keep paying attention, you will start to feel something." For your own information, let me give you some background on children who can't tune in on their hunger, appetite, and satiety.

As I pointed out in my September 1996 article in the *Journal of the American Dietetic Association*, "Internal Regulation and the Evolution of Normal Growth as the Basis for Prevention of obesity in childhood," children are born with the ability to eat the right amount of food to get the body that is right for them. The ability to self-regulate will be preserved if the people who feed them maintain a division of responsibility in feeding, trusting them to eat as much or as little as they want.

TUNING IN ON EATING

Your body knows how much you need to eat. It has some ways of telling you. Does anybody know what it feels like when your body needs food?

Your body needs a lot of different kinds of food. Usually, food tastes best when we don't have to eat the same thing all the time. Has anybody had the feeling that you want to eat something in particular? Have you ever really liked something but still not felt like eating it?

Your body knows when you have had enough. What does it feel like inside when you are ready to stop eating?

Let's do a little experiment to see if you can find any of those feelings inside of you. Let's experiment with this food (crackers, potato chips, strawberries, M&M's).

First, you need to close your eyes and relax. That way, you can settle down so other feelings and sensations go away for a while. While you relax, pay attention to how your breathing goes in and out. We will do that for 30 seconds; so take your time and settle down.

Now, open your eyes and pick up your food. Don't eat it yet. Just look at it and smell it and touch it. What does it feel like inside of you when you do that? Do you feel like you want to eat it? What does that feel like? Does anybody not want to eat it? What does that feel like?

Shut your eyes again to get settled down.

(About five breaths in and out.) Now open your eyes and look at your food. When you are ready, if you feel like it, eat the food. Pay close attention to what happens in your mouth and in your body. Does anybody want to say what that felt like? Did anybody have positive feelings, like you enjoyed it? Did anybody have negative feelings, like you didn't like eating this food?

Did anybody feel like you didn't want to swallow? You have a napkin, you can spit your food into that if you want to.

Shut your eyes again to get settled down. (About five seconds.) Now open them and look at your food again. Eat another bite, if you feel like it. What did you notice this time? Was it the same as before? Was it different?

All right, now sit quietly at your desk and eat as much of your food as you like. Pay attention to every bite of food. Chew it up and swallow it before you take another bite. What was that like for you? Did it feel like it was too fast? Too slow? Did you enjoy the food?

That's all. This is a little exercise to help you to be more aware of how your body helps you with your eating. If you pay attention, your body can do a better job of helping you.

What do you think makes it hard for you to know what goes on inside of you when you eat? What can you do to be more aware?

Self-regulation will be undermined if adults try to dictate the amounts or types of food that children eat. For more background and references on food regulation, see appendix E, "Children and Food Regulation."

Children who lack intuitive eating capabilities have real difficulty as they begin to move away from their parents and spend more time in the outside world. Children can't put it into words, but they are aware that they don't know how to eat, and their efforts to manage eating can turn into distorted or even disordered eating patterns. Internal capability can be rebuilt, but usually the child requires lessons that go beyond those that can be offered in the classroom. For a child to trust internal regulation, both school and home have to provide structure, give opportunities to learn, and trust the child to eat the right amount and type of food.

CURRICULA ON FOOD REGULATION

Generally, curricula that teach about food regulation do so from the point of view of stressing weight management. To manage weight, fat restriction is emphasized, as is increasing the child's physical activity. From the opposite perspective, programs for school-age children that are designed to prevent eating disorders stress avoidance of dieting and physical self-acceptance. Such programs often teach the Food Guide Pyramid and assume that if children eat off the pyramid, they will be able to manage their body weight.

Both sets of programs appear to have little impact on children's weight management behaviors. Children weigh the same, whether or not they have had school-based interventions for weight management.[5] Children who have been warned off restrained eating appear to have gone back to it within a couple of years of the intervention.[6]

Is the approach I recommend effective? I assume so, because what I teach is normal food regulation. The goal of my approach is not to get children to be thin or to warn them away from dieting. The goal of my approach is to support children's capability with tuning in on and respecting their internal regulators of hunger, appetite, and satiety. When children are in tune with their internal regulators, they eat and grow in a stable and consistent fashion, and they achieve the adult body that is right for them.

Respect for Diversity in Body Size and Shape

In the food acceptance unit, we talked about studying and accepting cultural diversity. Here, we will focus on accepting different body sizes and shapes. The theme of all the units is that "everybody's different" with respect to food preference, energy requirements, and body size and shape. Whenever you help children to trust their eating, you help them to trust and accept their bodies. Here, we are being more direct in emphasizing the goodness of children's bodies and how they work.

The issue of diversity teaches facts, but the most important lessons are attitudinal. By reinforcing the notion that "everybody's different" with respect to food preference, energy requirements, body size, shape, and physical capability, you can help children to correct contemptuous or disdainful attitudes toward themselves and other people.

TEACHING SIZE AND SHAPE ACCEPTANCE

Lessons on size and shape have to be handled with particular care so they don't single out or embarrass anyone. Given the struggles adults have in this area, it may not be easy for you to be relaxed and accepting about children and their bodies. In fact, if you have trouble accepting children of all sizes and shapes, this unit would be better taught by someone who is more relaxed about physical diversity.

Everybody *is* different. Some people are fat, some are thin, some are tall, some are short. Some people eat a lot and some people don't eat so much. In most cases the way people eat doesn't have much to do with how they are shaped. Today, children and even some adults think that they can eat or exercise to get their bodies to turn out the way they want them to. They can't. Size and shape are determined mostly by genetics, not by what they *do*.

In building physical self-esteem, the first task is for children to get a clear and accurate image of their own size and shape. A young child is interested in herself, and she will enjoy tracing around her outline on a big piece of paper,

measuring to see how tall she is, drawing pictures of herself and her family, writing stories about her eyes and hair and skin color and, yes, about her size and shape. I don't recommend weighing children. Given all the weight consciousness in our culture, it's too easy to get into value judgments and negative comparisons. Children can handle it, but adults can't.

Older children have the additional task of becoming more conscious of ideas and expectations about size and shape and making positive use of those ideas. The theme for the older school-age child is *industry*. Children at around ages 10 through 12 want to *achieve*, and they look to adults for ways to do that. Because older children are oriented toward doing and achieving, it seems natural to them that body size and shape can be done and achieved like other tasks. They assume they can pick out a particular body and get it through their own efforts. As a consequence, for older children it is important to emphasize the parts of the lesson that point out that size and shape are not optional. For preadolescents, it may be helpful to talk about what to expect concerning growth and development and to emphasize individual differences in times and rates of growing. Then turn their energies away from waiting and worrying about what nature has in mind for them and toward more productive avenues for doing and achieving. Developing skills with physical activity and cooking, for example, are both directions that can support and enhance their feelings of self-confidence.

CHILDREN HAVE THEIR OWN ISSUES WITH SIZE AND SHAPE ACCEPTANCE

It's important to remember that the topic of physical self-acceptance is quite different from the child's point of view than it is from our own. For instance, the preschooler and young school-age child begin to be conscious of their own and others' bodies. Often children ask, "Am I fat?" or "Am I skinny?" Adults get all upset about such questions because they immediately jump to the conclusion that "fat" or "skinny" is being used as a taunt, that the child is being made the target of teasing, and that it will scar her for life. Parents, teachers, and other caring adults are quick to say, "No, dear, you're not skinny, you're just slender." They may go on to say, "Everybody's different, some people are slender and some are fat." The really worried parent might say, "But don't worry about it, you'll grow out of it."

EVERYBODY'S DIFFERENT
Get children started thinking about natural differences in the sizes and shapes of people's bodies.

- Think of adults who are tall or thin or short or fat (this might be people on television or in movies).
- Talk about how people in different cultures vary in size and shape: Fulani people in northern Africa are very tall and slender. Pygmy people are very small.

Introduce the idea that different people naturally eat different amounts and that that is all right.

- Can you think of anybody who is small and slender who eats a lot?
- Can you think of anybody who is large and heavy who doesn't eat very much? Lots of times, thin people eat more than fat people.

Introduce the notion that there are natural differences in people's size, shape, eating, and activity. Point out that a person's size and shape are not optional. When people are babies, some babies are active and eat a lot, other babies are not so active and don't eat so much.

- Do you know somebody who is strong?
- Do you know somebody who can run fast?
- Do you know somebody who seems to feel best when moving around?
- Do you know somebody who seems to like sitting still?
- What are you like?

By now, the alert child participating in this conversation will have figured out that there is something really wrong with being skinny, especially if that child is looking for *information* rather than reassurance. It's like the old joke in which the little boy comes home and asks, "Where did I come from?" His resolute and prepared father, anticipating the moment, presents the whole sex education story, complete with charts and pictures and positive values. His puzzled son responds, "What does that have to do with it? Johnny said he was from New York and I want to know where I came from."

"Am I skinny?" could mean just that. Find out. The answer (if it fits) is "Well, you're pretty slender. But I wouldn't call you skinny because usually when people say that they are teasing. Why do you ask?" *Keep in mind* that "skinny" might be a pejorative term only in *your* mind.

For your child, it could be a simple descriptive term.

In his book *Walking across Egypt,* Clyde Edgerton told of Mattie Rigsbee telling her girlhood story of running angrily inside to tell her grandmother that Tom Sykes had said her legs were skinny. "Well, honey, they are a mite thin," commented her grandmother. What was her grandmother telling her? "Well, your legs are thin, but it doesn't worry me. You might as well get used to the idea."

The issue here is not striving for the ideal but accepting children the way they are and assuming they will do the same with themselves. Part of growing up is coming to terms with what nature has given. There is no reason the thin child or the fat child should feel bad about herself, but she does have to come to grips with her body and accepting herself just the way she is.

DEALING WITH CULTURAL ISSUES IN SIZE AND SHAPE ACCEPTANCE
For older children, the issue of physical self-esteem gets more intense as they start to grapple with cultural ideals. Often, children try to conform to the cultural ideal by dieting. In a Cincinnati study of grade 3 through 6 middle-income children, researchers found that 45 percent were dieting, some as young as the third grade. Newer studies have found the same thing, but this study asked about dieting behavior of the parents. It appeared children were more likely to become anxious and preoccupied with size, shape, and eating if those were issues for their parents.[7]

An article in *Girls' Life* magazine reinforces the point.[8] Most preadolescent readers said they were realistic and accepting of even less-than-perfect size and shape in themselves and their friends. However, they acknowledged that they still talk about the topic a lot. The author explained the discrepancy by pointing out that body size and shape talk is simply girl talk, similar to boy talk about sports.

The magazine's downplaying of the dieting concern may be self-serving, since the major content of *Girls' Life* seems to be clothes, weight, and boys, all topics that tend to focus concern on size and shape.* However, I can still go

---

*For girl-focused magazines that are broader in subject matter, check out *New Moon* for preadolescents and its older sister magazine and *HUES: Hear Us Emerging Sisters.* You can track down both by calling 800-381-4743.

along with the author's theory, to a point. I have noticed that most times, preadolescent dieting has more of a hobby quality to it than being anything too alarming. Girls talk about dieting, then they find something in the lunchroom they like and fall off their diets. Then they say, "Oh, I am so gross," and they giggle and squeal. They go to a party and "pig out" (which is, by the way, normal food-exploration behavior for kids that age and *not* binge eating), and they giggle and squeal again.

However, some children are dead serious about dieting. About a third of *Girls' Life* readers did have a negative body image. Of those, 80 percent or more reported being told by their moms to diet, work out, and quit eating junk food. Moms, out of their concern or fear for daughters, were inadvertently sending messages that were crushing the girls' self-confidence. A Massachusetts study looked at mothers of eating-disordered daughters. The mothers themselves often had distorted eating attitudes and behaviors. They were uncomfortable with their daughter's appearance and that thought that their daughters should lose weight.[9]

The part of you that is a teacher can now legitimately reach the conclusion that if a child gets a lot of family pressure about eating, size, and shape, there is only so much you can do to help her. The part of you that is a parent may be squirming by now, and I am sorry for that. However, I must be blunt: If the shoe fits, wear it. You are important to your daughter, and your attitude toward her will make an enormous difference in the way she feels about her body. However, it is virtually impossible to be accepting of your daughter's—or your son's—body if you can't be accepting of your own.

Afraid to Eat

In supporting children's eating capabilities and emphasizing acceptance of size diversity, you may be doing more for children than you realize. You will also be swimming against the tide. In her book *Afraid to Eat*, Frances Berg captures the dilemma of today's children as they grapple with their weight: "Instead of growing up with secure and healthy attitudes about their bodies, eating and themselves, many kids fear food and fear being fat." Berg stresses that it is a "national crisis" that attempts at dieting are common in the third grade and even earlier. She is right. Berg emphasizes that health goals for children need to emphasize normal eating, active living,

self-respect, and appreciation of size diversity. She's right. Berg points out that the backward (my word) U.S. health policy contributes to this crisis by emphasizing obesity and weight loss rather than maintaining nutritional status. Berg points out how seriously our health policy suffers, especially when compared with the Canadian Vitality program, which says "Eat well, be active, and feel good about yourself." Still again, she's right.

Although public health policy isn't a household issue, it permeates our thinking about eating, weight, and even what we know. As the results of periodic national nutrition surveys are released to the public, we are treated to headlines that decry the shocking increase in child and adolescent obesity. Those same surveys unearth even more startling findings that we rarely hear about—data about the extent to which our teenagers are starving themselves and suffering from nutritional deficiencies. While nutritional health of preadolescents remains pretty good, the quality of adolescent diets has markedly decreased to the point that teenage girls have the poorest nutrition of any age group in the United States. Most girls and many boys eat so poorly that they compromise their growth and development and their lifelong physical health. They eat so poorly that they can't think straight, their emotional stability is sabotaged, and their social development is obstructed. Why don't we hear about it? It isn't the priority. The priority is weight. Survey data about nutritional status is analyzed late and released quietly to the public, if at all.

U.S. public health policy identifies obesity as the nation's number one health concern, and dietary fat control for disease avoidance is number two. Eating well to build healthy strong bodies and minds is addressed only incidentally. The U.S. Centers for Disease Control publication *Guidelines for School Health Programs to Promote Lifelong Healthy Eating* identifies "healthy eating" using those priorities: weight management and dietary fat reduction. Many nutrition education curricula are written emphasizing these concerns. As a result, messages become the negative and avoidant ones I have been complaining about throughout this book.

EATING DISORDERS

Obsessive dieting becomes a public health policy concern only when carried to the extremes evident in eating disorders. Estimates vary on the incidence of eating disorders. Some sources say that 0.5 percent of people develop anorexia, and 3 percent develop bulimia. Frances Berg says that 1 in 10 teenage girls develop an eating disorder. Whatever the incidence, it is too high.

Policy makers don't seem to notice the contradiction of promoting dieting on the one hand and deploring eating disorders on the other. Is there a connection? In my experience, there is, but it may not be what you think. Dieting doesn't cause eating disorders, but it can make a child unconsciously choose distorted eating as a way of acting out overwhelming emotional and social distress. By way of explaining what I mean, let me give you an example.

Mary didn't know how to eat. She had been restricted by her mother ever since the doctor had pronounced her too fat at age 6 months. Under her mother's careful control, Mary had slimmed down and remained slim until she was 11. At that point, a family crisis put her mother out of commission. Not only did Mary's mother stop cooking, she stopped restricting Mary's food intake. Since she had grown up with external control, Mary had long since lost any natural ability to regulate her food intake. Lacking either external or internal control, Mary's eating became chaotic. She ate whenever and whatever she could, and she ate as much as she could hold. In a few months, she gained over 30 pounds. She went to a commercial weight loss clinic and dieted to force her weight down, but, as she put it, "The minute my weight hit bottom I started eating and gained it all back and more besides." I met her when she was 19 years old. By then she had become seriously bulimic.

Because she and her family had a lot of emotional problems, and because eating had been such an issue all along, Mary acted out her distress with eating. She had understandably gotten the idea that she had to be thin to be successful in life. Other children, who don't have the eating issues, might act out significant distress in other ways: by going defiantly dirty or by exorbitantly puncturing body parts or by becoming rebellious or promiscuous or by abusing alcohol or drugs. Generally, children unconsciously choose the issues that most concern their families as the ones they use to act out their upset and confusion. With Mary, eating was an obvious choice.

Other children who have lost touch with their internal regulators but are able to deal with their feelings more effectively and directly don't develop eating disorders. They do, however, have an eating problem when they get into middle and later grade school. At that point their world widens so that parents can no longer supervise what and how much they eat, and they are left with no tools for managing their eating. Many times children without internal controls overeat, the way Mary did. Other children resort to rigidly imposing the same rules that were used at home. A child may talk about "dieting" as a way of describing the rigid control she uses to try to manage her food intake.

Teaching about Nutrition

I have focused our lesson plans on *food* and *experience.* I haven't recommended any nutrition lessons. Nutrition lessons emphasize learning with the head, and they focus on nutrients in food and the impact of those nutrients on the body. Unfortunately, but too frequently, nutrition lessons open up the whole Pandora's box of rules. "Shoulds" and "oughts" crop up, along with the messages about avoidance.

Children do enjoy learning about nutrients, where they come from and what those nutrients do in the body. Children like learning that carrots contain vitamin A and that vitamin A can help them see in the dark. But children won't eat carrots because carrots contain vitamin A. They eat carrots because carrots are familiar and because they taste good.

For children, learning about nutrition is learning for its own sake, just like it's fine to learn how airplanes fly or where drinking water comes from. We don't expect children to use information about aerodynamics to fly their own airplanes or water purification to sanitize their own water. It's equally unrealistic to give them nutrition lessons and expect them to choose their own food and plan their own diets.

Adults, not children, are the ones who have to act on nutrition lessons and apply them to food selection. Even so-called kid-friendly nutrition messages, like "go, slow, and whoa foods" or "traffic light lists" (red-, yellow- and green-light food) are subjective and value laden and beyond a child's ability to comprehend. Kids are literal, black-and-white thinkers. A food is good or bad; it's either go or whoa, red or green. You eat it or you don't. In a child's mind, if it is on the table and the child likes it, she will eat it until she gets enough or the supplies run out. Kids automatically eat moderately, but for them there is no such thing as *deciding* to eat moderately.

If certain foods are "slow" or "yellow light" foods—foods to eat occasionally or in moderation—then adults are the ones who have to see to that. For instance, consider my controversial and alarming dessert recommendation. I encourage adults to put the child's portion of dessert by her plate when the table is set and allow her to eat it when she wants it: before, during, or after the meal. Once that serving is gone, however, no more dessert. I don't recommend letting children have unlimited quantities of dessert. Most children can't be moderate with sweets; adults need to help them. The principle is that while children push themselves along to like new foods, they also take the easy way out when it is offered. Although it takes many tries to learn to like a new vegetable, with a new dessert, you generally get one-trial learning.

Help in Other Places

Raising your healthy eater is not strictly a do-it-yourself project. Many people will help you feed your child. According to the Agricultural Research Service (*Research News—USDA*), on any given day nearly half of 3- to 5-year-olds consumed some food or drink outside the home, most often at someone else's house. Roughly two-thirds of children over age 6 ate elsewhere, most often at the school cafeteria. If you make arrangements for other dependable and loving adults to feed your child, you are executing your responsibilities in feeding and your child will feel secure and provided for. You are wise to depend on other people to help expose your child to a variety of food. Moreover, you *have* to depend on others to teach her to eat in a variety of social settings. That is all to the good.

When she eats at a friend's house or at school, your child may be offered foods she doesn't like. She needs to know how to politely say "no, thank you." She may be asked to use unfamiliar dishes or serving methods. She needs to know how to observe what everyone else does and follow along. In other words, you can give her a little coaching so she can learn to manage.

For the most part, children can cope, and they take *pride* in coping. At times, however,

you may have to be your child's advocate, as one mother found with a situation in her son's school lunchroom. He was being traumatized by the rule that he had to eat everything on his plate. She hesitated for a long time before she talked with his teacher. The teacher couldn't change the rule, so the mother went to the school lunch supervisor. The supervisor said she couldn't change the rule either because it came from the administration.

The principal knew where the rule came from, and he didn't see any problem with it. He was a bean counter. He didn't like having children throw away food. Like a lot of people, he assumed that the solution to the problem of food waste was to make children clean their plates. The mother raised his consciousness. She explained the principles of food acceptance to him, and pointed out that when children are coerced into eating they eat less well, not better. Most important, she told him how miserable her son was, and *that* made an impression.

Together, the principal and the mother talked with the school lunch supervisor, who recommended they go to the offer-versus-serve policy, which would allow children to turn down two food items at each lunch. That would relieve school lunch workers of having to put food on children's plates whether they wanted it or not. The principal agreed, and the policy was changed. Beyond that, the principle and supervisor agreed not to force children to eat food that they had taken. The mother managed to remain positive and diplomatic throughout, for which I admired her. She wanted her child to continue to participate in the school lunch program, so she knew she couldn't alienate anyone.

CHILD CARE AND HEAD START
In chapter 3, you learned about child care and Head Start in some detail. A good Child Care Food Program or Head Start program that observes and maintains a division of responsibility in feeding can help your child grow up with respect to eating. These programs are good about exposing children to a variety of foods and work with providers to help them observe and maintain a division of responsibility in feeding. However, with staff turnovers, training difficulties, and today's eating attitudes and behaviors being what they are, at times you may see a provider who is more controlling than trusting. Deal with it. Raise the issue with the teacher or child care provider, and if you

don't get results, talk with the nutrition coordinator or the field consultant. Workers in these programs are familiar with my concepts, and you will be able to get support in applying them.

Fat avoidance in the Child Care Food Program: Only recently, without saying much of anything to anybody else in the nutrition community, the U.S. Department of Agriculture made it the policy of the Child Care Food Program (CCFP) to restrict the fat in the diets of preschool children. For children over age 2, the CCFP manuals and cookbooks specify keeping fat to below 30 percent of total calories.

In my view, this is unnecessary and dangerous. In chapter 3, you learned my recommendations for children and fat consumption. In appendix H, "Children, Dietary Fat, and Heart Disease: You Don't Have to Panic," you can learn why I made those recommendations. It is very difficult to reduce dietary fat for children without overdoing it, and if you overdo it, children may not eat and grow well. Pennsylvania State researchers did computer modeling to calculate what day care children might eat of typical low-fat menus. They included favorite foods in their calculations and estimated child-sized portions. To lower fat in their imaginary menus, researchers used typical fat-lowering strategies: 1) They used mostly lean meats, 2) they used skim milk, 3) they used low-fat food preparation techniques, and 4) they avoided any added butter, margarine, or salad dressing.

Researchers found that it was easy to force fat intakes down too low. For the 4- and 5-year-olds, the limit was to use only one fat-lowering strategy, using skim milk, for instance, or using mainly lean meats, but not both. If more than one fat-lowering strategy was used, the percentage of fat calories fell to 20 percent or below and the children's diets were inadequate in calories and other nutrients. For the 2- and 3-year-olds, fat-lowering strategies were even riskier: using any fat restriction strategy at all made it very difficult to meet nutritional recommendations.[12]

SCHOOL NUTRITION
The National School Lunch Program (NSLP) is obligated to offer children a third of their daily nutritional requirements at lunchtime. Many programs offer breakfast as well. Children who can't afford to buy school breakfast or lunch are eligible for free or low-cost meals.

NSLP can help you feed your child and help you raise your healthy eater. School lunch will expose your child to foods you don't prepare at home. It can also help your child learn to eat in an institutional setting—to eat food that is not catered specifically to her likes and dislikes in a big room with lots of other people. NSLP programs and their philosophies on feeding children vary from give-them-what-they-will-eat at the one extreme to school-nutrition-as-education at the other. The first type of program makes pizza, chicken nuggets, and tacos the mainstay of the menu. The second type makes an effort to introduce children to a variety of food and helps them to increase their mastery with eating.

Some energetic and creative programs that take the educational view even provide menu bars for children and teach them to serve themselves from a variety of wholesome foods. Often these programs collaborate with teachers, who introduce children to the food in the classroom and help them gain comfort through studying, tasting, cooking, and even growing food. These programs work. Children regularly learn to like many new foods and take pleasure in their mastery.

As in child care, the best school nutrition programs are in schools that take food and nutrition seriously as an important part of the program day. In addition to teaching children about foods and exposing them to new foods, school nutrition works best when adults pass on to children their own belief that mealtime is important and their conviction that children can learn to like what is served in school lunch. By attitude, example, limit setting, and telling, adults make it clear to children that it is their responsibility to eat until they are satisfied so they can concentrate on the business of learning as well as meet their physical needs. Most important, when parents and teachers take feeding themselves seriously, children will too. When school staff and teachers eat in the cafeteria, it gives the children the message that lunchtime is important.

Of the many ways that schools support nutrition programs, one of the most important is giving children enough time to eat. In addressing the hurry and chaos of lunchrooms, some schools have realized that rushing children through to get them out to recess is part of the problem. In a Rockford, Illinois, elementary school, children who had recess first and lunch afterward settled down more, took more time with their food, and ate better.[10] Boys particularly wasted 15 percent less food when recess came before the meal. Not surprisingly, children had fewer stomachaches and less dizziness during noon recess when they ate afterward rather than before. Any teacher would expect children to perform better in afternoon classes if they had eaten better at lunchtime.

Even if the program in your child's school is a chaotic, give-them-what-they-will-eat program, your child will benefit. She will be offered nutritious food, prepared differently from the way it is prepared at home, and she will get the opportunity to learn to eat in an unfamiliar setting. I might add that it is often a challenging setting. I am amazed at how children manage to eat anything at all given the hurry and commotion that goes on in many school lunchrooms—but they do. To allow your child to be as comfortable and successful as possible, here are the features to work toward in a school nutrition program:

- Children are greeted pleasantly by lunchroom personnel.
- Adults take an interest in children and may even know their names.
- Children are given the opportunity to say "yes, please" and "no, thank you."
- Children are not forced to take anything they don't want.
- Children are not forced to eat anything they have taken.
- The physical setting is pleasant.
- Lunchroom supervisors are pleasant and positive.
- Children are given enough time to eat.
- Children are not forced to clean their plates.

Supporting the feeding program: It is fashionable to be critical of feeding programs, and particularly of school lunch. Before you let a child hear your criticism, consider this. What would happen if you were the family cook and your spouse said to your child, "What he makes isn't very good. I don't think you should have to eat that." I would expect that you would be absolutely burned up about it, for starters, and that your child wouldn't eat. When administrators, teachers, and parents are openly critical of the school lunch program, the same thing happens. If adults don't support each other, children lose. They don't challenge themselves to learn and grow.

School nutrition programs produce many meals with little money and a skeleton staff.

The fact that so many do it at all, let alone do it well, is nothing short of astonishing. The expectations placed on school lunch programs keep increasing, and the money available to them keeps decreasing. To make ends meet, many programs have resorted to selling what they call "a la carte" foods—brand-name tacos or pizzas or prepackaged entrées. Unlike the so-called "reimbursable meals" that have to provide a child a third of her daily nutritional requirement and add up to 30 percent fat or less, a la carte foods have to do nothing of the sort. They just have to have sales appeal for the children. Because they are familiar, higher in fat, and often carry the brand names that seems to be so important to children, they have more sales appeal than the generic offerings. Most school nutrition managers do their level best to make sure that a la carte offerings are nutritious, but that is because they care about children's nutrition, not because they are mandated to do so.

The upshot is that school nutrition programs end up competing with themselves for the child's nutritional favor. It is as if you put on a lovely meal of tuna noodle casserole and also said to your child, "Would you rather have this or would you rather we ordered out to [Your Favorite] Pizza Place for pizza?" I'll lay you odds that your child would go for the pizza rather than the casserole. When a favorite food is readily available, children don't push themselves along to learn to like the alternative. It is not good for a child to be courted or treated like a customer when it comes to food. It puts her in the adult's role of making the menu decisions and keeps her from increasing her food acceptance.

What can you do to support positive school nutrition programs? Get involved in a supportive way. Talk to the manager, not to your children. For starters, see if you can keep a la carte food out of grade schools and middle schools. Children in the early grades are still developing their food habits, and the easy availability of alternative foods limits their growth. A la carte foods are not so bad in high school, because teenagers have already developed their food habits and are figuring out ways of managing their own nutritional world. Adolescents explore and take risks, and many times they don't eat very well. That is just what they do, and beyond offering good food at predictable times, there isn't much we can do to change it. Except wait. Eventually, children go back to the eating habits they learned when they were younger. In the meantime, don't feel you have to pander to your teenager's food preferences. If you pay for her school lunch, pay for the reimbursable meal, and if your child wants to eat from the more expensive a la carte menu, let her pay the margin herself.

Fat avoidance in the school lunch program:
The National School Lunch Program is handicapped by the U.S. Department of Agriculture regulations that mandate restriction of the fat in menus to 30 percent of calories. Always the target of public scrutiny and malcontent, the NSLP instituted the fat restriction in response to considerable public pressure. Ironically, participation in the program decreased when the fat content was reduced,[3] presumably because the menus were not as appealing to the children. In the past, some programs have used way too much fat, and in those cases reductions were in order. Now the fat is often way too low. A more reasonable figure would be 35 percent, both from the point of view of appeal in eating as well as ease in cooking. However, my wishing won't make it so: the regulation is 30 percent, and for the time being we are stuck with it.

Because children are such wizards at confounding adults' attempts to control them, fat restriction at school appears not to have had much impact on children's fat intake overall. In a school lunch study in Nebraska, children in an experimental school were given low-fat, low-sodium menus. Their food intake was compared with that of children in another school that had regularly salted food with a higher fat content. Although the study was declared successful in limiting children's fat intake, to me it seemed that success was in the eye of the beholder. Children in the low-fat school ate more fat than they were scheduled to eat, children in the high-fat school ate less fat than they were served. The difference between the two schools was only 2 percent. Children in the low-fat school ate 31 percent of their calories as fat, whereas children in the high-fat school ate 33 percent. Differences in sodium weren't much to write home about either. The children in the experimental group ate 631 milligrams of sodium at lunch, whereas children in the control group ate 742 milligrams.[11]

Another goal of the Nebraska study was to slim down fat children by feeding them less dietary fat and by keeping them more active in school physical education programs. Again, the children were ahead of the researchers. They simply compensated at home for the changes at school. They ate more fat, exercised less, and after two years they were no fatter or thinner than when they began.[5]

Despite the negative results in the carefully conducted Nebraska study, there is still a strong conviction among child obesity specialists that school nutrition and physical education programs should be modified to control obesity. The strategies don't work, and they are potentially harmful. If children get the idea that school lunch and physical education programs are trying to repair them, they will be turned off to both.

What to Do Next

"So," you may say. "Why are you telling me all this?" Because half the battle is knowing the problem. If you know the problem, I am sure you'll figure out how to make some improvements.

"So," you may say, "what *do* you expect me to do about it?" Ah, I thought you would never ask! Do as much—or as little—as your time and interest allow. Look for opportunities in your child care setting, your child's grade school, your child's scout troop, or your PTA. Consider talking with schedule makers about timing practices and events to stay away from family dinnertime. You might talk with your child care provider or your child's teacher and give them a copy of this chapter or buy them this book. Once you and the teacher get your signals straight, you might volunteer to teach a class on nutrition.

If you have the time and energy, approach the principal, the school lunch director, the school nurse, or the school social worker. (This is a social work issue because mental health professionals are concerned about kids and eating disorders.) You can ask for help from the director of your state Nutrition Education and Training Program (NETP), a fine federally funded program sponsored by the U.S. Department of Agriculture with the mandate to sponsor and support nutrition education programs. You can activate the parent-teacher organization and make your case before the school board.

Many states have a health and wellness team called the Comprehensive School Health Program whose stated goal is not only to teach students positive health behaviors but also to support those behaviors in the total school environment. Having nutritious food available in vending machines and at concession stands would be an example of an integrated effort that would support healthful eating. Since the national Parent Teacher Association (PTA) actively promotes the Comprehensive School Health Program, you could become involved through the PTA. I hope that whatever your avenue of involvement, you will insist on teaching children positive eating attitudes and behaviors and supporting physical self-esteem. You don't have to settle for teaching children the Food Guide Pyramid.

I'm sure you'll think of other ways to help children with their eating. Keep in mind that you don't have to go on a campaign to make a contribution. Your very *attitude* can make a difference. If you are relaxed and positive about children and their bodies, if you love good food, enjoy eating, and make feeding yourself a priority, your child and the children around you will benefit.

What is the bottom line? Children love learning about food and nutrition, but they do not benefit from being taught formulas and they do not benefit from being taught avoidance. No child ever ate according to a formula. Children eat because they enjoy it, just as their grown-ups do.

Selected References

1. Lytle, L. A., A. L. Eldridge, K. Kotz, J. Piper, S. Williams, and B. Kalina. 1997. Children's interpretation of nutrition messages. *Journal of Nutrition Education* 29: 128–136.
2. Lytle, L., and C. Achterberg. 1995. Changing the diet of America's children: What works and why? *Journal of Nutrition Education* 27: 250–260.
3. Crockett, S. J., and L. S. Sims. 1995. Environmental influences on children's eating. *Journal of Nutrition Education* 27: 235, 249.
4. Perry, C. L., D. B. Bishop, G. Taylor, D. M. Murray, R. W. Mays, B. S. Dudovitz, M. Smyth, and M. Story. 1998. Changing fruit and vegetable consumption among children: The 5-a-Day Power Plus program in Saint Paul, Minnesota. *American Journal of Public Health* 88: 603–660.
5. Donnelly, J. E., D. J. Jacobsen, and J. E. Whatley. 1995. Obesity and metabolic fitness: Effects of a school intervention of nutrition and physical activity. *Food and Nutrition News*, 7–10. Chicago: National Live Stock and Meat Board.
6. Smolak, L., M. P. Levine, and F. Schermer. 1998. A controlled evaluation of an elementary school primary prevention program for eating problems. *Journal of Psychosomatic Research* 44: 339–353.
7. Maloney, M. J., J. McGuire, S. R. Daniels, and B. Specker. 1989. Dieting behavior and eating attitudes in children. *Pediatrics* 84: 482–489.
8. Bokram, K. 1998. Who's making you fat? *Girls' Life* 4 (6): 52–55.
9. Pike, K. M., and J. Rodin. 1991. Mothers, daughters and disordered eating. *Journal of Abnormal Psychology* 100 (2): 198–204.
10. Getlinger, M. J., C. V. Laughlin, E. Bell, C. Akre, and B. H. Arjmandi. 1996. Food waste is reduced when elementary-school children have recess before lunch. *Journal of the American Dietetic Association* 96: 906–908.
11. Whatley, J. E., J. E. Donnelly, D. J. Jacobsen, J. O. Hill, and M. K. Carlson. 1996. Energy and macronutrient consumption of elementary school children served modified lower fat and sodium lunches or standard higher fat and sodium lunches. *Journal of the American College of Nutrition* 15: 602–607.
12. Sigman-Grant, M., S. Zimmerman, and P. M. Kris-Etherton. 1993. Dietary approaches for reducing fat intake of preschool-aged children. *Pediatrics* 91: 955–960.

APPENDIXES

Appendix A   What Surveys Say about Our Eating   202
Appendix B   The Dietary Guidelines and Why
              They Are Rule Bound   204
Appendix C   Grazing, Cue Sensitivity, and Your
              Weight   205
Appendix D   To Diet or Not to Diet—That Is the
              Question   206
Appendix E   Children and Food Regulation   208
Appendix F   Children and Food Acceptance   210
Appendix G   Dietary Fat and Heart Disease: It's
              Not as Bad as You Think   211
Appendix H   Children, Dietary Fat, and Heart
              Disease: You Don't Have to Panic   214
Appendix I   Sodium in Your Diet   217
Appendix J   A Primer on Dietary Fat   219
Appendix K   Resources Available from Ellyn Satter
              Associates   221

Appendix
A
What Surveys Say about Our Eating

The American Dietetic Association Survey of Dietary Habits, first done in 1991 and repeated in 1993, 1995, and 1997, shows that consumers are having a difficult time living up to current standards of eating and food selection. In response to questions about whether they were doing all they could to achieve balanced nutrition and a healthy diet, only 25 percent of people fit into the "I am already doing it" category (see chapter 4, "Choosing Food for Your Family"). For 35 percent, the attitude was "I know I should but . . . ," and the attitude of the 40 percent of people in the third group was "Don't bother me." The gap between what people felt they should do with their eating and what they were actually able to do made it clear that paying attention to nutrition makes many people feel guilty and anxious about eating. How bad were they feeling? In the "I know I should but . . ." group, the gap was a whopping 34 percent. In the "I'm already doing it" group, the gap was 15 percent. The "don't bother me" group was the most comfortable with their eating: The gap was only 9 percent. The moral of the story? If your eating is driving you nuts, set more realistic standards.

The "already doing it" people cooked from scratch, purchased low-fat or fat-free food, actively sought nutrition and diet information, and read nutritional labels. The "I should but" people agreed about the importance of diet, but they didn't want to give up the food they liked and thought a healthy diet took too much time. The "don't bother me" people didn't consider diet and nutrition to be as important as the people in the other two groups. They ate out often and skipped meals.[1]

Interestingly, for the "don't bother me" group, attitudes about food selection and dieting were still positive. They just weren't perfectionists. In my view, the "don't bother me" attitudes are healthiest. When asked to rate the importance of nutrition on a scale of 1 to 7, 62 percent of the "don't bother me" group

assigned a score of 5 or more. I could settle for that. When asked how careful they are in selecting what they ate to achieve a healthy diet, 89 percent assigned a score of 4 or more out of 7. That sounds reasonable to me. Eating is, after all, only one of life's great issues. Conversely, 60 percent of the "already doing it" group checked the box that said it is important to check every food item for nutritional content. That makes eating quite a chore!

In spite of the advice that bombards consumers about following the nutrition rules, and in spite of the fact that some consumers have made following rules their nutritional priority, most still seek pleasure and predictability. A 1998 university-sponsored national survey indicated clearly that for most consumers, taste is still the most important influence on food choices, followed by cost and convenience.[2] The question, of course, is whether consumers feel comfortable with making taste the priority. The gaps we just talked about between nutritional goals and actual behavior indicate that no, they do not. Certainly, nutrition professionals do not feel comfortable with these priorities, as indicated by the discussion comment in the 1998 survey article that, given the importance assigned to taste by consumers, nutrition educators need to "stress the good taste of healthful foods."

The assumption, of course, is that there is a contradiction between good nutrition and good taste, a deeply embedded and erroneous attitude held not only by nutritionists but also by the public at large. Over half of respondents in an ADA-commissioned Gallup poll said that eating a healthy diet is too much work. Although they reported eating to be enjoyable, when health was factored in, 36 percent asserted that the fun was taken out of eating and that they feel guilty about eating the foods they like.[3]

Whether it is because of the policy itself or due to the misunderstanding and "overzealous application" blamed on consumers by many policy makers, current nutrition policy distorts the public understanding of nutrition principles. Despite all the controversy and the emphasis on avoidance to prevent disease, nutrition enthusiasts and moderates alike agree that the nutritional bottom line is positive: to sustain life and support vitality. The question, of course, is whether overall nutritional status is being undermined by the emphasis on avoidance. Attitudinally, at least, the over-all nutrition emphasis is suffering. A 1998 survey by the Food Marketing Institute showed that the primary nutritional concern for a whopping 59 percent of respondents was dietary fat avoidance (up from 27 percent in 1988), with nutritional value of food assigned priority by only 12 percent of respondents and a "desire to be healthy and eat what's good for us" a paltry 3 percent.[4]

While fat restriction originated as a disease-avoidance tactic, in the minds of many professionals and consumers, fat avoidance has become synonymous with weight management. Fat restriction as a means for energy restriction continues to be hotly debated, one piece of epidemiological research is clear: as percentage of fat in the diet has gone down, body weights have gone up.[5]

Despite all the conflict and interference, our commitment to family meals remains strong. According to a Food Marketing Institute–Better Homes and Gardens survey, parents and children eat dinner together an average of five times per week. When asked why they believed family dinners to be important, survey respondents said they felt strongly that eating meals together strengthens family ties and unity and that children who have family dinners eat a healthier diet. They felt that eating together gave important opportunities for family communication and promoted a better family atmosphere, including giving a sense of stability and togetherness.[6]

Selected References

1. American Dietetic Association. 1997. *Survey of American Dietary Habits*. Chicago: American Dietetic Association.
2. Glanz, K., M. Basil, E. Maibach, J. Goldberg, and D. Snyder. 1998. Why Americans eat what they do: Taste, nutrition, cost, convenience, and weight control concerns as influences on food consumption. *Journal of the American Dietetic Association* 98:1118–1126.
3. Wellman, N. 1990. The good and the bad: How Americans are making food choices. *Nutrition News* 53: 1–3.
4. Nature of concern about nutritional content, 1989–1998. Trends in the United States. *Consumer Attitudes and the Supermarket*, 1998. 72. Washington, D.C.: Food Marketing Institute.
5. Lichtenstein, A. H., E. Kennedy, P. Barrier, D. Danford, N. Ernst, S. Grundy, G. A. Leveille, L. Van Horn, C. L. Williams, and S. L. Booth. 1998. Dietary fat consumption and health. *Nutrition Reviews* 56: S3–S19.
6. Hoban, T. J. 1995. Americans speak up for dinnertime. *MealWatch*. 1, 4–5. Washington, D.C.: Better Homes and Gardens and Food Marketing Institute.

Appendix
B
The Dietary Guidelines and Why They Are Rule Bound

Rules can be helpful if they give us advice or free us from having to make the same decisions over and over again. Rules can be flexible if we can choose to use them or not, depending on the situation and how we feel. Rules can be informative when they set standards of behavior, like the old Basic Four Food Guide did in defining the minimum to eat to get a nutritionally adequate diet. But rules become destructive when they are controlling, when they emphasize the shoulds and oughts. These rules are controlling because they define down to the last morsel what to eat, and then they take away choice by overstating the health hazards of failing to follow the rules.

Eat a variety of foods: Well, okay. I can live with that. Variety is good. The rules come in when the guidelines instruct us in detail what that variety should consist of. We are told which foods to eat and how much of them to eat. The rules may help you decide what to put on the table, but they do not help you decide what to eat. When you *eat*, you need to go by how you feel inside.

Balance the food you eat with physical activity; maintain or improve your weight: Activity is good. It takes care of your body and helps you to regulate your food intake. But this message says to balance out activity and food regulation with your head, a method that is inferior to your intuitive capability. Furthermore, it mandates weight reduction efforts by using standards that classify most of us as overweight. In reality, you came from your Creator with the ability to automatically balance food intake with your physical needs and to maintain a preferred and stable body weight. This weight may or may not be what the Dietary Guidelines say it should be.

Choose a diet with plenty of grain products, vegetables, and fruits: Certainly these are healthful foods, but the catch with the recommendation is that it is external and controlling. You are being told to eat a lot of these foods—more than you need for nutritional adequacy and perhaps more than you *want.* You are to eat these foods in certain amounts whether you are hungry for them or not and whether they taste good to you or not.

Choose a diet low in fat, saturated fat, and cholesterol: This is certainly a rule, and a rigid, hard-to-follow one at that. The guidelines say to restrict fat to 30 percent of calories and to keep saturated fat to less than 10 percent of calories. Not only are these directives unintelligible to everyone but trained dietitians, but also this is the food-as-medicine attitude I complained about in chapter 1. It has everything to do with avoidance and nothing to do with using fat to make food taste good.

Choose a diet that's moderate in sugars: I can agree with that. I am for moderate. The problem with this guideline is in the eye of the beholder. We are so shell-shocked with all the limitations that we tend to think of moderation as deprivation.

Choose a diet that's moderate in salt and sodium: Again, I won't quibble with moderation. Neither the Dietary Guidelines nor the Food Guide Pyramid says how much sodium is moderate. They do say, though, that the maximum need for sodium is 2,400 milligrams per day, and that amount has become the recommended limit in general practice. That isn't moderate; it's low. Keeping sodium that low puts extreme constraints on food selection.

If you drink alcoholic beverages, do so in moderation: Even I can't quibble with this recommendation!

To get a copy of the Dietary Guidelines for yourself, call your university extension office in your county and ask for a copy of *Nutrition and Your Health: Dietary Guidelines for Americans,* Home and Garden Bulletin No. 232. There will be a small charge. This is a worthwhile investment for the nutrition information it contains. However, remember it is served generously seasoned with negativity and control. If reading it makes you feel guilty and bad about your eating, put it away.

Appendix
C
Grazing, Cue Sensitivity, and Your Weight

You have within you the ability to eat the right amount of food to maintain a consistent body weight. However, depending on your internal food-regulating apparatus, you'll need to give yourself more or less situational help to be able to regulate well. It depends on whether you are more *external* or *internal* in the way you eat. As the eating folks say, it depends on your cue *responsiveness*.[1]

If you are more external—more cue responsive—you will be enticed to eat when food is available, even if you aren't hungry and even if eating is far from your mind. If you are more internal and less cue responsive, you will be interested in that food only when you are hungry.

Being cue responsive doesn't have anything to do with being fat or thin. In every weight category, there are some people who are externally responsive and some who are not. Being cue responsive can be an inborn quality or it can be acquired. Some babies are willing to eat when they aren't hungry simply because they enjoy eating; others are not. Undereating can make you more likely to eat when food is available. People who undereat, whether by choice or circumstance, become preoccupied with food and prone to overeat when they get a chance.

Being externally responsive *may* make it more challenging to maintain a stable body weight. I say "may" because it appears that for some people differences in metabolism correct for being externally responsive. Some people who eat more because food is available and appealing simply squander the extra calories. They burn or fidget them off. Others just seem to get fat.

By now, you probably know whether you are internal or external. If you are highly external, to help you regulate, have predictable meals and snacks and keep food put away between times. If you are internal, you won't need that structure so much—at least not to help you regulate. (Structure will still help you get a nutritionally adequate diet.) If you are external and can eat all day and not gain an ounce, then lucky you! But your spouse or child may not be so lucky, and you will be helping them regulate if you go along with structure.

Selected Reference

1. Rodin, J. 1981. Current status of the internal-external hypothesis for obesity: What went wrong? *American Psychologist* 36 (4): 361–372.

Appendix
D
To Diet or Not to Diet—
That Is the Question

The arguments for and against weight-reduction dieting break down along two familiar themes: *trust* and *control*. By now you've probably caught on that I am in the *trust* camp. In an article for the September 1996 issue of the *Journal of the American Dietetic Association (JADA)* , I emphasized supporting a stable body weight and avoiding influences that can destabilize weight.[1] Among those destabilizing influences is weight-reduction dieting. For more detail and more references, refer to the journal article. Here, I offer a brief summary.

I think in terms of *trust* with respect to body weight. Given appropriate supports of the type I discuss in this book (and in all my work), people weigh what is right for them. The currently prevailing thought, from the *control* camp, says that weight has to be managed and forced. But the trust and control people agree on some things. Everybody agrees that dieting doesn't work. Everybody agrees that when people lose weight, they sooner or later gain it back again. Most agree, in fact, that weight-reduction dieting can promote additional weight gain and the fattening process. Is any amount of overweight so bad for you that you should keep trying to lose weight, knowing the very high odds that you will gain it back? The *control* folks say yes; the *trust* people say no.

Doctors and other medical people are mostly in the *control* camp. They are guided in their thinking by a large working group of the National Institutes of Health called the National Task Force on the Prevention and Treatment of Obesity. In 1994 the task force published a review concluding that weight cycling is not harmful. In fact, the review stated, weight cycling is better than no weight loss at all.[2] Given this illogical conclusion, the National Task Force was strongly criticized for biased reporting and conflict of interest: each of the members in some way received funding and support from the diet industry.

The National Task Force arrived at their conclusions in spite of the well-established fact that weight loss tends to erode lean body tissue—muscles and organ tissue—and weight regain tends to restore fat. Furthermore, the weight gaining and losing process tends to be disruptive of the body's attempts to maintain metabolic and regulatory balance. Ample evidence suggests that weight-reduction dieting is counterproductive and even destructive. Convincing evidence indicates that being moderately fat is not bad and may even be better than being moderately thin. Glenn Gaesser and others maintain that it is only at extremely high weights—50 to 100 percent or more above "normal"—that health is compromised. For an exhaustive review of the evidence, see Gaesser's book *Big Fat Lies*. However, ignore Gaesser's advice on following a 20 percent fat diet. Gaesser is an exercise physiologist, not a nutritionist, and he added that advice to satisfy his publisher. He didn't think through the issue carefully or research his recommendations.

A January 1997 American Dietetic Association position paper published in the *Journal of the American Dietetic Association* emphasized maintaining a stable weight and developing the positive health behaviors of eating and exercising consistently, sustainably, and well. These achievable goals, said the JADA article, can significantly enhance health without weight loss. However, this same article reserved its emphasis on stabilizing weight for those who conformed to such a stringent definition of "normal" that 25 percent of us are considered overweight. Acceptable weight was defined as a weight-to-height ratio, expressed as a Body Mass Index (BMI) of 27, the point at which there is a moderate increase in health risk, but only for men. Recently, another National Institutes of Health Committee, also a *nutritional enthusiast* organization, set the cut-off for overweight at a BMI of 25. The committee had no new information; they were relying on all the same articles Gaesser read for *Big Fat Lies*. They were just interpreting them differently. Setting the cutoff for overweight at a BMI of 25 means that 50 percent of us would be considered fat.

Fortunately, rather than taking it to heart, many people were angered by the recommendation. Furthermore, the media took it lightly. In his August 2, 1998, newspaper column, Dave Barry commented in his usual tongue-in-cheek way that this change was intended to correct the alarming discovery that "a shocking *two-thirds* of Americans were within federal weight guidelines." Likening the Committee to the Internal Revenue Service, "which has done such a fine job that only nine U.S. citizens are in full compliance with all tax regulations," Barry observed that such a high figure of conformity was "a flagrant violation of federal guidelines regarding federal guidelines."

Having the commonly accepted standards for weight set so low means that many people who are simply maintaining a high normal weight are labeled as overweight and, therefore, in need of treatment. Whether or not we as individuals choose to buy into those standards depends on highly individual cost/benefit balances. Some people put such an extreme value on lower weight that they are willing to sacrifice to achieve it. For some, the sacrifice is relatively low; some people who maintain a body weight lower than constitutionally normal for them can do so with only modest changes in eating and exercise. They have high energy requirements to start with, their bodies cooperate by letting go of weight, and they attempt only modest weight shifts. Others

have to maintain near-starvation eating and near-exhaustion activity to achieve weight goals. Little wonder that people with durable weights and a great need to be thin are likely to periodically binge eat and may even develop eating disorders. Overwhelming craving for food, especially high-fat, high-sugar food, is simply part of the enormous biological pressure to restore calorie balance and body weight.

Thus, we're confronted with a problem that can't be solved. Being fat is bad and being thin is bad, and it doesn't work to try to lose weight but we're supposed to do it anyway. What to do? Why not set aside weight loss as an outcome goal and instead define the problem in a way it can be solved?

You don't have to be thin to be healthy. You *can* take good care of yourself with eating. You *can* take good care of yourself with activity. And you *can* let yourself weigh what you will in response to these positive behaviors. Healthy weight is what you maintain without too much trouble.

Selected References

1. Satter, E. 1996. Internal regulation and the evolution of normal growth as the basis for prevention of obesity in childhood. *Journal of the American Dietetic Association* 9: 860–864.
2. NIH Task Force on the Prevention and Treatment of Obesity. 1994. Weight cycling. *Journal of the American Medical Association* 272 (15): 1196–1202.

Appendix
E
Children and Food Regulation

Children know how much they need to eat, and virtually from birth they are resilient and resourceful regulators. At the University of Iowa, Fomon's group showed that when infants over age 6 weeks were fed either over-concentrated formula or overly dilute formula, they simply ate less of the concentrated or more of the dilute and grew consistently.[1] Adair followed formula- and solid-food intake of a little boy demand-fed from age 1 week to 9 months. She found that although the infant ate three times as much some days as others, and even though his food intake was lower than 90 percent of other babies, his growth was consistent and average. When he started eating solid foods, he took less formula and continued to regulate well.[2]

Birch and colleagues at the University of Illinois found that the amount children ate varied throughout the day,[3] and Beal found that children vary from year to year in their overall food intake as well as the composition of their intake.[4] Some years, for instance, they ate less fat, and other years they ate more. Even premature babies can regulate. Saunders found that medically stable babies weighing as little as 3 1/3 pounds were able to give signs to their care providers indicating when they were hungry and when they were full, and they grew well when they were fed on demand.[5] You can't predict how much children will eat. Children of all ages who look alike and act alike may vary from one another in their calorie requirement by as much as 40 percent.6

Although children are good regulators, their ability to regulate can be impaired by the way they are treated with regard to eating. Johnson and Birch experimented with children's food regulation abilities by giving them snacks before meals and then observing how much they ate. Most children who ate high-calorie snacks automatically ate less at lunch than children who had been given low-calorie snacks. However, some of the children in the eating experiment didn't compensate: they ate the same at mealtime, whether or not they had had a snack. Those who didn't adjust their intake were children whose eating was over-controlled at home: parents told them what and how much to eat.[3] Sometimes this over-control shows up in indirect ways. A 16-year longitudinal study conducted in the San Francisco Bay Area in California tried to identify differences between infants who became fat as teenagers and those who remained slim. The two groups were highly similar in many ways: with respect to family composition, calorie intake, and food habits, to name a few. However, infants who became fat as teenagers were more likely to have had eating problems as preschoolers, and they were more likely to have had parents who were worried that their children would grow up to be fat.[7] From my clinical experience, I reason that these early eating problems came about when parents were overcontrolling and children were reacting. Furthermore, parents and children often have feeding struggles when parents try to restrict the amounts children eat. Eating struggles with parents can be so upsetting for children that they lose track of their internal regulators and have trouble eating the amount of food that is right for them.

The point? Children know how much they need to eat, but they need help from adults if they are to act on and retain that capability. Children need to be able to tune in on what goes on inside of them and be aware of how hungry or how full they are. If adults are too active and controlling in feeding, what children experience is interference with their own sensations. Sometimes children go along with pressure from the outside and eat more or less than they really want. Sometimes they fight against that pressure and, again, eat more or less than they really want. Either way, they lose sight of how much they need and potentially make errors in regulation. They eat too much or too little, and get too fat or too thin.

Selected References

1. Fomon, S. J., L. J. Filer Jr., L. N. Thomas, T. A. Anderson, and S. E. Nelson. 1975. Influence of formula concentration on caloric intake and growth of normal infants. *Acta Paediatrica Scandanavica* 64: 172–181.

2. Adair, L. C. 1984. The infant's ability to self-regulate caloric intake: A case study. *Journal of the American Dietetic Association* 84 (5): 543–546.

3. Birch, L. L., S. L. Johnson, G. Andresen, J. C. Peters, and M. C. Schulte. 1991. The variability of young children's energy intake. *New England Journal of Medicine* 324: 232–235.

4. Beal, V. A. 1961. Dietary intake of individuals followed through infancy and childhood. *American Journal of Public Health* 51 (8): 1107–1117.

5. Saunders, R. B., C. B. Friedman, and P. R. Stramoski. 1990. Feeding preterm infants: Schedule or demand? *Journal of Obstetric, Gynecologic, and Neonatal Nursing* 20: 212–218.

6. National Research Council. 1989. *Recommended Dietary Allowances*, 10th ed. Washington, D.C.: National Academy Press.

7. Crawford, P. B., and L. R. Shapiro. 1991. How obesity develops: A new look at nature and nurture. *Obesity and Health* (now *Healthy Weight Journal*), edited by F. M. Berg, 40–41. Hettinger, N.D.: Healthy Living Institute.

Appendix

F

Children and Food Acceptance

Children want to learn to eat new food, and they automatically eat a variety. At the University of Illinois, Birch and her group demonstrated that toddlers and preschoolers are naturally *neophobic*.[1] That is, they don't like new food. But they will taste food, and the more often they taste it, the more they like it. But bribing or any sort of pressure, even "positive" pressure, slows the learning process. Birch and colleagues found that preschoolers who were rewarded with a trip to the playground for trying a new juice were less likely to try that juice the next time they were offered it than children who had simply been allowed to experiment with it on their own.

A process that Rolls called sensory *specific* satiety explains much of children's erratic eating behavior.[2] Children (and other people) tire of even favorite food and choose otherwise. In support of Rolls's theory, Birch found that children were more likely than adults to eat in response to their appetites: how food tastes to them at any given time.[3] Children also like high-sugar foods, and they like what is familiar. Children push themselves along to learn to like new food, but they also take the easy way out when it is offered. A parent is offering the child the easy way by making sweets too readily available or by offering only familiar foods. In Toronto, Pelchat and Pliner found that children who were reluctant to try new food had mothers who offered only foods that children readily accepted and short-order cooked for their children.[4]

So even positive, cleverly designed pressure doesn't work to help children accept new food, and limiting the menu to foods children readily accept doesn't work. What does work? Being there. Children do more and dare more with eating when they eat with familiar and trusted adults who make conversation and are good and positive company.[1]

The point? Children want to grow up with respect to their eating, just as they do with everything else in their lives. But they need help from adults if they are to act on and retain that capability. Children watch their parents eat certain foods and assume, even if they don't yet eat them, that "some day I will eat that." Their assumption and their desire to grow up can be squashed by adults' behaving at either, or both, of the two extremes: by being too demanding or too protective. Children need adults to be supportive and companionable, to show them what it means to grow up with respect to food and to give them opportunities to experiment and master. They don't need to be motivated—they come already motivated.

Selected References

1. Birch, L. L., and J. A. Fisher. 1995. Appetite and eating behavior in children. *Pediatric Clinics of North America* 42 (4): 931–953.
2. Rolls, B. J. 1986. Sensory specific satiety. *Nutrition Reviews* 44: 93–101.
3. Birch, L. L. 1979. Preschool children's food preferences and consumption patterns. *Journal of Nutrition Education* 11: 189–192.
4. Pelchat, M. L., and P. Pliner. 1986. Antecedents and correlates of feeding problems in young children. *Journal of Nutrition Education* 18 (1): 23–28.

Appendix
G
Dietary Fat and Heart Disease: It's Not as Bad as You Think

There is enough disagreement about the correlation between dietary fat and heart disease to make prevention only a *hope*, not a *guarantee*. Despite the extent to which health professionals, scientists, and educators back the fat restrictions of the Dietary Guidelines, the strength of the link between diet and atherosclerosis is debatable. The debate goes back a long way and is quite involved.

Ancel Keys of the University of Minnesota is credited with spawning the dietary fat/heart disease connection with his 1953 seven-country epidemiological survey in which he found an association between dietary saturated fat and heart disease mortality.[1] Clinical studies in the 1960s demonstrated that saturated fat raised blood cholesterol.[2] One piece of the puzzle remained: could reductions in dietary fat reduce mortality from heart disease? In the 1970s, results from three major studies were interpreted to mean that the connection existed: the Framingham Study,[3] the Multiple Risk Factor Intervention Trial (MRFIT),[4] and the Coronary Primary Prevention Trial or Lipid Research Clinics (CPPT or LRC).[5] Reports from all three studies indicated that middle-aged men with high blood cholesterol were roughly twice as likely to die of heart attacks than those with low blood cholesterol. Reported in that way, as relative differences, those were alarming figures. However, a look at the actual numbers in the three studies gave a less alarming view of the risk of high blood cholesterol. The *actual* reduction in death rate for the men with lower blood cholesterol was from 1.4 to 0.7 deaths per 1,000 men per year. That is a small difference—so small, in fact, that given the low death rates in both treated and untreated subjects, it was hard to distinguish between deaths associated with high blood cholesterol and those resulting from mere chance.

MRFIT and CPPT were intervention trials done with high-risk men between the ages of 35 and 59 who tried to lower their blood cholesterol with diet, exercise, and smoking cessation. In addition, the CPPT administered a cholesterol-lowering drug. Results showed that it was extremely difficult, despite energetic intervention and even with drug therapy, to demonstrate an association between reduced blood cholesterol and lower mortality from heart disease. However, despite the weakness of the evidence, and despite the fact that the MRFIT and CPPT research was done on middle-aged, high-risk men, researchers declared their trials a success, asserting that they provided proof that a high intake of saturated fat was a cause of heart disease.

These are the studies, and the numbers, that form the basis of our current nutrition policy: the Dietary Guidelines and the Food Guide Pyramid. It is in the *interpretation* of the numbers that the dietary enthusiasts and dietary moderates diverge. The enthusiasts, who are currently directing nutrition policy and get the limelight, insist that the results are significant enough to warrant putting us all on modified-fat, low-cholesterol diets. The moderates, who are heard only if you happen to read one of their dissenting articles, look at the same research and disagree.[6,7,8] Moderates insist that such weak evidence supports dietary change only for people who are actually found to be at high risk of heart disease. Current thinking has redefined the culprit as low density lipoprotein (LDL) cholesterol, but the division in thinking between the two schools of thought remains.

Even though results from those original studies were modest and the significance of the differences open to question, today's research doesn't go back and retest the connection between dietary fats, blood cholesterol, and heart disease. Because the studies were so large and so expensive, it is unlikely that retesting will ever be done. Instead, current research takes the connection at face value and attempts to refine aspects of the equation by doing studies designed to establish, for instance, whether the heart disease diet should be low in fat or moderate in fat with an emphasis on monounsaturated fat;[9] or by investigating the impact on blood lipids of particular fats like fish oils or olive oil or fatty acids like stearic acid[10] or cholesterol-lowering medications;[11] or by evaluating the fat equations for particular groups (for whom the connections appear to be quite different), such as women[12] or distance runners.[13]

Whatever the fine-tuning of the dietary fat recommendations, applying them and getting convincing results has been extraordinarily difficult. Even patients in carefully supervised clinical studies have considerable trouble adhering to the modified-fat, low-cholesterol diet, and when they do, they have a modest and variable response: on the average, a decrease in cholesterol of 3 to 4 percent[14] with a presumed decrease in incidence of heart disease of 13 percent for each 10 percent blood cholesterol is reduced.[11] Some people respond well to dietary changes; others respond poorly.[15] Do the changes help? Again, it is a matter of interpretation. In reporting their results, researchers tend to describe small changes like a 13 percent decrease in incidence (or 20 percent or 30 percent) by using words like "a sharp decrease." When *you* interpret these numbers, remember that changes from any intervention are likely to be small and that the word "sharp" was used to describe the "50 percent decrease" in relative mortality found in the original studies, the studies in which deaths were reduced in absolute numbers from 1.4 to 0.7 per 1,000 individuals per year.

Community and work-site interventions show that, although it is difficult to change diet, it is less difficult to make people wary about eating. Clinical research involves intensive education and follow-up throughout the course of the intervention. Community or work-site interventions are much less intensive. People participating in these interventions have not changed their eating behaviors, although they have become more aware and concerned about the connection between diet and disease.[16,17]

Heart disease is a leading cause of death and disability in the older portion of the American population. It is not, however, the epidemic that many people fear. That perception seems to have arisen from a problem in measurement. In the late 1960s, statistics showed an alarming increase in death rates from heart disease. It was a false alarm. More careful examination of the data some years later showed the age-adjusted mortality from heart disease actually declined between 1940 and 1960.[19] The source of the error? Categories for causes of death had changed and more deaths were attributed to coronary heart disease than before and fewer to other diseases of the heart. To go even further back, repeating Keys's epidemiological research with all 21 countries for which data was available showed a far weaker association between diet and heart disease mortality.[18] However, correcting the errors in measurement and research did not correct the thinking—heart disease was still considered a national emergency.

The conclusion? There may be a connection between dietary fat and heart disease, but it is not as lethal as we thought. Fat is not the only suspect. Marginal intakes of other nutrients, such as folic acid, vitamin B6, beta carotene, vitamin C, and vitamin E, may also be linked with heart disease.[19] Also, there are many nondietary risk factors for heart disease.

If you have a *particular* risk of heart disease, get individual guidance. See a dietitian, have your eating patterns respectfully evaluated, and do the least you can to get the results you want. Don't forget about activity as a way of increasing your high density lipoproteins (your good cholesterol). As you make changes, have your blood lipids tested to see if you are getting results. You may respond to diet and exercise, or you may not. If your doctor recommends drugs, read all the fine print. Remember that the drugs are tested by enthusiasts who are funded by drug companies and that drugs often have significant negative side effects.

I trust by now that your head is spinning, as is mine. More research will be ballyhooed, and much of it will be contradictory to what we presently think we know. You can't be running around purging and refilling your pantry shelves every time you hear about a new study. (Well, I guess you can. It depends on how you want to spend your time.) What to do instead? Put your emphasis on dietary variety, including a variety of fats and fatty foods. Be honest about what you love and don't feel you have to give it up. And prepare to be surprised. The mystery of heart disease is a long way from being solved.

Selected References

1. Keys, A. 1953. Atherosclerosis: A problem in newer public health. *Journal of Mt. Sinai Hospital* 20: 118–139.
2. Hegsted, D. M., R. B. McGandy, M. L. Myers, and F. J. Stare. 1965. Quantitative effects of dietary fat on serum cholesterol in man. *American Journal of Clinical Nutrition* 17: 281–295.
3. Kannel, W. B., W. P. Castelli, T. Gordon, and P. M. McNamara. 1971. Serum cholesterol, lipoproteins and risk for coronary heart disease: The Framingham Study. *Annals of Internal Medicine* 74: 1–12.
4. Martin, M. J., S. B. Hulley, W. S. Browner, L. H. Kuller, and D. Wentworth. 1986. Serum cholesterol, blood pressure and mortality: Implications from a cohort of 361,662 men. *Lancet* 2: 933–936.
5. Lipid Research Clinics Program. 1984. The Lipid Research Clinics Coronary Primary Prevention Trial results II: the relationship of reduction in incidence of coronary heart disease to cholesterol lowering. *Journal of the American Medical Association* 251: 365–374.
6. Harper, A. E. 1996. Dietary guidelines in perspective. *Journal of Nutrition* 126 (suppl.): 1042S–1048S.
7. Muldoon, M. F., S. B. Manuck, and K. A. Matthews. 1990. Lowering cholesterol concentrations and mortality: A quantitative review of primary prevention trials. *British Medical Journal* 301: 309–314.
8. Howell, W. H., D. J. McNamara, M. A. Tosca, B. T. Smith, and J. A. Gaines. 1997. Plasma lipid and lipoprotein responses to dietary fat and cholesterol: A meta-analysis. *American Journal of Clinical Nutrition* 65: 1747–1764.
9. Katan, M. B., S. M. Grundy, and W. C. Willett. 1997. Beyond low-fat diets. *New England Journal of Medicine* 337: 563–566.
10. Grundy, S. M. 1994. Influence of stearic acid on cholesterol metabolism relative to other long-chain fatty acids. *American Journal of Clinical Nutrition* 60 (6 suppl.): 986S–990S.
11. Gould, A. L., J. E. Rossouw, N. C. Santanello, J. F. Heyse, and C. D. Furberg. 1995. Cholesterol reduction yields clinical benefit: A new look at old data. *Circulation* 91: 2274–2282.
12. Bush, T. L. 1990. The epidemiology of cardiovascular disease in postmenopausal women. *Annals of the New York Academy of Science* 592: 263–271.
13. Leddy, J., P. Horvath, J. Rowland, and D. Pendergast. 1997. Effect of a high- or a low-fat diet on cardiovascular risk factors in male and female runners. *Medicine and Science in Sports and Exercise* 29: 17–25.
14. Brunner, E., I. White, M. Thorogood, A. Bristow, D. Curle, and M. Marmot. 1997. Can dietary interventions change diet and cardiovascular risk factors? A meta-analysis of randomized controlled trials. *American Journal of Public Health* 87: 1415–1422.
15. Krauss, R. M. 1997. Understanding the basis for variation in response to cholesterol-lowering diets. *American Journal of Clinical Nutrition* 65: 885–886.
16. Luepker, R. V., D. R. Jacobs, A. R. Folsom, et al. 1988. Cardiovascular risk factor change 1973–74 versus 1980–82: The Minnesota Heart Survey. *Journal of Clinical Epidemiology* 41: 825–833.
17. Frank, J. W., D. M. Reed, J. S. Grove, and R. Benfante. 1992. Will lowering population levels of serum cholesterol affect total mortality? *Journal of Clinical Epidemiology* 45: 333–346.
18. Yerushalmy, J. H., H. E. 1957. Fat in the diet and mortality from heart disease: A methodological note. *New York State Journal of Medicine* 2243–2354:
19. Kwiterovich, P. O., Jr. 1997. The effect of dietary fat, antioxidants and pro-oxidants on blood lipids, lipoproteins and atherosclerosis. *Journal of the American Dietetic Association* 97: S31–S41.

Appendix

H

Children, Dietary Fat, and Heart Disease: You Don't Have to Panic

At this writing, there are no generally accepted Dietary Guidelines for children about fat intake. There is a movement in that direction, and the arguments have begun. The enthusiasts say to reduce fat in children's diets by the time they are 2 years old,[1] the compromisers say by 5 years old,[2] and the moderates say not until after puberty.[3,4,5] The justification given for extending the guidelines to young children is that fat restriction is effective in preventing heart disease in adults and that it will be even more effective if it is begun at age 2 years. This argument leaves something to be desired since, as I pointed out in appendix G, "Dietary Fat and Heart Disease: It's Not as Bad as You Think," dietary changes are only marginally effective.

The atherosclerotic process begins in childhood, warn the enthusiasts. Well, yes and no. Almost all children, regardless of national origin, diet, and sex, do develop fatty streaks in their major arteries.[6] Since children everywhere, on every kind of diet, develop fatty streaks, it is unclear what can be done about it. These fatty streaks are reversible and do not necessarily progress to the hardening and plaque formation that is characteristic of heart disease. It is only after puberty that the hardening process continues and then only for some people, and only after age 30 does the process become significant.[7]

If hardening of the arteries starts in childhood, it must be slow. Heart disease, for the most part, is a disease of aging. Eighty percent of deaths from heart disease occur after age 65.[8] The alarming and often-repeated figure that "53 percent of people over age 50 die of heart disease" implies that heart disease presents a great risk of *premature* death. However, when you break the numbers down by age ranges, it appears that old people are the ones who are most likely to die of heart disease. Only 1 percent of women aged 50 to 55 die of heart disease, 2 percent at ages 60 to 65, 6 percent at 70 to 75, 20 percent at ages 80 to 85, and 45 percent over age 85.[9]

People who develop heart disease when they are young are, for the most part, people born with errors in fat metabolism, called *familial hyperlipidemia*, which give them early hardening of the arteries. Their disease process is quite different from that of other people. The someone we know who died of a heart attack at age 30 was probably a victim of familial hyperlipidemia. Even children who have high blood cholesterol are not likely to be at risk because most children who have high blood cholesterol grow out of it.[10]

The Canadians are much more sensible than we are about dietary guidelines for children. They say that adult fat recommendations should be applied only after puberty. The Canadian Pediatric Society/Health Canada report pointed out what even the enthusiasts acknowledge, that there was no clear evidence. No long-term testing has been done to see if modified-fat, low-cholesterol diets in childhood reduce heart disease in adults, nor, given the complexity and expense of such studies, is it likely to be done. As a consequence, the Canadians decided it was impossible and even risky to set rigid guidelines for what and how much children should eat.[5]

The safety of applying the Guidelines to young children is a major point of contention in the United States. The moderates say that it is dangerous to try to restrict children's fat intake and show clinical evidence of poor growth in many children put on such regimens by parents who were trying to do the "right" thing.11 The enthusiasts say that it is only overzealous parents who cause such problems and that, if the diet is intelligently applied, children will grow just fine. For their evidence, enthusiasts show intensively supervised clinical interventions in which parents and children were provided with laborious instruction and follow-up.[12] The truth of the matter is that applying the Dietary Guidelines with all the complicated fat instructions is complex, difficult to do, and easy to screw up. If you screw up, your efforts don't do any good, and they may even do harm.

Children are already eating only 33 percent of their calories as fat.[13] Getting them to eat 30 percent or less without interfering with their intake of energy or other nutrients involves a significant increase in precision, attention to detail, and risk of error. Pennsylvania State researchers doing computer modeling of children's diets found that using more than one fat-lowering strategy produced deficient diets, particularly for children under age 2. Strategies included using low-fat meat and milk, doing low-fat cooking, and avoiding added fats at the table.[14] If your child has a particularly high risk of heart disease, and if you and your doctor have determined that she needs a special diet, get careful and informed dietary guidance from a registered dietitian to avoid the likelihood of nutritional deficiencies and poor growth.

Most people, however, are not in the high-risk category. Most of us are simply trying to be responsible and practical in feeding our children. For the most part, neither the moderates nor the enthusiasts are too practical about children and how they eat. They argue about the formula for managing the fat in children's diets, but neither group seems to realize that no child ever ate according to a formula. The moderates have the edge, however, because they are more flexible, which is always a good idea when dealing with children.

I am sad to say it, but current nutritional politics being what they are, when the Dietary Guidelines for children come out, they are likely to reflect the enthusiast point of view. Right now, there are many sets of guidelines. The U.S. Department of Agriculture has already gone ahead on its own and is recommending fat restriction after age 2 in the Child Care Nutrition Program. In January 1999, the American Dietetic Association published its position paper on children and dietary fat; it is from the enthusiast camp. (My name is on it, but only because I wasn't given the opportunity to remove it.) The American Academy of Pediatrics is meeting to reconsider theirs, and early signs indicate its statement is likely to be from the enthusiast camp as well.

The National Cholesterol Education Program has long taken the position that children's diets should be restricted, and they are making a lot of noise with their Eat Smart school curriculum for teaching low-fat nutrition classes. The American Heart Association, with its huge advertising budget, has been in the fat-modification business since the 1960s. When the Dietary Guidelines for children are released to the media, it will seem like news, it will be with great fanfare, and it could scare you. Don't worry, it won't be news. It will be a political event, not a nutritional event. Stay calm. Be positive. Feed your child well. Emphasize variety. Wait to see what happens next. If something you hear about "eating for health" makes you and your child afraid of food, it won't help.

Selected References

1. NCEP expert panel on blood cholesterol levels in children and adolescents. 1992. National Cholesterol Education Program (NCEP): Highlights of the report of the expert panel on blood cholesterol levels in children and adolescents. *Pediatrics* 89 (3): 495–501.

2. American Academy of Pediatrics, and Committee on Nutrition. 1992. Statement on Cholesterol. *Pediatrics* 90 (3): 469–473.

3. Olson, R. E. 1995. The dietary recommendations of the American Academy of Pediatrics. *American Journal of Clinical Nutrition* 61: 271–273.

4. Newman, T. B., A. M. Garber, N. A. Holzman, and S. B. Hulley. 1995. Problems with the report of the expert panel on blood cholesterol levels in children and adolescents. *Archives of Pediatric and Adolescent Medicine* 149: 241–247.

5. Canadian Paediatric Society, and Health Canada. 1993. Nutrition Recommendations Update: Dietary Fat and Children. *Report of the Joint Working Group of the Canadian Paediatric Society and Health Canada.*

6. Tejada, C. J., J. P. Strong, M. R. Montenegro, C. Restrepo, and L. A. Solberg. 1968. Distribution of coronary and aortic atherosclerosis by geographic location, race and sex. *Laboratory Investigation* 18: 509–526.

7. Pathobiological Determinants of Atherosclerosis in Youth (PDAY) Research Group. 1990. Relationship of atherosclerosis in young men to serum lipoprotein cholesterol concentrations and smoking. A preliminary report. *Journal of the American Medical Association* 264: 3018–3024.

8. Harper, A. E. 1996. Dietary guidelines in perspective. *Journal of Nutrition* 126 (suppl.): 1042S–1048S.

9. Bush, T. L. 1990. The epidemiology of cardiovascular disease in postmenopausal women. *Annals of the New York Academy of Science* 592: 263–271.

10. Lauer, R. M., and W. R. Clarke. 1990. Use of cholesterol measurements in childhood for the prediction of adult hypercholesterolemia: The Muscatine study. *Journal of the American Medical Association* 264: 3034–3038.

11. Lifshitz, F., and O. Tarim. 1993. Nutrition dwarfing. *Current Problems in Pediatrics* 23: 322–336.

12. The Writing Group for the DISC Collaborative Research Group. 1995. Efficacy and safety of lowering dietary intake of fat and cholesterol in children with elevated low-density lipoprotein cholesterol. *Journal of the American Medical Association* 273: 1429–1435.

13. Lytle, L. A., M. K. Ebzery, T. Nicklas, D. Montgomery, M. Zive, M. Evans, P. Snyder, M. Nickaman, S. H. Kelder, D. Reed, E. Busch, and P. Mitchell. 1996. Nutrient intakes of third graders: Results from the Child and Adolescent Trial for Cardiovascular Health (CATCH) baseline survey. *Journal of Nutrition Education* 28: 338–347.

14. Sigman-Grant, M., S. Zimmerman, and P. M. Kris-Etherton. 1993. Dietary approaches for reducing fat intake of preschool-aged children. *Pediatrics* 91: 955–960.

Appendix

I

Sodium in Your Diet

Official nutrition policy (the Dietary Guidelines) implies that we should keep our sodium intake down to 2,400 milligrams per day, or about 6,000 milligrams of salt (sodium chloride). That implication has been taken as a guideline and has been applied as the standard for the daily values you see on nutrition labels. That's pretty low. A teaspoon of salt contains 2,132 milligrams of sodium. Our usual sodium intake is about 4,000 to 6,000 milligrams per day. Getting sodium intake down to 2,400 milligrams per day seems like a small difference, but it is actually a significant reduction. To force your sodium intake down to the recommended level of 2,400 milligrams per day, you would have to virtually eliminate canned foods like soups, vegetables, meats, and mixed dinners. You would have to completely avoid luncheon meats and cured foods like ham, bacon, and smoked turkey breasts. Furthermore, you would have to limit the salt in cooking and not add salt *after* cooking. Such limitations restrict dietary choices to the point of making it hard to get a meal on the table, and *that* has a serious impact on nutrition and feeding a family. My cooking strategies are based on keeping sodium intake around 3,000 to 4,000 milligrams per day, still a modest amount.

As with fat, there is a heated debate about whether the restrictions should be applied to everyone or only to people who have a particular vulnerability to high blood pressure. One huge U.S. population study found no relationship between diet, sodium intake, blood pressure, and heart disease and concluded that routine, population-wide sodium reductions are not justified.[1] A literature review found a relationship between urinary sodium excretion (which is usually about the same as dietary intake) and blood pressure and recommended the opposite.[2] Still another analysis of 56 research studies showed some blood pressure reduction with a 2,000 milligram per day reduction in urinary sodium intake excretion

with older, hypertensive people but no change for people with normal blood pressure whose excretion went down by almost 3,000 milligrams per day.[3] As with the fat issue, the debate about sodium is at least as much about politics as it is about nutrition. If you are interested, read "The (Political) Science of Salt."[4]

As usual, lacking clear direction, we may as well steer a course between the extremes of "too little" and "too much." To be moderate but not fanatic, don't try for the 2,400 milligrams of sodium per day that is the implied standard. A more reasonable target level is 3,000 to 4,000 milligrams. There is no evidence that an extra 1,000 milligrams or so per day of sodium makes any health difference. However, allowing that small increase makes a *big* difference with food selection and cooking. The higher sodium target level lets you use salt in cooking; it lets you use canned soups in moderation, eat canned vegetables and meats, and eat salty snacks occasionally. If you are worried about salt, put the emphasis on *occasionally*. Since 75 to 80 percent of our sodium comes from processed foods like snacks and canned and frozen mixed dinners rather than from the salt shaker, cooking from scratch at home and holding down on salty snacks automatically cuts down significantly on salt intake.

This middle-ground approach to salt intake gives a practical, reasonable, and still modest approach to cooking for a family. Young children don't seem to miss a lot of salt if they aren't introduced to it. If you want more salt, you can add it at the table. However, if you find yourself regularly salting food at the table, it may be that you are being too stingy with salt in your cooking. You are likely to use more salt when you cook without salt and add salt at the table than if you add salt when you cook.

If you have high blood pressure, your daily salt intake is a medical matter. About 10 to 25 percent of people suffering from high blood pressure improve when they strictly limit their salt intake—to about 1,000 milligrams per day. Keep in mind, however, that just because drastically cutting down on salt makes blood pressure go down it doesn't follow that salt made it go up in the first place. Excess sodium may not even be the blood-pressure culprit, but rather, insufficient potassium and calcium. It has long been recognized that we can help prevent high blood pressure by consuming enough potassium (from a variety of fruits and vegetables) and calcium (from dairy products). I prefer the calcium and potassium theory because it encourages seeking food, not *avoiding* it.

Like a lot of other current nutritional issues, even this positive and encouraging information has been medicalized and taken to extremes. You will hear about the DASH eating plan (Dietary Approaches to Stop Hypertension), which had people eat three servings of low-fat dairy products and 8 to 10 servings of fruits and vegetables per day. On the diet, people with mild hypertension had a decrease in blood pressure by 5.5/3.0 (systolic/diastolic) milligrams of mercury; those with more pronounced hypertension had a decrease of 11.4/5.5. Blood pressure, in other words, went down modestly, "as much as some medications for hypertension."[5] Drinking 2 to 3 glasses of milk and eating 4 to 5 servings of fruits and vegetables a day may be practical; a diet with 8 to 10 servings of fruits and vegetables is extreme. Do you need to go to the extreme to get the calcium and potassium benefit for your blood pressure? Probably not. Do you want to? It is up to you, but beware of the going-without then making-up-for-lost-time cycling (restraint and disinhibition) that is frequently a part of going to extremes.

Consistency in sodium intake is important, particularly for people with weakened hearts. In a condition called congestive heart disease, the heart doesn't circulate blood to the kidneys well, and sodium, and therefore fluid, accumulates in the tissues. The same holds true for kidney patients. Maintaining a diet lower in sodium, especially in conjunction with diuretics, relieves fluid retention and strain on the heart. When someone is hospitalized for congestive heart disease, sodium is strictly limited to 1,000 to 2,000 milligrams per day. When they improve or go home, the diet is liberalized to 3,000 to 4,000 milligrams per day.

Heart patients who don't have congestive heart disease benefit from moderating sodium intake, but they don't have to be on rigid sodium restriction.

Now, here is the important point. For someone with congestive heart disease, diuretic medications are adjusted to balance out the sodium in the diet. For the medication to work consistently and well, the sodium in the diet has to be moderate and reasonably steady. Thus, it is more important to be *consistent* about sodium intake and to avoid extremes than to try to be low and fail.

But this is not a medical nutrition textbook, and you are not likely to be that person with congestive heart disease. So why am I making a point about all this? Because much of the scare about sodium comes from the someone we know who is ill. Rigid sodium restriction is not a priority for healthy people. Furthermore, for people with congestive heart disease, it is not sodium intake that causes the problem. It is the weakening of the heart muscle, from heart attacks or simply from aging, that creates the problem.

Selected References

1. Alderman, M. H., H. Cohen, and S. Madhavan. 1998. Dietary sodium intake and mortality: The National Health and Nutrition Examination Survey. *Lancet* 351: 781–785.
2. Elliott, P., J. Stamler, R. Nichols, A. R. Dyer, R. Stamler, and H. Kesterloot. 1996. Intersalt revisited: Further analyses of 24-hour sodium excretion and blood pressure within and across populations. *British Medical Journal* 312: 1249–1253.
3. Midgley, J. P., A. G. Matthew, C. M. Greenwood, and A. G. Logan. 1996. Effect of reduced dietary sodium on blood pressure. *Journal of the American Medical Association* 275: 1590–1597.
4. Taubes, G. 1998. The (Political) Science of Salt. *Science* 281: 899–907.
5. Appel, L. J., T. J. Moore, E. Obarzanek, W. M. Vollmer, L. P. Svetkey, F. M. Sacks, G. A. Bray, T. M. Vogt, J. A. Cutler, M. M. Windhauser, P. Lin, and N. Karanka. 1997. A clinical trial of the effects of dietary patterns on blood pressure. *New England Journal of Medicine* 336: 1117–1124.

Appendix

J

A Primer on Dietary Fat

This lesson in fat chemistry goes beyond what you really need to know. I include it because you may be curious and because I think that understanding the technical terms could help you be more relaxed about eating fat. What do the terms *saturated, monounsaturated, and polyunsaturated* fat really mean? It all has to do with fat chemistry. Fat is made up of fatty acids, which, in turn, are chains of carbon atoms with hydrogens hooked on. Some carbons in fats have as many hydrogens hooked onto them as they possibly can. Those are called saturated fats. Some fatty acids have double bonds between the hydrogen atoms with fewer carbons hooked on. Those are unsaturated. (That means they are not "saturated" with hydrogen.) Fatty acids with one double bond are called "mono" unsaturated fatty acids; those with several double bonds are the "poly" unsaturated fats.

The fat and heart disease theory says that saturated fats raise blood cholesterol more than unsaturated fats, and high blood cholesterol is correlated with cardiovascular disease. The Dietary Guidelines and the Food Guide Pyramid say to hold total fat down to 30 percent of calories consumed and to decrease saturated fat and emphasize unsaturated fat. The "Step 1" diet recommended by the National Cholesterol Education Program and others gets even more prescriptive by recommending roughly a 10–10–10 ratio: 10 percent or less of saturated fat, about 10% of polyunsaturated fat and 10 to 15 percent of monounsaturated fat. Clearly, you have to be a registered dietitian to make good use of that information, but we will do the best we can.

Along with the percentages come the general directive to cut down on animal fat and emphasize vegetable oils, presumably because the former are saturated and the latter unsaturated. It ain't necessarily so. Using my computerized nutrition calculating program, Food Processor, let's examine that generalization. The table below summarizes the percentage of calories from saturated, monounsaturated, and polyunsaturated fat in common oils and hard fats.

Using this table, you can examine the thinking on the fat-and-heart-disease issue. Are animal fats all bad? Not really. Our favorite animal fats, butter and cream, do have most of their fat in the form of saturated fat—but not all. The fats in butter and cream are about 30 percent monounsaturated and 5 percent polyunsaturated. And what about the universally deplored lard, a fat that by its very name implies sloth? The fat in lard is a desirable 40 percent monounsaturated and 15 percent polyunsaturated. Most people who use chicken and goose fat fear it is entirely reprehensible, but these poultry fats turn out to have a very respectable fat profile. Furthermore, about 25 percent of the saturated fat in red meat and poultry and 10 percent of the saturated fat in butter and cream is stearic acid. Studies show that rather than raising blood cholesterol, stearic acid is neutral—it neither raises nor lowers blood cholesterol.[1]

The vegetable-oils-are-good generalization doesn't hold with nut oils. Coconut oil is particularly saturated. Palm oil isn't as saturated and has some monounsaturated and polyunsaturated fats. The generalization also doesn't hold with vegetable oils like those in solid shortenings and stick margarines that have been *hydrogenated*. *Hydrogenated* means saturated. To make them solid, the oils have been changed chemically by "saturating" them with hydrogen atoms, which makes them raise blood cholesterol much the same way naturally saturated fatty acids do. To go on, unsaturated fat, according to recent evidence, can be bad for you if is in the *trans* form (as opposed to the *cis* form).[1] Where do you get *trans* fatty acids? In vegetable shortenings and products baked with them, most stick margarines, in the filling of sandwich cookies, in cake mixes, and in most of the products that proudly proclaim "all vegetable shortening!"

219

PERCENTAGE OF CALORIES FROM SATURATED, MONOUNSATURATED, AND POLYUNSATURATED FATS IN COMMON OILS AND HARD FATS

	Saturated	Monounsaturated	Polyunsaturated
High monounsaturated fats			
Olive oil	14	74	8
Canola oil	7	62	27
Peanut oil	17	52	26
High polyunsaturated fats			
Safflower oil	9	12	74
Sunflower oil	12	16	67
Corn oil	14	24	59
Soybean oil	14	23	58
Sesame oil	14	40	42
Walnut oil	9	23	63
Animal fats			
Butter	62	30	4
Lard	40	42	14
Tallow (suet)	50	42	4
Chicken fat	30	45	21
Goose fat	28	57	11
Nut oils			
Coconut oil	88	6	2
Palm oil	49	37	9

As if the story weren't complicated enough, recent research indicates that not even all unsaturated fats are the same. Monounsaturated fats lower total blood cholesterol without also lowering high-density lipoprotein (HDL), or good cholesterol. Polyunsaturated fat lowers HDL as well. Based on current research, I would encourage you to make your primary oil one of the monounsaturates: olive, canola, or peanut oil; for taste or other qualities that you prize, use the other oils. However, don't bet the farm on it. A few years back, we thought the high polyunsaturated fats were best.

Do you see why I encourage you to emphasize variety? If you have a high blood cholesterol level that needs to be treated by diet, get professional help. Don't settle for having your whole eating life turned upside down by a general chart of "good" or "bad" foods. See a registered dietitian, and while you are there, make sure she recommends changes in your diet based on the chemistry of the fat you actually eat, not some list of good and bad foods. Wave this table at her, if you need to, and tell her Ellyn Satter sent you. When you add up everything you eat, you may find that the food

you love is just fine—even the steak or the refried beans made with lard.

So are you going to march right down to the grocery store and buy some lard? Or are you, like a shopper I overheard the other day, going to smirk and point and say, "I guess it's been a long time since we ate *that*!" It depends on how daring you are. There is a certain political correctness these days about grease. At a recent holiday party, I got into a discussion about fat, of all things. One of my companions smugly announced that he was looking for the perfect olive oil. Refusing to pander to his superior attitude, I announced that lard was my favorite fat. To my surprise, my other companion put his bid in for suet—beef tallow. He had grown up in Britain and said there is nothing like shaved suet for making flaky pie crust.

Selected Reference

1. Kris-Etherton, P. M., and S. Yu. 1997. Individual Fatty acid effects on plasma lipids and lipoproteins: Human studies. *American Journal of Clinical Nutrition* 65: 1628S–1644S.

Appendix
K
Resources Available from
Ellyn Satter Associates

Child of Mine: Feeding with Love and Good Sense. Bull Publishing Co., Palo Alto, CA. A warm, supportive and entertaining book for parents about basic nutrition for infants and young children. Is also used as a solid nutrition reference for professionals. *Child of Mine* teaches about breast and bottle feeding, calories and normal growth through preschool.

How to Get Your Kid to Eat...But Not Too Much. Bull Publishing Co., Palo Alto, CA, 1987. This is *the* book about feeding dynamics. Based on a solid understanding of child development and parent-child relationships, *How to Get Your Kid to Eat* firmly builds the bridge between nutrition and feeding. A must-have reference for anyone who works with parents, children and feeding.

ELLYN SATTER'S FEEDING WITH LOVE AND GOOD SENSE: Video and Teacher's Guide. These live action videotapes of real situations touch, move, startle, upset and inform parents and child care workers and help them take a look at their own feeding behavior. Sometimes feeding goes well, sometimes it doesn't. The hour-long videotape shows what makes the difference. Lesson plans teach nutrition and feeding by observation and experience. Each 15-minute segment comes with a lesson plan, audio script and six reproducible masters. The information on these tapes is based on Ellyn Satter's two books.
The Infant. Babies know how much they need to eat, and parents read their messages.
The Older Baby. Babies learn to eat solid foods and talk to parents.
The Toddler. Toddlers need to explore, but they also need support and limits.
The Preschooler. Preschoolers want to get better at everything--eating included.

ELLYN SATTER'S NUTRITION AND FEEDING FOR INFANTS AND CHILDREN: Handout Masters. Distilled from the pages of both *Child of Mine* and *How to Get Your Kid to Eat*, these informative, readable and engaging handouts are ready for copying and distribution to parents in nutrition, health and education settings. Equally valuable for training nutrition workers, each of the 56 handout masters is two 8 1/2 by 11 pages long. Topics have been selected on the basis of questions most often raised by parents about growth, feeding and nutrition. Feeding behavior is emphasized with nutrition information embedded in the question driven format. Indexed and cross referenced, these handout masters provide an accessible road map to the complexity of feeding infants and young children. Titles include *Being a Role Model for Your Child's Eating, Breastfeeding Your Baby, If Your Baby Doesn't Eat Enough, What is Normal Growth? If Your Preschooler Seems Fat, If Your Child Won't Eat Vegetables, Should Your Child Drink Milk?* Registered purchasers may make up to 300 copies of each master. Subsets available.

Ellyn Satter's Montana FEEDING RELATIONSHIP Training Package. Ellyn Satter gives in-depth staff training on feeding children and preventing feeding problems. Includes five hours of professional quality videos of lecture, demonstration and audience participation. Handouts include a multi-page training outline and materials, references, and informational handouts for parents.

FEEDING WITH LOVE AND GOOD SENSE: Intensive Workshop Training for professionals in evaluating and solving childhood feeding problems that integrates the principles of nutrition, feeding, child development and parenting. Specific problems covered in the workshop are: the child who eats poorly; the finicky child; and the obese child. For health, education, child care and mental health professionals.

FEEDING WITH LOVE AND GOOD SENSE: Training Manual This 150 page training manual for the *Feeding with Love and Good Sense* intensive workshop serves as an in-depth resource handbook. The clinician doing secondary intervention with childhood feeding problems will find essential tools, including guidelines for assessment and treatment, examples of written evaluations, letters to parents and physicians, teaching materials and annotated bibliographies.

TREATING THE DIETING CASUALTY:
Intensive Workshop Professional training that teaches a step-by-step approach to teaching positive, orderly eating based on internal regulators. This workshop teaches an in-depth, theoretically sound understanding of eating attitudes and behaviors and approaches to treatment. For health, education and mental health professionals.

TREATING THE DIETING CASUALTY:
Training Manual This 150 page training manual for the *Treating the Dieting Casualty* intensive workshop serves as an in-depth resource handbook for working with adults whose eating is out of control. Included in the manual are evaluation and treatment protocols, guidelines for communicating with other professionals, standard eating and eating disorders tests, outlines of principles of cognitive and behavioral management and annotated bibliographies.

For a current catalog and price list, call Ellyn Satter Associates, 800-808-7976 or see Ellyn Satter's website at **www.ellynsatter.com**

QUANTITY DISCOUNTS
ON
Secrets of Feeding a Healthy Family

| 30% discount on 10+ books | $11.87 each |
| 60% discount on cartons of 34 books | 6.78 each |

If you found *Secrets* helpful, others will to. Why not order a carton to use for training and resource material, or sell copies of *Secrets* for a fund-raiser for your organization?

Call Kelcy Press to order quantities 877-844-0857

Or write Kelcy Press at   PO Box 46457
                            Madison, WI 53744-6457

Also available through Ellyn Satter Associates 800-808-7976

INDEX

References to the major treatment of a topic are printed in bold.
References to recipes are printed in italic.

Allergies, 61–62, 76, 117
Anxiety about eating, 4, 7, 17, 18, 49
Appetite, 24, 39–40, 189. *See also*
    Hunger, appetite, and satiety
Apples
    apple custard, *142*
    applesauce, *144*
    cooking, 143
Appliances, small, 159–160
Attitudes
    toward body weight, **12**, 191–193
    toward eating, 11–13, 51, 179,
        202–203
        acquisition of, 6–7
        adjustment of, 4
        healthy, 6, 51
        negative, 11–12, 13, 17–18, 20
        positive, 22, 51

Bacon, 85, 139
    greens and, *139*
Bacteria in foods, 13, 75, 81, 156–157
Barriers, to cooking, 2, 54–55
Beans
    black beans and rice, *110–111*
    cooking, 109
    dry, 61, 109
    flavoring, 111
Beef
    cooking methods, 89
    ragout, *106–107*
    stew, 107
    stroganoff, *90*
    Swiss steak, *88*
    See also Hamburger; Ground beef
Behavior
    eating
        erratic, 41, 42
        healthy, 6–7
        normal, 5
    feeding. *See* Feeding, behavior
    mealtime, 25, 55–56. *See also* Table
        manners
Body image, 181, 182, 191–193
Body weight, attitudes toward, **12**, 30.
    See also Obesity; Fatness
Books
    for children, 180
    cookbooks, 121–122, 180
    by Ellyn Satter, 221–222
Bread, 26, 37, 168–169
Bread pudding, *143*
Breads, cereal, rice, and pasta group,
    57–58
Breakfast, 53, 59, 72
Broccoli
    chowder, *84*
    gingered, *136*
Broth, preparation of, 105

Browning meat, 81, 107
Butter, 65, 74
    herbed, *133*
    mustard, *133*
Buttermilk, 142

Cabbage, and carrots, *135*
Calcium
    intake, 62
    sources of, **63**
Candy, 9, 64
Canned goods, 126–127, 168, 169
Capabilities. *See* Eating capabilities
Carrots
    and cabbage, *135*
    glazed, *135*
Casserole
    generic, *119–121*
    hamburger, *80–81*
    tuna noodle, *78*
Catering to children, 36–37, 54–55
Centipede, 51
Cheese, 62–63
    cream cheese spread, *134*
    cheese sauce, *133*
    See also Dairy products
Chicken
    and food safety, 83
    jambalaya, *114–115*
    lemon, *98*
    marinated stir-fry, *112–113*
    mock fried, 98
    poaching, 105
    and rice, *82–83*
    shopping for, 169–170
    soup, *104*
    See also Poultry
Child care, 46
Child Care Food Program, 46, 195–196
Children
    and body weight, 193
    and dietary fat, 62, 66, 196, 198,
        214–215
    and dieting, 193
    and eating capabilities, 7–8, 39–42,
        180–181, 184–185
    and eating out, 148–149
    eating-troubled, 8–10, 20–22
    and finickiness, 5, 6, 21–22, 38–39
    and food acceptance, 42, 185, 210
    and food regulation, 6, 39–40,
        188–191, 208
    and grazing, 38
    and meal preparation, 44, 75–76,
        129, 153–154
    and meals, 5–6
    and nutrition education, 178–199
    and nutrition rules, 182
    and overeating, 9, 25, 40

    and serving sizes, 67
    and undereating, 9, 25
Cholesterol
    effect on blood cholesterol, 60–61
    in eggs, 60, 87
Choosing food, 36–37, **48–68**
Cobbler, fruit, *142*
Coleslaw, poppyseed, *135*
Control
    reasons for, **10–13**
    vs. trust, 8–9, 51
Convenience foods, 118, 154
Cookbooks, 121–122, 180
Cooking classes, 121
Corn
    pudding, *140*
    scalloped, *135*
Coupons, 167–168
Crisp, fruit, *143*
Cucumber salad, sweet-sour, *134*
Cue sensitivity, 205. *See also* Hunger,
    appetite, and satiety
Custard
    apple, *142*
    pumpkin, *134*
Cutting boards, 156
Cycle menu
    strategies for planning, 152–153
    table, 151

Dairy products, 62–63, 170, 172–173
Deprivation, feelings of, 25–26
Dessert, 76
Dietary Guidelines, **18**, 50, 204
Dieting, weight reduction, 18–19, 30,
    206–207
Dieting casualties, 18–20
Dietitians, 45, 220
Disease avoidance, 20, 50
Disinhibition, and restraint, **28**, 65
Diversity, in size and shape, 191–193
Division of responsibility, 6, **34–36**, 180
Dressing, poppyseed, *135*
Dried foods, 128
Dumplings, 105

Eating attitudes. *See* Attitudes, toward
    eating
Eating behavior. *See* Behavior, eating
Eating capabilities, **39–42**
    acquisition of, **7–8**
    adults and, 8
    loss of, **8–10**
    teaching, 180, **184–185**
    See also Skills, eating
Eating disorders, 193–194
Eating out, 148–149
Education. *See* Nutrition education
Efficiency in the kitchen, **74–75**

Egg dishes
  spaghetti carbonara, *86–87*
  spinach-feta frittata, *97*
Eggs, 60–61, 87
  heart disease and, 60–61
  shopping for, 172–173
  storage of, 173
Enthusiasts, vs. moderates, 18, 28,
    66–67
Equipment, for cooking and serving,
    76, 159–160. *See also* Knives

Fast food, 146–147
Fat, content of foods, 170
Fat, dietary, 219–220
  amount of, 73, 133
  avoidance of, 18, 65
  in children's diets, 66
  concern about, 18, 29
  and heart disease, 211–212
  in meat, poultry, and fish, 170
  restriction of, 64–65
  types of, 65, 73–74, 220
Fatness, 30, 40, 191–193. *See also* Body
    weight; Obesity
Fats and oils, 26, 64–65
  amount of, 73, 133
  types of, 73
Feeding
  relationship, 32–46
  tasks, **36–39**
Feeding behavior, 38–39
  dependability in, 23
  lore, 11
  problems, 20–22, 40, 54–57
    evaluation of, 35
    finickiness, 5, 6, 21–22, 38–39
    overcautiousness, 185–186
    panhandling, 37
Feelings, about eating, 18, **24**, 190
Fiber, dietary, 58, 152
Finickiness, 5, 6, 21–22, 38–39
Fish, 61, 93
  fried, *116–117*
  herb-baked fish, *92*
  sautéing, 117
  shopping for, 93, 170
  Wisconsin fish boil, *100*
Flour, sifting, 105
Food, as medicine, **12–13**
Food acceptance, 42, 58, 185–188
  and cultural issues, 187
  teaching, 185–188
Food Guide Pyramid, 18, **50**, 57–65
  teaching to children, 181–182
Food regulation, 188–191, 205, 208
  lessons, 184, 188–189
Food safety. *See* Safety
Food selection, 36–37, **48–68**
Food storage, 154, 173
Food thermometer, 95
Freezers, 155
Fried foods, 26
Frittata, *97*
Frozen foods. *See* Fruits; Vegetables

Fruit
  with brown cream sauce, *144*
  cobbler, *142*
  crisp, *143*
Fruits, 58–59
  canned, 126–127, 168
  dried, 128
  fresh, 125–126, 170–171
  frozen, 127–128
  seasonal, 125–126, 171–172
Frying foods, 116
Fullness, stages of, **24**, 189. *See also*
    Hunger, appetite, and satiety

Garlic, 107
  and olive oil, *133–134*
Good eater, definition of, 179
Grab-and-dump meals, **118**
Grains, 169
Gravy, how to make, 101
Grazing, 23–24, 38, 205
Greens
  and bacon, *139*
  keeping fresh, 137, 171
  preparation of, 137
Grocery shopping, **163–177**
  for baked goods, 168–169
  for canned goods, 168
  for dairy products, 172–173
  for eggs, 172–173
  for fish, poultry, and meat, 169–170
  P&E system, 163
  for produce, 170–172
Grocery stores, 164–165
Ground beef
  browning, 81
  freezing, 81
  safety of, 81
  See also Hamburger
Growth, physical, 7–8, 41
Guilt, about eating, 18

Hamburger
  casserole, *80–81*
  meat loaf, *94*
  See also Ground beef
Hamburgers, *101*
Hand washing, 155–156
Head Start, 46, 195–196
Health clinics, 45
Health foods, 13, 169
Healthy eater, **6–7**, 179
Heart disease
  and dietary fat, 211–212, 214–215
  and eggs, 60–61
Hunger, 56–57
Hunger, appetite, and satiety, **24**, 29,
    30, 56, 188–189

Ice cream scoops, 94, 95
Infants, feeding, 34, 36, 37
Ingredients
  equivalents for
    fatty foods, 120
    protein foods, 120

starchy foods, 119
  pre-prepared, 153, 154
Internal regulators, **24–25**, 188–189, 205

Jambalaya, *114–115*
Juice, 37, 58, 59, 62
Junk food, 29, 49

Knives, 158–159

Leftovers, 75, 148
Limit setting, 56–57, 150
Love of eating, **25**. *See also* Pleasure in
    eating
Low-fat foods, 29, 65–66
Lunch, 72

Manners. *See* Table manners
Margarine, 74
Marinating, 112
Mastery expectations, 38
Meals
  convenient, **118**, 154
  grab-and-dump, **118**
  importance of, 23, 53
  parental involvement in, 37–38, 44,
    56
  planning, 23, 53–55, **146–160**
    sadistic, 37
  pre-prepared, **75**
  schedule of, 23–24, 37–38
  serving, 150
  vegetarian, 152
Mealtime behavior, 25, 55–56. *See also*
    Table manners
Meat, 59–60
  browning, 81, 107
Meatballs, 94, 96
Meat loaf, *94*
Media, and nutrition issues, 52
Menu planning. *See* Meals, planning
Microwave
  chunky applesauce, *144*
  cooking, 132, 144
  thawing, 75
Milk, 37, 62–63, 172. *See also* Dairy
    products
Moderates, vs. enthusiasts, 66–67
Mostaccioli with spinach and feta, *91*

National School Lunch Program,
    196–198
Natural foods, 13, 169
Noodles. *See* Pasta
Normal eating, 5, 179
Nurturing, 2
Nutrition education, **179–199**
  effectiveness of, 183–184
  food acceptance lessons, 187–188
  food regulation lessons, 188
  respect for diversity, 191–193
Nutritional requirements, **57**
Nuts, 61

Obesity, 6. *See also* Body weight

Oil
  olive oil
    with garlic, *133–134*
    grades of, 74
  peanut oil, 117
  sesame oil, 113
  See also Fats and oils
Organic foods, 13
Organization
  of storage space, 154–155
  of work space, 153–154
Overcontrol. *See* Control
Overeating, 9, 25, 40, 65

Panhandling (on-demand feeding), 37
Pasta
  cooking, 79
  macaroni-tomato-hamburger
    casserole, *80*
  mostaccioli with spinach and
    feta, *91*
  spaghetti carbonara, *86–87*
  spaghetti and meatballs, *96*
  tuna noodle casserole, *78*
Peach crisp, 143
Peanut butter, 61
Peanut oil, 117
Peas, herbed, *140*
Peppers, sweet, 142
Permission to eat, **28–29**
Pineapple upside-down cake, 144
Planning meals, 23, 37, 53–55, **146–160**
Plant proteins, 61
Pleasure in eating, 2, 25
Plum cobbler, 142
Poaching, 105
Pork
  chops, *99*
  shopping for, 169–170
Potatoes, 57
  mashed, *138–139*
  oven-fried, *141*
  sweet, *99*
  varieties of, 139
Pot roast, 89
Pots and pans, 159
Poultry, 61, 169–170. *See also* Chicken
Pre-prepared meals, **75**
Priorities, 4, 7, 19, 53
  distorted, 19–20
  people as, 4
Produce, 170–171, 173. *See also* Fruits;
  Vegetables
Pumpkin custard, *134*

Ratatouille, *141–142*
Recipe listing, 77
Regulation of food intake, 188–191,
  205, 208
Resources, 221–222
Responsibility, division of, 6, **34–36**, 180

Restaurants. *See* Eating out
Restrained feeding, 8
Restraint and disinhibition, **28**, 65
Rice
  black beans and, *110–111*
  chicken and, *82*
  cooking methods, 111
  jambalaya, *114–115*
  shopping for, 169
  types of, 111
Role modeling, for children's eating, **4**,
  17, 30

Safety
  and chicken, 83
  and eggs, 87
  and fish, 93
  and food handling, 13, 75, 155–157
  and ground beef, 81
  in the kitchen, 153, 158–159
Salad
  coleslaw, *135*
  green, *137*
  spinach, *136–137*
  sweet-sour cucumber, *134–135*
Salad greens, 137, 171
Salt, 29, 64, 66, 217
  amount of, 73, 133, 217
  restriction of, 64, 73
Satiety, **24**, 189. *See also* Hunger,
  appetite, and satiety
Sautéing, 74, 109, 117
Schedule, of meals, 23–24
School nutrition programs, 46. *See also*
  National School Lunch Program
Serving sizes, **67**
Sesame oil, 113
Shopping. *See* Grocery shopping
Skills, eating, 6, 36, 40, 42. *See also*
  Eating capabilities
Snacks, 37, 56, 150
Sodium. *See* Salt
Soft drinks, 62
Soup
  broccoli chowder, *84*
  chicken, *104*
  chicken and dumpling, *105*
  minestrone, *108–109*
Spaghetti
  carbonara, *86–87*
  and meatballs, *96*
Spinach
  creamed, *139*
  and feta frittata, *97*
  mostaccioli and feta, *91*
  salad, *136*
Sprouts, 157
Squash, summer, *140*
Staples, 154–155, 166–167, 169, 174–177
Steak
  cooking methods, 89

Salisbury, 95
Swiss, 88
Sugar, 29, 63–64
Supermarket. *See* Grocery store
Support
  for children with feeding problems,
    40
  for nutrition professionals, 221–222
  for older children, 44
  for parents, 44–46, 195–196, 221–222
  for school feeding programs,
    197–198
Sweet potatoes, *99*
Sweets, 63–64
Swiss steak, *88*

Table manners, 25, 39, 55–56, 186
Taste, **25–26**, 54
Thawing frozen foods, 75
Time management, 149–150, 153
Toddlers, 34, 37, 43, 56
  and fat restriction, 62
Tomatoes
  stewed, *139*
  with vinaigrette, *138*
Trust, **22**, **30**
  vs. control, 8–9, 51
Tuna
  canned, 79
  tuna noodle casserole, *78*

Undereating, 9, 25, 40
Utensils, 159–160

Value-added foods, 128, 154, 165–166.
  See also Meals, convenient
Variety, of food, **26–28**, 36, 40–41
Vegetables, 58–59
  canned, 126–127, 132, 168
  dried, 128
  fresh, 125–126, 129, 170–171
  frozen, 127–128, 131–132
  high-starch and low-starch, 130–131
  oven-roasted, *141*
  preparation of, 129–131
  sautéing, 109
  seasonal, 125–126, 171–172
  See also specific types
Vegetarian diet, 60, 152
Vinaigrette, *138*

Washing
  greens, 137
  hands, 155–156
  produce, 157
Weight attitudes, 12

Yams, *99*
Yogurt, 62–63. *See also* Dairy products